Eva Herschey
103,92 $

ATLAS OF LASER VOICE SURGERY

ATLAS OF LASER VOICE SURGERY

Jean Abitbol, M.D.
With Contributions from
C. A. Timsit, M.D., and J. J. Maimaran, M. D.

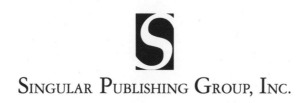

SINGULAR PUBLISHING GROUP, INC.

Singular Publishing Group, Inc.
4284 41st Street
San Diego, California 92105-1197

© 1995 by Singular Publishing Group, Inc.

Typeset in 11/15 New Century Schoolbook by So Cal Graphics
Printed in Hong Kong by Paramount Printing Company

All rights, including that of transition reserved. No part of this publication may be reproduced, stored in a retrieval system or transmitted in any form or by means, electronic, mechanical, recording, or otherwise, without the prior written permission of the publisher.

Library of Congress Cataloging-in-Publication Data
Abitbol, Jean
    Atlas of Laser Voice Surgery / Jean Abitbol.
      p.   cm.
      Includes bibliographical references and index.
      ISBN 1-56593-190-4
    1. Voice disorders — Laser surgery — Atlases.   I. Title
      [DNLM: 1. Laryngeal Diseases — surgery — atlases.   2. Vocal Cords —
      surgery — atlases. 3. Laser Surgery — atlases. WV 17 A149a 1994]
RF516.A26 1994
617.5'33059 — dc20
DNLM/DLC
for Library of Congress   94-6939
                                                                                CIP

CONTENTS

Preface vii
Acknowledgments vii
Introduction xiii

CHAPTER 1 **Laser** 1

History 2
Laser Concept 4
Components of a Surgical Laser 7
Laser-Tissue Interaction 7
Laser Safety and Limitations 18
What Kind of Laser for Phonosurgery? 21

CHAPTER 2 **Larynx** 41

Embryology 42
Anatomy and Physiology 71
Exploration of Normal Voice 78

CHAPTER 3 **Micro-Laryngoscopy** 107

Indications and Preoperative Procedures 108
Surgical Instruments and Procedures 108
Complications of Laryngoscopy 118
Anesthetic Techniques 118
Complications of CO_2 Laser Surgery 123

CHAPTER 4 **Laryngeal Pathologies** 125

Nodules 126
Polyps 154
Cysts 173
Granulomas 196
Papillomas 207
Vascular Pathology 221
Vocal Fold Hemorrhage 242
Reinke's Edema 250
Chronic Laryngitis 281
Malignant Tumors 300
Paralysis of the Vocal Folds 336
Sub-ankylosis of the Cricoarytenoid Joint 354
Hernia of the False Vocal Folds or Laryngocele 357

CHAPTER 4 Laryngeal Pathologies *(continued)*

Epiglottic and Vallecular Cysts   363
Laryngeal Stenosis   366
Congenital Laryngeal Web   371
Anterior Post-traumatic Web   380
Sulcus Vocalis   387
Changing the Vocal Pitch   394
Miscellaneous Lesions   401
Multiple Lesions   410

CHAPTER 5 Conclusions   417

Personal Experience   418
Indications, Contraindications, Complications, Cautions, Advantages and Disadvantages   421
What to Avoid   427
A Team Operates, Not a Surgeon   433
Key Rules   435

Bibliography   437
Voice Exploration   438
Filmography   445
Laser Phonosurgery and Anesthesia   445

Index   455

PREFACE

The *Atlas of Voice Surgery* proposes to take you on a journey into the world of the laser, the universe of voice, and their semantic meeting point: laser voice surgery. Color photographs, graphic tables, and all knowledge of voice and "Laser-eye" microsurgery will be entertained and interpreted.

For centuries, inquiring minds have asked: how is the human voice produced? How is light converted to a coherent beam? The mystery of light has intrigued humans throughout recorded history. The forces of wavelength, distance and velocity, an unnatural phenomenon to prehistoric humans, remain extant today. Light waves are electrical in nature and differ from mechanical sound waves. The laser beam is a physical and reproductive element. Voice is personal and is bestowed with personality. Each human being bears his or her own imprintable voice. Surgery to the vocal fold anatomy does not necessarily modify its individuality. Voice and laser surgery identify the marriage of art and science in dynamic flux.

This book is written for otolaryngologists, voice therapists, students, and vocalists. A better understanding of voice production and laser microsurgery, accompanied by color photographs and figures, are provided.

Two novel techniques, Laser and phonosurgery, are particularized. For some of my colleagues, the words are irreconcilable and paradoxical. Fifteen years of experience with laser, in 5,035 cases, will be shared in this book to demonstrate their compatibility. If surgical success cannot be measured just by "the sound of voice," then laser burns of the vocal folds and ligament by the third millennia are inexcusable. Is it not the poor worker who blames his tools? The laser is unmatched in accuracy and safety in secure hands. Frozen section sampling and analysis are practice following laser surgery. Examples of total recovery of the vocal fold anatomy, after laser microsurgery, are manifested in the color photographs.

The laser concept was developed by Einstein. Chapter 1 enlightens us of his revolutionary genius.

Phonosurgery demands a meticulous inspection of the anatomy of the larynx, vocal cord vibration, and physiology and is found in Chapter 2. The following chapter describes anesthesia and the laryngoscopic technique for surgery. Chapter 4 offers 350 photographs with 40 precise pathological conditions and their pre-, per-, and postoperative states. Chapter 5 offers the reader the benefit of 15 years of personal experience and more than 5,000 cases of laser phonosurgery. "What to do" and "What to avoid" are carefully recalled to prepare the practitioner.

Surgery of the voice is an art and a science. A limiting margin can hardly be defined.

ACKNOWLEDGMENTS

I wish to express my sincerest gratitude to the following people who were directly or indirectly instrumental in the production of the *Atlas of Laser Voice Surgery*.

To my co-workers: Dr. C.A. Timsit and Dr. J.J. Maimaran.

Dr. Claude Alexandre Timsit and Otolaryngologist, Paris, President of Medispace, was a main contributor. When I invited him to assist us with the chapter "Steps of Phonosurgery" and the "Larynx Anatomy" with his marvellous drawings, I did not expect such a personal and enthusiastic period. The author is indebted to Dr. Timsit for countless hours of support, suggestions, editorial assistance, and above all, proofreadings. His input has enhanced this book.

Dr. Jean-Jacques Maimaran, Otolaryngologist, Paris: He assembled and organized the photographs, figures, data, and references. His faithful assistance these last 10 years in and out of the operating room is a sign of an exceptional generosity and friendship.

Dr. Henri Chevallier, Anesthesiologist, Paris: He took care of almost all the patients who underwent Laser surgery. He helped to make precise the accuracy and safety of the laser technique. Without him, laser phonosurgery as presented in this book would not have been possible. Through him I want to acknowledge the surgical team.

Dr. Archibald Felgeres, Anatomo-pathologist, Paris.

Caroline Abitbol, my sister, a photographer, for her help and her beautiful slides.

To Dr. W. J. Gould, Chairman Emeritus and Founder of the Voice Foundation in New York, Clinical Professor of Otolaryngology, New York University, who passed away February 5th 1994. He instilled in me the faith of voice science and inspired me further and further in my research. He was not only a Master teacher, but a friend who knew how to listen, to comprehend, to galvanize the energy to excel.

To Dr. Robert T. Sataloff, Professor of Otolaryngology, Thomas Jefferson University, Director, Jefferson Arts Medicine Center, Chairman of the Voice Foundation, Philadelphia, Pennsylvania, who more than anyone else encouraged me to write and publish my work. Without him and Dr. Singh, of Singular Publishing Group, this book would be still in the world of the imagination. Bob is a humanist, a scientist, and an artist.

I acknowledge the Voice Foundation and its exceptional team, H. Von Leden, D. Brewer, P. Moore. J. Casper, P. Woo, D. M. Bless, and J. Kahane.

I would like to manifest my friendship and my appreciation to the following colleagues who promote laser phonosurgery: Herbert Dedo, Charles Vaughn, Stanley Blaugrund, Krzysztof Izdebski, and Vasant H. Oswald.

M. Hirano, Professor and Chairman of Otolaryngology-Head and Neck Surgery, Kurume University, Kurume, Japan, whose pioneering work in voice inspired us to increase our research in this field. His objectivity and rigor are an example for all of us.

Dr. R. Feder, associate professor UCLA, helped me discover Laser phonosurgery in the early 1980s. More than a colleague, he became a friend.

To Professor F. Paquelin who guided me at the beginning of this work, and Professors Y. Lallemand, C. Freche, and J. Bouche.

To Professors G. Jako and Strong from Boston, Narong Nimsakul from Bangkok, Kazuhiko Atsumi from Tokyo, B. Aronoff from Dallas Texas, E.W. Friedman from New York, and Theodore H. Maiman who are pioneers in laser surgery.

To Dr. Raymond Sultan, Head of the digestive laser unit of Stell Hospital, from Paris, Founder of the European Laser Association. He was the perfect advisor. Ray and Anne-Marie, his wife, knew how to restrain my enthusiasm when overzealous and inject it into myself when frustrated and discouraged. His professionalism, his honesty, and his suggestions were made without reservation.

Professor Isaac Kaplan from Bellingson Hospital, Tel Aviv, Israel, has created the International Laser Society. He is a pioneer in laser surgery, a "Laser Philosopher" arriving with his wife Macha, from the Holy Land, and has merit as a holy man .

To Dr. Charly Presgurvic who guided my first steps in medicine and taught me that if medicine is a particulate of science, it is only the emerging part of the iceberg.

To Serge Golse, M.D., who, with warm feelings and wisdom, has helped me since the beginning of my career.

To Yves Gauguet and his wife, Aliki, who made me realize that between science and art is an imaginary world in which voice is the impalpable instrument of the emotional being.

Special thanks: to Dr. Louis Katz, M.D., F.A.C.P., New York, for his assistance and his suggestions; to S. Benzaquen from Bemas and Sharplan Industry for their twofold contribution: in surgery, by their laser, and in the book by their slides; to Coherent Laser for their slides and particularly J. Stevenson from Cambridge (England) and T. Brunner from Palo Alto (USA); to Jose Taieb, a video-engineer, for his computerized system which helped me set up the video-dynamic-vocal-exploration. To Christian Boutmy (Micro-France) for his collaboration in creating and realizing the laser laryngoscopy instruments. To Valerie Prevost, my secretary, whose efforts to prepare the manuscript are most appreciated. The author is indebted to the publisher, Singular Publishing Group, Inc., for the encouragement, patience, and efforts necessary to realize this book.

The acknowledgments would not be complete without mentioning the sympathetic complicity of my patients; my students who taught me that nothing is ever taken for granted; the speech therapists: Rachel Houdin, Sylvie Drai-Jacquin, and André Allali; and the singers and singing teachers: Fiamma Izzo (coloratura), Mady Mesple (soprano coloratura), Francis Bardot (tenor), Yva Barthelemy, Schuyler Hamilton, Charles Aznavour and Liza Minelli who taught me how to experience the adventure of voice.

DEDICATION

To my wife Beatrice, my son Patrick, and my daughter Delphine
to whom I owe very much for creating the environment that was
indispensable to conceive such a book

with love

and my parents Charles and Liza Abitbol, my sisters Caroline and Betty,
my niece Candice, my nephew Thierry, my mother-in-law Helene Blankiet,
my father-in-law Michel Blankiet, and my uncle Leon Tuszynski.

I

Introduction

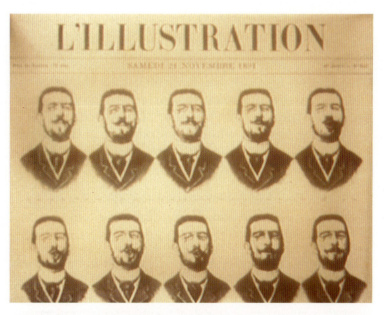

PLATE I.1: Voice production as depicted on the cover of the journal *L'Illustration*, November 21, 1901

He stated that the glottis is the sole vocal organ; the trachea furnishes only the air.

1681–1737: Gliandomenico Santorini published the first picture of the larynx in situ from above.

1682–1771: Giovanni Battista Morgagni related the changes in function and in the voice to specific pathologic changes in the larynx. He is considered the second founder of our specialty. In the larynx, he described the oblique fibers of the thyroarytenoid muscles, the cuneiform cartilages, the epiglottic glands, the pharyngo-epiglottic ligaments, the ventricles, and the ventricular bands.

1693–1769: Antoine Ferrein described numerous experiments on human cadaver larynges. He was the first to use the term "vocal cords." He observed that the tones vary with the speed of the vibrations.

1708–1777: Albrecht von Haller realized that vocal resonance was related to the cavities of the nose, throat, and sinuses.

1801–1858: Johannes Muller proclaimed the myoelastic theory of phonation in 1839. He confirmed that the voice is produced by the airstream that originates in the lungs and sets the vocal folds in vibration. He proved that the vocal folds are passive, while the airstream is the active element in the production of sound.

1813–1878: Claude Bernard demonstrated two fascicles in the same nerve for opening and closing the vocal fold.

1850–1906: Manuel Garcia, after having destroyed his voice by vocal stress and abuse, devoted himself to teaching to protect other singers from the same problems. He published in 1847 a "Traité Complet de l'Art du Chant." On March 13, 1855, he presented a report on the "Physiological Observations of the Human Voice" in which he described a method of looking at his own larynx and visualizing the phonating organ using a small dental mirror to reflect the sunlight.

Introduction

980–1037: Avicenna, the Persian, wrote the *Quanum*, in which he devoted a whole chapter to the production of voice and voice disturbances.

936–1013: First description of Laryngotomy by Abdul Quasinu.

1452–1519: Leonardo Da Vinci gave information about anatomy, physiology, and pathology of the human voice. In his textbook *Quaderni d'Anatomia* (1500), he included several drawings of the organ of voice production or larynx. He produced tones from the larynx of a goose by squeezing the lungs. The experiment was not repeated until 1741 (by Antoine Ferrein). Da Vinci noted the difference between waves and vibrations, which was not rediscovered before 1911 when Giesswein described the same phenomenon. Da Vinci also postulated the waveform of a string which was not rediscovered until 1860 by Melde. In addition, Da Vinci described articulation, the structures of the mouth, lips, and teeth, and assigned phonetic terms to different sounds.

1514–1565: Andreas Vesalius found errors in Galen's book: he discovered two separate arytenoid cartilages rather than one.

1523–1563: Gabrielle Fallopio coined the term "cricoid" for the second major laryngeal cartilage. He also offered a more accurate presentation of the laryngeal muscles.

1537–1619: Hieronymus Fabricius ab Aquapendente wrote three books on the larynx and the organs of communication, including a treatise that he called "De Larynge Vocis Instrumento."

1550–1624: Caspar Bauhinus described accurately and named the three pairs of extrinsic and five pairs of intrinsic laryngeal muscles.

1613–1688: Claude Perrault in "Oeuvres Diverses de Physique et de Mécanique" explained voice production using laws of mechanics.

1621–1675: Thomas Willis presented a definite description of the origin of the superior laryngeal nerve.

1634–1707: Dennis Dodart presented a paper, "Memoire sur les Causes de la Voix de l'Homme," in which he ascribed the production of the voice to the movement of the vocal lips.

DEFINITIONS OF PHONOSURGERY

The term phonosurgery was first introduced by Von Leden. It represents one of the multiple aspects of otolaryngology practice. The goal of this surgery is to restore a normal voice. Phonosurgery is also called "plastic surgery of the vocal organ." It refers to any surgical technique the aim of which is the improvement of voice.

PHONOSURGERY: A CHRONOLOGY OF EVENTS, INSIGHTS, AND DISCOVERIES

The History Of Larynx And Voice

2900 BC:	Memorial stone of King Aha depicting operation on the larynx. Tomb of Sakkara.
131–220AD:	Claudius Galen, founder of Laryngology, godfather of phoniatrics and voice science, was the first to describe the larynx with its three major cartilages and paired muscles. He first identified the larynx as the instrument of voice.
320:	St. Blaise was familiar with techniques of tracheostomy and became famous for his treatment of throat diseases.
535–538:	First picture of the vocal organ on a mosaic, Church of St. Apollinaris, Ravenna.
850–923:	Rhazes "The Experienced" referred to the afflictions of voice and hoarseness. He related changes in the voice to the laryngeal lining, recurrent nerves, laryngeal muscles, respiratory system, and brain.
990:	Aly Abass described the dual function of respiration and phonation of the larynx. He stated that the voice is produced by blowing air from the chest through the closed larynx.

1906: Marey introduced stroboscopy in cinematography, enabling slow-motion visualization of the vocal folds.

The History of Phonosurgery

1850: Ludwig Turck adapted the Garcia technique in a few patients.

1870: Johann Nepomuk Czermak popularized this indirect visualization of the larynx throughout Europe.

1895: Alfred Kirstein developed the art of direct laryngoscopy, setting the stage for the beginning of laryngeal surgery.

1911: Wilhelm Brunings presented a new technique for the relief of aphonia in patients with unilateral vocal fold paralysis; he described the injection of paraffin into the paralyzed vocal fold. Later, Alfred Seifert described the same injection by a percutaneous approach.

1915: To restore voice after hemithyroidectomy, Erwin Payr designed an ingenious trapdoor procedure using thyroid cartilage, which forced the paralyzed vocal fold medially

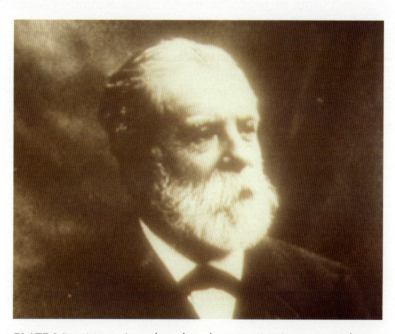

PLATE I.2: Marey introduced stroboscopy in cinematography.

for better approximation. The rectangular flap of thyroid cartilage remained hinged posteriorly and the anterior end was pressed inward, so the patient's voice was restored.

1924: Charles Frazier attempted to cure paralysis of the laryngeal nerve by anastomosing it to the descending ramus of the hypoglossal nerve. By 1926, he reported improvement in 6 out of 10 patients in the *Journal of Surgery, Gynecology, and Obstetrics*.

1942: Yrjo Meurman reported the implantation of a sliver of autogenous costal cartilage for medializing the paralyzed vocal fold.

1950: Basic anatomic and physiologic studies by Paul Moore and Hans Von Leden at Northwestern University set the foundation for phonosurgery.

1954: Rosemarie Albrecht first described the microscopic visualization of the vocal folds. Without doubt, the adaptation of the surgical microscope for magnification of the laryngeal interior was the most important element in the evolution of phonosurgery.

1955: Odd Opheim presented a modification of Meurman's technique in which he implanted a section of cartilage from the ipsilateral thyroid alae.

1957: Godfrey Arnold described two successful vocal fold injections using diced autogenous cartilage from the nasal septum in place of paraffin. The same technique was used by Von Leden. Injection of bovine bone dust (Goff), tantalum powder (Lewi), and silicone (Rubin) followed, and then the successful use of Teflon paste, which has given new hope to patients with unilateral vocal fold paralysis. In spite of a high success rate, some problems associated with Teflon injection led laryngologists to search for other appropriate filler substances, such as bovine collagen and autogenous fat.

1960: The development of objective measures of laryngeal function at the Institute of Laryngology and Voice Disorders in Los Angeles was an important element for accurate evaluation of the surgical results.

1962: Geza Jako developed an improved laryngoscope for binocular diagnosis and bimanual surgery. He developed a series of microlaryngeal instruments with the firm

	Stürner in Würsburg. His skill and vision resulted in instrumentation that has not changed significantly in the past 20 years.
1962–1968:	Oskar Kleinsasser adapted a Zeiss microscope with a 400 mm focal lens that permitted the facile use of the long-handled laryngeal instruments for precision surgery on the vocal folds. In 1968, he published a comprehensive book of microlaryngoscopy, *Mikrolaryngoskopie und Endolaryngeale Mikrochirurgie,* with magnificent photographs of the larynx in health and disease.
1963:	Ryozo Asai described the first laryngoplasty, which represented an entirely new approach for the restoration of voice after laryngectomy. Several other procedures have been devised to create a tracheopharyngeal fistula and deflect the air from the trachea into the esophagus for improved vocalization (J. Conify, T. Calcaterra, L. Miehlke).
1968:	Miehlke and Berendes are the only surgeons who have reported success with an autologous graft of the recurrent laryngeal nerve with a branch of the greater auricular nerve. It was the first successful use of such a technique.
1969:	Patrick Doyle reported the first cases of functional recovery of the recurrent laryngeal nerve in six patients on whom he had operated within 5 days of their injury.
1969:	*Surgical Techniques for the Vocal Rehabilitation in the* Publication of *Post-Laryngectomized Patients* (J.J. Conley, New York).
1969:	P. Kluyskans of Gand University in Belgium performed the first case of a larynx homo-transplantation in humans, with a follow-up of 4½ months.
1970:	Hans Von Leden began to inject a local anesthetic into the laryngeal nerves of patients with spastic dysphonia.
1970:	The professional liability crisis in the United States hampered further development of these new surgical modalities for esthetic changes in voice. The risk of legal redress increased exponentially; and most, if not all, professional liability insurance contracts excluded coverage of any procedure that was not generally accepted by the medical profession in the community. Under these circumstances, it is not surprising that highly skilled European and Japanese surgeons assumed the leadership in surgery for an esthetic improvement of the voice.

1974: Nobuhiko Isshiki described surgical techniques for altering the framework of the larynx, leading to changes in length, tension, and mass of the vocal folds and thereby permitting a true transformation of the patient's voice. Working on the thyroid cartilage to achieve the vocal fold change was an Isshiki master idea. Since his original description of four types of thyroplasty Isshiki has modified some of these basic steps to improve the functional results. He also has designed a series of new procedures to achieve this objective.

1975: Working at the University of Kyoto like Isshiki, Minoru Hirano devoted himself to the study of the human voice and published a report on the basic and clinical applications of phono-physiology and surgery.

1975: Harvey Tucker transplanted a nerve/muscle pedicle consisting of the branch of the ansa hypoglossi nerve to the anterior belly of the omohyoid muscle, together with the surrounding muscular segment, directly into the posterior cricoarytenoid muscle. Four years later, he reported success in 40 of a series of 45 cases.

1976: Herbert Dedo decided to sever the recurrent laryngeal nerve to relieve disabling spasticity. His first patient recovered her voice, and a successful procedure for the relief of spastic dysphonia was born.

1983: Advancement of the anterior commissure to tighten the vocal ligament and strengthen the voice in patients with bowed vocal folds or weak voices was described by Le Jeune. This procedure was also used for raising the vocal pitch by mobilizing a midline strip of thyroid cartilage. The everted upper end was held in position with a sliver of tantalum foil.

1986: Andrew Blitzer and Mitchell Brinn injected a solution of botulinum toxin into the vocalis muscle to relieve spasticity. A significant improvement in voice was obtained that lasted several months.

1987: Le Jeune developed an elaborate caliper for measuring the tension of the vocal ligament and described a modification of the original procedure for additional extension of the vocal cords.

1989: James Koufman enhanced the anterior advancement technique by silastic implants between the thyroarytenoid muscles and the thyroid alae for patients with bowed vocal folds.

REFERENCES

von Leden, H. (1992). The history of phono-surgery. In W. R. Gould, R. Sataloff, & J. R. Spiegel (Eds.), *Voice surgery* (pp. 3–65). New York: C. V. Mosby.

von Leden, H. (1991). The history of phono-surgery. In C. N. Ford & D. M. Bless (Eds.), *Phono-surgery: Assessment and surgical management of voice disorders* (pp. 3–24). New York: Raven Press.

Weir, N. (1990). *Otolaryngology: An illustrated history*. London: Butterworths.

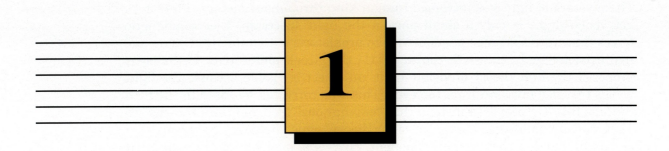

Laser

HISTORY

The mystery of light has intrigued human kind throughout history (Plate 1.1). Yet visible light is only a small part of the light spectrum. Electromagnetic forces that were a strange phenomenon to prehistoric man millions of years ago still exist today. In the sixth century B.C., the Greek philosopher Pythagorus proposed the first theory of visible light: an object is visible because the light waves traveled outward from the eyes. This was corrected by Plato in the fifth century B.C. He proposed instead that "emanations" occurred from the sun. In 1704, Newton published his "corpuscular theory" which held that light consisted of rapidly moving particles; an opponent, Huygens, maintained that the light was a series of waves. J.C. Maxwell, an English physicist, developed the first

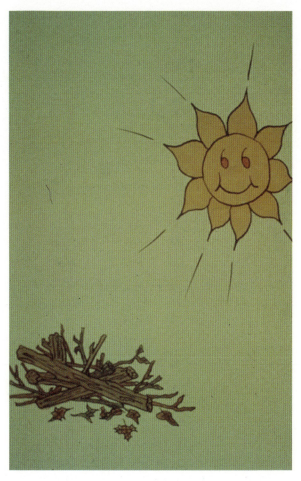 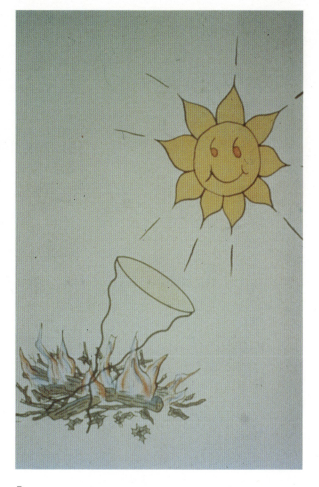

A B
PLATE 1.1: The same picture illuminated with an unfocused beam (**A**) and a focused beam (**B**).

electromagnetic theory of light. Light waves, he said, were electrical in nature and different from the mechanical nature of sound waves (Plates 1.2, 1.3, and 1.4). Many of phenomena of light, such as propagation, reflection, refraction, interference, diffraction, and polarization were explained by the electromagnetic waves theory. But the absorption and emission of light by matter remained unexplained until Hertz proposed the photoelectric emission theory in 1887 in which photoelectric emission is independent of the intensity of light but dependent on the wavelength of the incident light. This incident light induces the ejection of electrons from conductors of light. These effects were explained by Einstein in 1905 as the absorption of light energy by matter. Einstein also extended the Planck Theory which held that light energy transferred by matter must be transferred in discrete units, or "quanta." According to Max Planck's theory, "Light is corpuscular in nature but apparently travels in electromagnetic waves emitting radiant energy by tiny packages of energy called quanta"; it was published on December 14th, in 1900, at the German Physics Society in Berlin. Einstein later postulated that the energy of a light photon was proportional to the frequency of light. The equation between "quanta" and "wavelength" is:

$$e = h\eta$$

where e = energy of the quantum, η = wavelength, and h = Planck's constant.

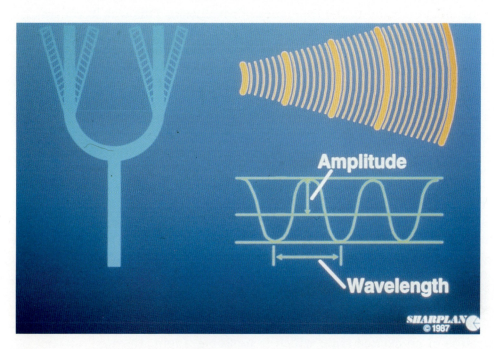

PLATE 1.2: Wavelength of sound.

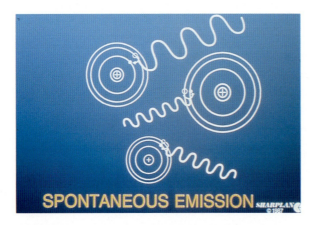 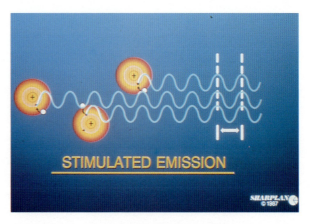

PLATE 1.3: Spontaneous emission of light.   **PLATE 1.4:** Stimulated emission of light.

LASER CONCEPT

But how did Einstein arrive at his revolutionary theory?

If the electromagnetic theory is true, electrons must continually emit energy as they revolve around the nucleus or spiral inward toward the center of the atom and collapse into the nucleus. The same theory predicts that all atoms emit a continuous spectrum because the frequency of radiation emitted by the revolving electrons must be equal to the frequency of revolution. This was in contradiction to the line spectra that had been observed. For the first postulate of the atomic theory, Bohr held that: Electrons can revolve around the nucleus of an atom in certain stable orbits without emitting radiant energy. The second postulate held that an electron makes a transition from a stable orbit to a lower energy level orbit by emitting a photon; the photon emitted has an energy equal to the difference between the two orbits; and the photon is the emission of radiant energy (Plate 1.5). Bohr's model explains only the emission spectra of an atom; it does not predict what energy level elements and molecules should have or the emission they should give off. To explain this, quantum mechanics is required. Quantum mechanics predicts the energy levels and explains the frequency of light observed in the atomic spectrum. In 1919, Einstein presented "Zur Quantum Theorie der Stralung'" (the Quantum Theory of Radiations). In the theory, electrons, atoms, molecules, and photons interact with electromagnetic radiation by quantum units in three types of radiation transitions: absorption, spontaneous emission, and stimulated emission (see Plates 1.6, 1.3, and 1.4). Absorption of a photon occurs when an electron goes up from a lower orbit to a higher orbit.

The electron is in an excited state which is unstable. Light, thermal, electrical, or optical energy can induce this kind of excited state.

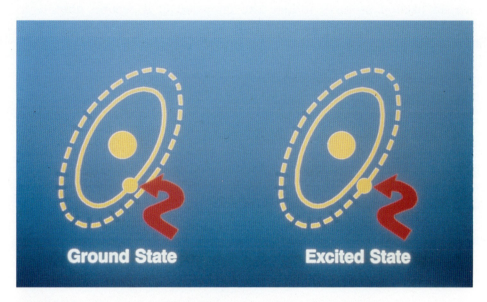

PLATE 1.5: Illustration of electrons in ground and excited states.

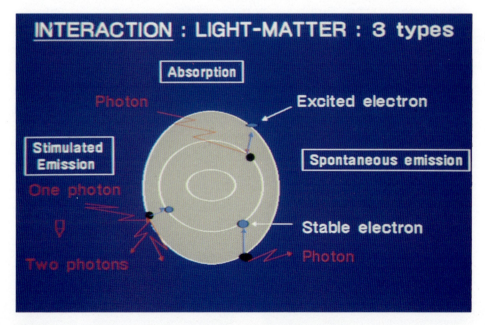

PLATE 1.6: Three types of interaction of light with matter.

Spontaneous emission of a photon occurs when the electron goes down to its stable orbit. Stimulated emission was the ingenious idea of Albert Einstein. He first voiced the hypothesis that one photon of a specific wavelength could interact with an excited atom to induce the emission of a second photon. Laser-produced light operates on that principle: in a stimulated emission, the second photon emitted from the excited atom has the same frequency, phase, and direction as the incident photon absorbed and immediately released. On this principle, the Laser was born. LASER is an acronym for *Light Amplification by the Stimulated Emission of Radiation*.

Light

Lasers produce a beam that has four fundamental characteristics: intensity (tremendous energy in a very focused, narrow beam), coherence (Plate 1.7) (in phase spatially and temporally), high collimation (light waves are parallel with minimal divergence and thus minimal dissipation of energy), and monochromaticity (uniform wavelength). The last characteristic is fundamental from a surgical point of view. The components of human tissue absorb wavelength selectively depending on their hydration, temperature, color, and thickness.

Amplification

Before the active medium of a laser is excited, it has more stable than unstable atoms. During amplification, it will become a tremendous source of energy. The electromagnetic emission released by stimulated emission is amplified by an external power source to produce an intense beam that will excite the atoms, leading to an excited state and allowing the emission of photons from the atoms. In essence, it creates a chain reaction in the active medium of a laser.

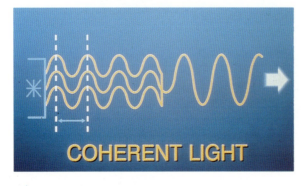

A

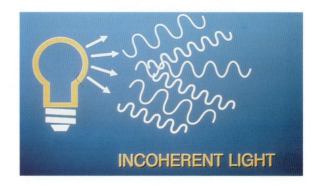

B

PLATE 1.7: **A.** Coherent light. **B.** Incoherent light.

Stimulated Emission of Radiation

We have already described stimulated emission. Radiation emitted from a laser consists of a spectrum of wavelengths ranging from 200 (ultraviolet) to 10,000 (infrared) nanometers (nm). The five types of surgical Lasers in current use emit around 500 nm (Argon Laser), 1060 nm (Neodymium Yttrium-Aluminium-Garnet Laser or Nd-Yag), 532 nm (KTP), 640 nm (Dye Laser), and 10,600 nm (the CO_2 Laser, the most important in surgery).

COMPONENTS OF A SURGICAL LASER

As illustrated Plates 1.8, 1.9, and 1.10, there are three components: an active medium of laser, a power source to pump energy, and an optical chamber which has a total reflector mirror on one side and a partial reflector mirror on the other side where the laser is emitted.

LASER TISSUE INTERACTION

Characteristics of laser-tissue interaction are numerous and specific. There are four primary interactions between laser and tissue (Plates 1.11, 1.12, 1.13, and 1.14):

- Reflection: Laser is not absorbed and does not go through the tissue.
- Transmission: Laser is not absorbed and goes through the tissue.
- Absorption: Laser is absorbed by the tissue.
- Scatter or dispersion: Laser is partially absorbed and transmitted and scattered by the tissue.

All four of these interactions may be mixed, depending on the type of laser and tissue.

Each type of laser interacts with tissue in a specific way, producing characteristic patterns of heat conduction, coagulation, ablation, and charring. Knowledge of laser physics and typical tissue interactions allows the surgeon to select the laser best suited to the task at hand. The properties of CO_2 lasers are particularly well suited to laryngeal surgery. The CO_2 lasers produce a cone-shaped impact which has three characteristic levels including, from the center to the outer layer, an area of charring, a region of tissue desiccation, and an outer layer of edema. (Plate 1.15).

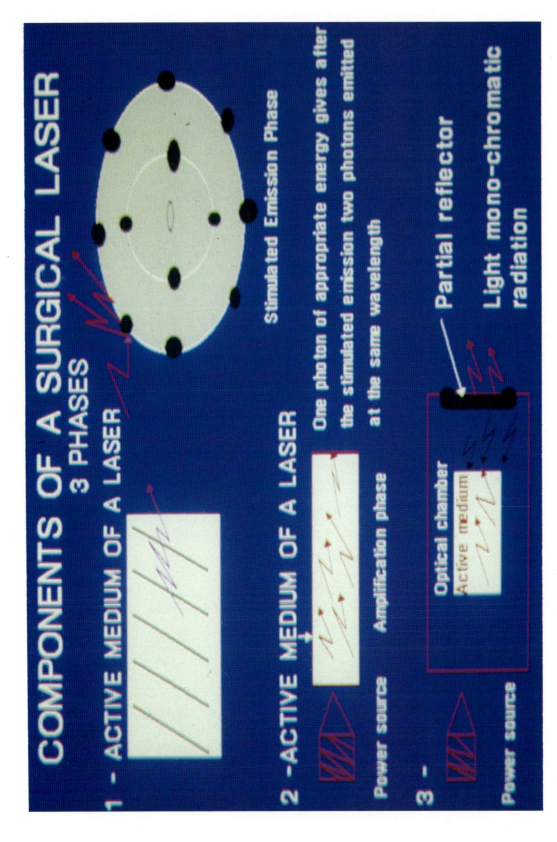

PLATE 1.8: Components of a surgical laser.

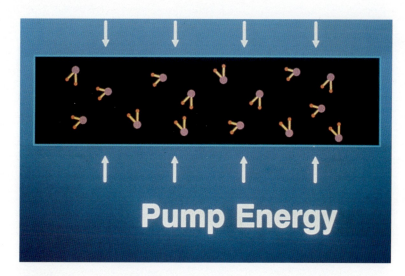

PLATE 1.9: CO_2 laser machine concepts: pump energy.

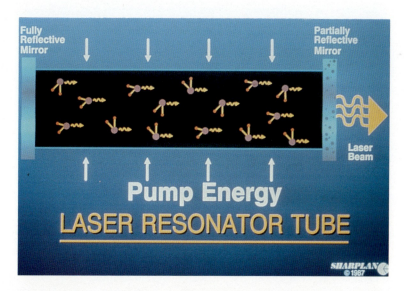

PLATE 1.10: CO_2 laser machine concept: optical chamber, laser resonator tube.

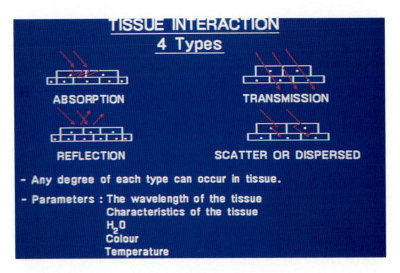

PLATE 1.11: Four types of laser-tissue interaction.

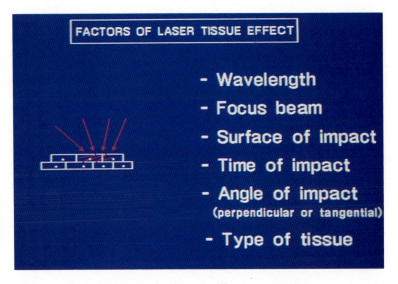

PLATE 1.12: Factors in the laser's effects on tissues.

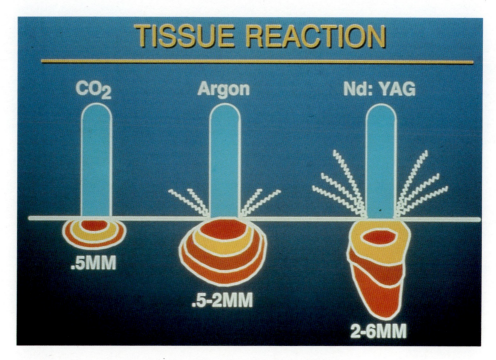

PLATE 1.13: Tissue reaction with different types of lasers.

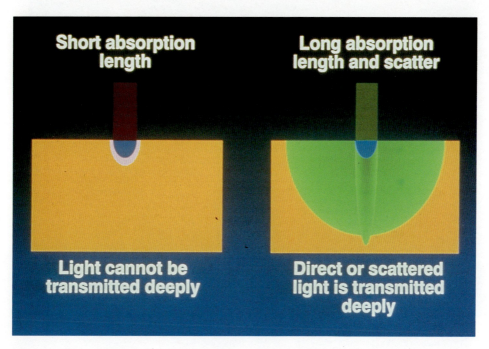

PLATE 1.14: Absorption length and laser transmission characteristics.

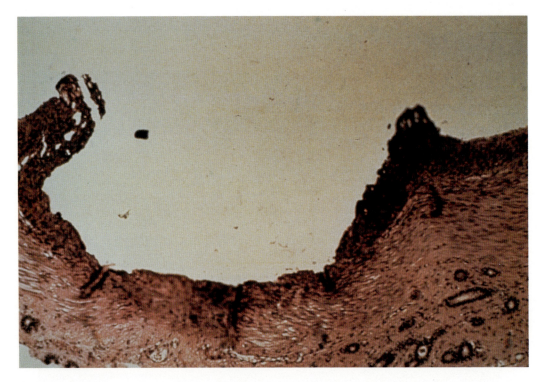

A

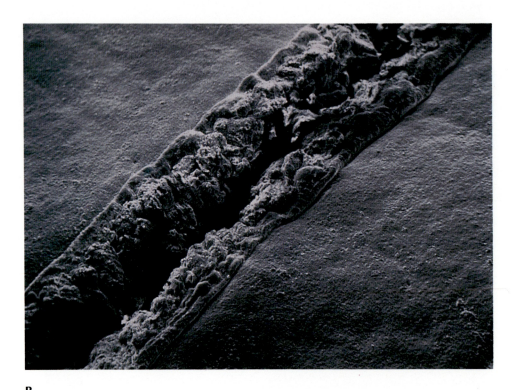

B
PLATE 1-15: Two examples of the histological effects of CO_2 laser.

Electronmicrographic studies in soft tissue show that, with a spot size of 130 microns, a power of 50 Watts, and an exposure of 1 second, CO_2 laser impact creates a cone-shaped lesion that is 450 microns deep and 230 microns wide (30 microns for the center area of charring, 100 microns for the intermediate desiccated tissue layer, and 100 microns on the outer layer of the edematous tissue).

Beside wavelength, laser tissue interaction depends of the mode of impact of the CO_2 Laser. It operates either in a continuous fire, a pulsed mode fire, or a Q-switched mode. (Plates 1.16 and 1.17)

In the continuous-fire mode, photons are emitted in a constant and stable delivery of energy and intensity. A constant power source to keep the active medium in an excited state to stimulate emission is necessary. In a pulsed mode, an intermittent power source such as a flash-lamp is used. It provides sudden bursts of energy to the active medium. Pulsed mode laser develops a higher energy in a very short time. If a continuous wave laser delivers easily 25 Watts, a pulsed mode Laser will deliver up to 2,000 Watts at each pulse, between the pulses, there is almost no energy (Plates 1.18, 1.19, 1.20, and 1.21). That is why a pulsed CO_2 laser provides a more acute, deeper cutting effect with less thermal damage than the continuous fire mode for the same diameter impact spot. The Q-switched mode can be associated with either a continuous or pulsed mode. It is a technical adaptation that provides a fast shutter positioned in the active medium and the partial reflector of the chamber. The pump is activated when the shutter is closed. Energy increase in the chamber. Suddenly, the shutter opens, and this excess excitation is delivered in a very short time: 10^{-6} to 10^{-9} second. The power can reach 10,000 to 100,000 watts in a picosecond. (Plates 1.22, 1.23, and 1.24).

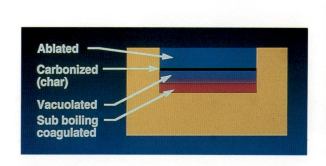

A B

PLATE 1.16: Zones of damage with low pulse energy.

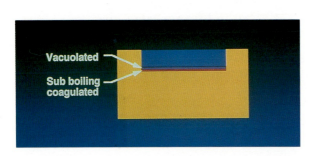

PLATE 1.17: Zones of damage with high pulse energy.

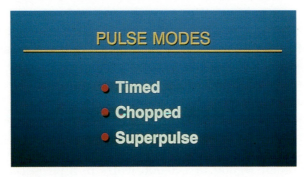

PLATE 1.18: Pulse modes.

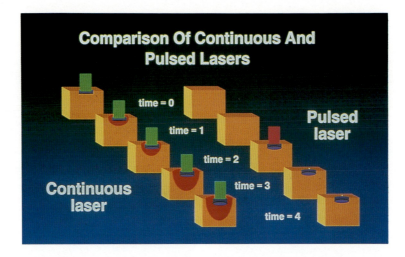

PLATE 1.19: Comparison of continuous and pulsed lasers.

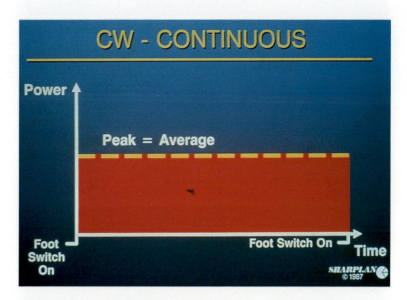

PLATE 1.20: Continuous wave.

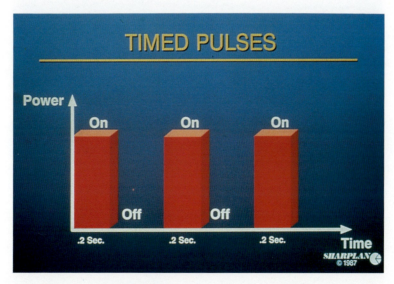

PLATE 1.21: Timed pulses.

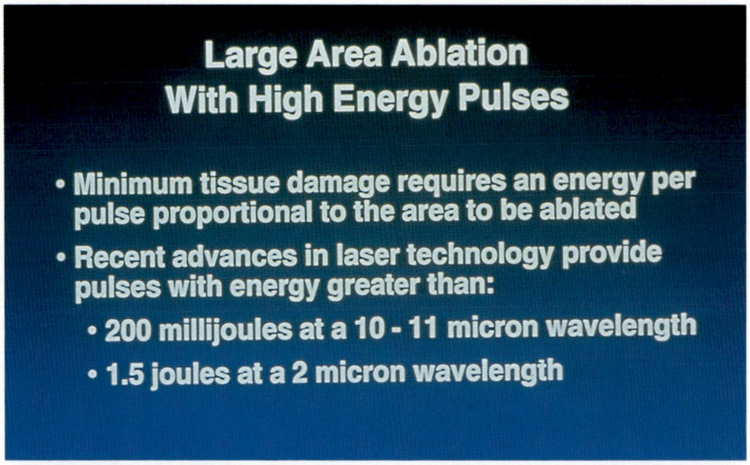

Large Area Ablation With High Energy Pulses

- Minimum tissue damage requires an energy per pulse proportional to the area to be ablated
- Recent advances in laser technology provide pulses with energy greater than:
    - 200 millijoules at a 10 - 11 micron wavelength
    - 1.5 joules at a 2 micron wavelength

PLATE 1.22: Ablation with high energy pulses.

A Pulsed Laser Can Be Adjusted To Cut Or Coagulate

- Smaller spot, higher energy gives char free cutting
- Larger spot, lower energy gives coagulation
- Intermediate settings can be used
- Continuous operation may be possible

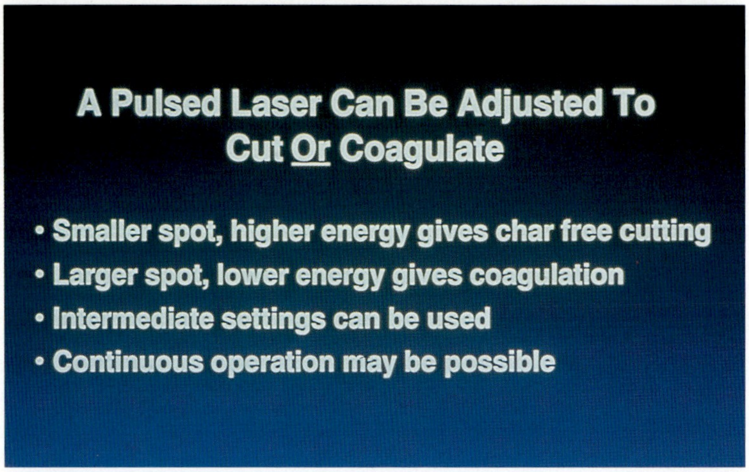

PLATE 1.23: A pulse laser can cut or coagulate.

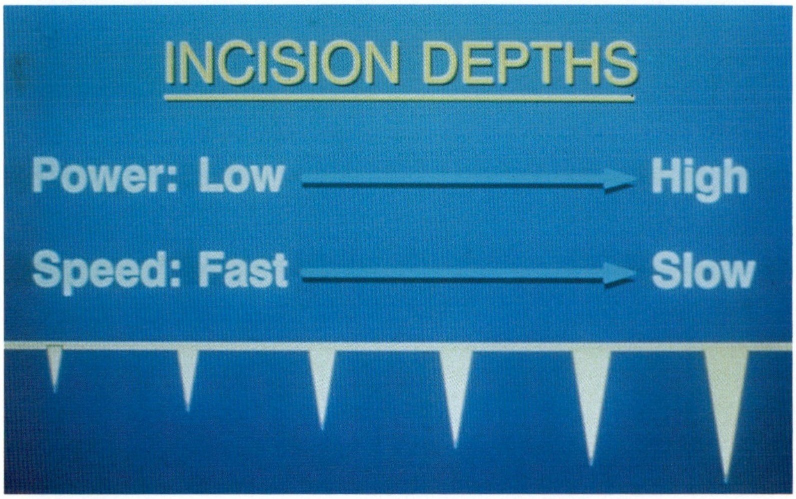

INCISION DEPTHS

Power: Low ⟶ High

Speed: Fast ⟶ Slow

PLATE 1.24: Incision depths depend on power and speed.

The key words in Laser-tissue interaction are the power-density per second, the amount of energy absorbed by a specific unit of tissue area per second:

$$P = \frac{\text{Laser power output (watts)}}{\pi R^2 \text{ (cm}^2\text{) per second.}}$$

(Plates 1.25, and 1.26)

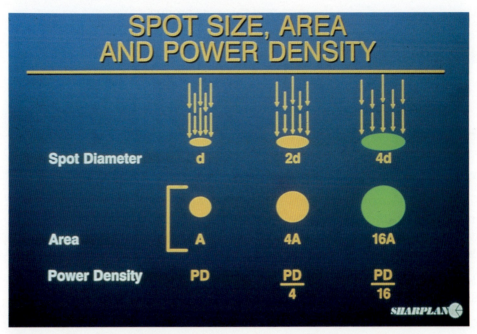

PLATE 1.25: The relationship between spot size area and power density.

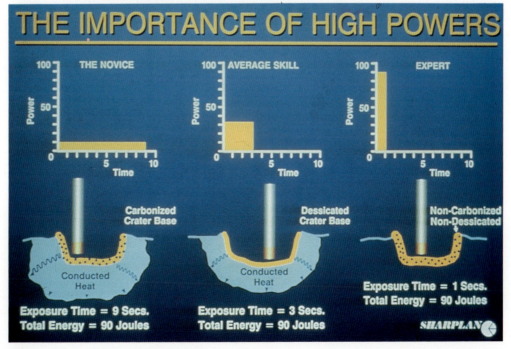

PLATE 1.26: Types of laser impacts.

LASER SAFETY AND LIMITATIONS

The increasing use of lasers requires more professionals to become familiar with the potential hazards associated with the misuse of this new product of modern science.

Laser Hazards

The basic hazards from laser equipment can be categorized as follows:

Laser Radiations

Eye (Plate 1.27)

- Corneal and/or retinal burns, depending on laser wavelength, are possible from acute exposure. Corneal or lenticular opacities (cataracts) or retinal injuries may also be possible from chronic exposure to excessive levels of radiation.

- Ocular hazards generally depend on which structure absorbs the most radiant energy per volume of tissue.

- Retinal effects are possible when the laser emission wavelength occurs in the visible and near infrared spectral regions (0.4 to 1.4 μm). Such light directly entering the eye can be focused to a very small image on the retina. Laser emissions in the ultraviolet and far infrared spectral regions (outside 0.4 to 1.4 μm) may produce ocular effects at the cornea or the lens.

Skin

- Skin burns are possible from acute exposure to high levels of optical radiation. At some specific ultraviolet wavelengths, skin carcinogenesis may occur.

- Skin effects, usually considered of secondary importance, become greater with the use of lasers emitting in the ultraviolet spectral region. Erythema and skin cancers are possible in the 0.2–0.28 μm wavelength range; increased pigmentation and photosensitivity may occur between 0.28–0.40 μm; and skin burns and excessive dry skin effects between 0.7–1.0 μm.

Chemical Hazards and Plume

Laser-induced reactions can release hazardous particulate and gaseous products.

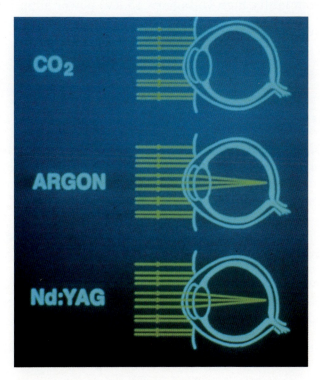

PLATE 1.27: Laser safety and limits for eye penetration.

Plume, or the smoke produced by CO_2 laser, can induce two kinds of reaction. The first reaction is the plume radiation. In our experience, it is not significant. The second reaction is the release of particulate matter, which may affect the tracheobronchial tree of the patient if there is no cuff. It also may affect the surgeon if he does not wear a mask (ideally, 95% efficiency for particles of 0.3 mm). Viruses, such Human Papilloma Virus, may be inhaled during laser surgery for papillomas.

Electrical Hazards

Lethal electrical hazards may be present, particularly in high-powered laser systems. Three fatal accidents associated with lasers have been reported due to accidental electrocution. These occurred when safety procedures were not carefully followed.

Secondary Hazards

Secondary hazards include:

- Cryogenic coolant hazards from some research lasers
- Excessive noise exposure from some very high energy lasers

- X radiation from faulty high voltage (> 15 kV) power supplies
- Explosions caused by faulty optical pump lamps
- Fire hazards

Laser Safety Standards

The most common classification of laser hazards is based on the intensity of the beam emitted from the laser and describes the capability of a laser or a laser system to produce injury to personnel. The higher the classification number, the greater the potential hazard.

Class 1: A laser or laser system that cannot, under normal operating conditions, produce a hazard.

Class 2: Low power visible lasers or laser systems that do not normally present a hazard, but have some potential for hazard if viewed directly for extended periods of time.

Class 3a: A laser or laser system that normally would not produce a hazard if viewed for only momentary periods with the unaided eye but may present a hazard if viewed using collecting optics.

Class 3b: A laser or laser system that can produce a hazard if viewed directly. This includes intra-beam viewing of specular reflections. Except for the high-power Class 3b lasers, this class of laser will not produce a hazardous diffuse reflection.

Class 4: A laser or laser system that can produce a hazard not only from direct or specular reflection, but also from a diffuse reflection. Such lasers may present both fire and skin hazards.

Safety in Carbon Dioxide Laser Surgery

The introduction of the carbon dioxide laser as a surgical tool by Strong and Jako in 1972 necessitated adjustments and precautions in operating room setup and in the administration of anesthetics, especially in surgery on the laryngotracheal airway and the intraoral cavity. Because these interventions are performed under general endotracheal anesthesia, protection of the endotracheal tube and adjustment in the provision of anesthetics are necessary to prevent an inadvertent laser-ignition explosion caused by internal laser heat. The Oswal-Hunton metal tracheal tube is very interesting and not traumatic.

Safety measures and precautions are employed to protect patients and operating room personnel from direct or reflected laser burns. The patient's eyes are carefully covered; the patient's face is covered with a wet towel; and a wet green gauze is used to protect the subglottic area, the endotracheal tube, and the nontarget area of the larynx. Protective glasses are used by all operating room personnel, because the carbon dioxide laser beam is absorbed by the cornea, plastic, glass, and water. The surgeon's eyes are protected by the microscope's optics. A suction device also is used to evacuate laser smoke during the procedure to allow visualization of the operative field. These precautions prevent most laser accidents.

Safety in Combination Laser Surgery

Combination laser units usually utilize CO_2 and Nd-Yag lasers, which are both Class 4 lasers. Safety precautions when using Class 4 lasers include:

- The laser site and dangerous areas must be controlled and unnecessary time spent in these areas must be prevented.

- Unnecessary reflections should be avoided.

- Protective eyewear must be used in the dangerous areas. It is essential to wear the right type of protective glasses.

- If possible, the beam path should be screened off.

- Laser warning signs must be posted on the doors to the laser room.

The patient's eye must also be protected against facial burns by a moistened cloth, if anesthetized, and by protective glasses if not anesthetized. Instruments used during laser operations should be anti-reflective to prevent dangerous reflections. Laser radiation also should not be used around inflammable or explosive gases, liquids, or other such materials. Finally, because of the potentially lethal voltages inside the console, only trained service personnel should be allowed to open the doors or other covers of the device.

WHAT KIND OF LASER FOR PHONOSURGERY?

History

Lasers can be used to incise, vaporize, coagulate, or penetrate (for phonosurgery, the site is the vocal fold structure — Plate 1.28). The idea of using light for surgery predates the laser. In 1946, Gerd Meyer Schwickerath treated detached retinas and eye tumors with the sun. Laser, as a surgical tool, was first proposed in 1958 by Schawlow and Townedes. Maiman built the first Ruby Laser in 1960 using a wavelength of 690 nm. Infrared emission laser action using pure carbon dioxide was first reported in 1964 by Patel et al.

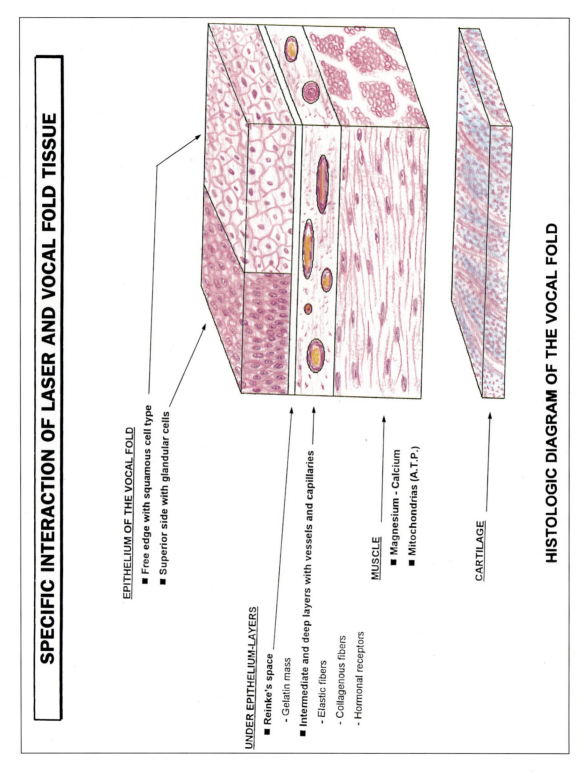

PLATE 1.28: Factors in the effect of lasers on tissues.

A high power laser using a mixture of carbon dioxide, nitrogen, and helium and operating continuously at 10,600 nm was reported by Patel et al. in 1965.

Preliminary studies using a 20 watt laboratory CO_2 Laser for liver surgery on dogs were reported by Yahr and Strully in 1966. Their results were encouraging and led to the development of an endoscopic system, which was reported by Polanyi in 1970. Laser application to laryngeal microsurgery began with the work of Jako in 1967 on a cadaver larynx. Other experimental studies were done on dogs. Clinical application started in 1972 when Strong and Jako presented their report of clinical use of the CO_2 Laser on 12 patients.

Characteristics of Lasers

Strong absorption by water means small penetration. Living tissue contains a large amount of water; therefore, absorption of CO_2 Laser emissions is maximum in the superficial layers of tissue. It causes a defect by evaporation of tissue fluids and burning of organic material. A small proportion of the energy of Laser light penetrates deeper, partly by absorption but mostly by conduction. This causes a zone of devitalized cells due to thermal damage. The depth of this scarring, which is covered by black particles, is due to carbonization and is proportional to the energy, density, and temperature of the tissue (Plates 1.29, 1.30, 1.31, and 1.32).

Energy density depends on the time of exposure to the laser, the energy delivered, handspeed, diameter of the focal point, and the angle of delivery.

Types of Lasers

The five main types of lasers used in surgery are the CO_2, Argon, Nd-Yag, KTP, and Dye Lasers (Plates 1.33 and 1.34). Wavelengths differ among these laser instruments along with their depth of tissue penetration, absorption effects, and the temporal behavior of the beam emitted (continuous, super-pulsed or ultra-pulsed). When tissues are exposed to the laser beam, the temperature increases suddenly at the focal point of the beam, decreasing on the edge according to the Gaussian shape. 60° Centigrade (C) is reached in less than a second with protein denaturation and coagulation; at 100° C, evaporation of intra-cellular water occurs, causing shrinkage of tissue; at 150° C, evaporization of tissue occurs (Plates 1.13, 1.14, 1.35, and 1.36).

CO_2 Laser

Carbon dioxide laser or CO_2 laser is a gaseous laser. It employs a mixture of carbon dioxide, nitrogen, and helium. Most CO_2 Lasers are sealed. When empty, the gas cannot be replenished. There are two main technologies:

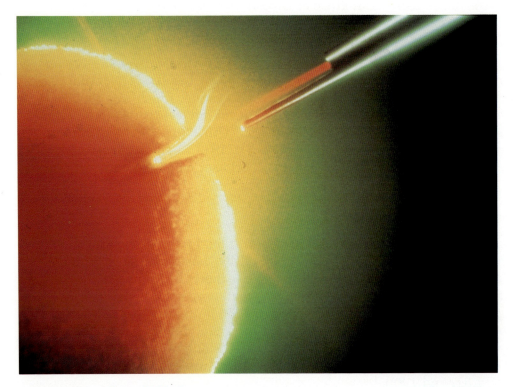

PLATE 1.29: Effect of CO_2 laser.

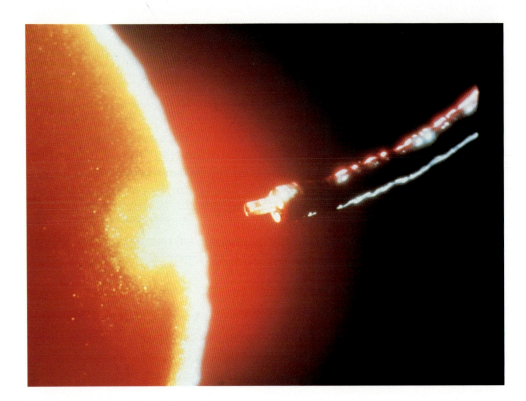

PLATE 1.30: Effect of Nd-Yag laser.

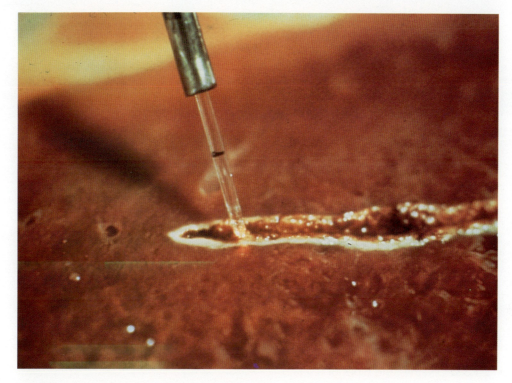

PLATE 1.31: Effect of sapphire Nd-Yag laser.

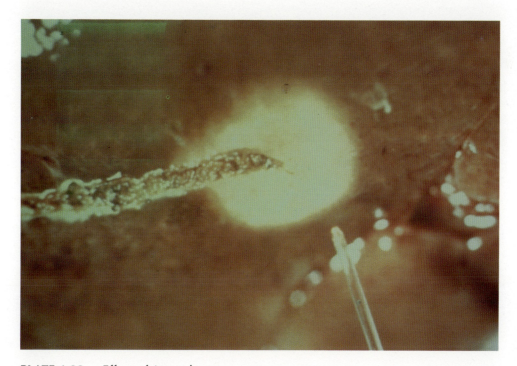

PLATE 1.32: Effect of Argon laser.

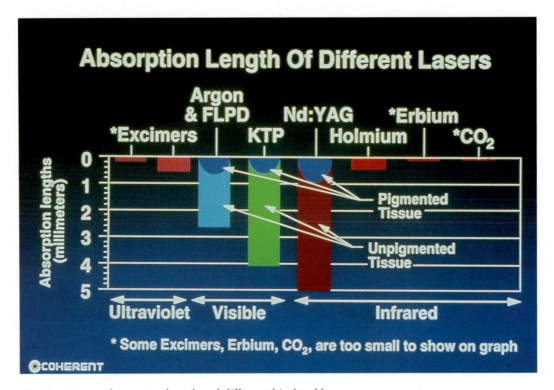

NAME	COLOR	WAVELENGTH
Excimers	Ultraviolet	200-400 nm
Argon	Blue	488 nm
	Green	515 nm
532 Yag	Green	532 nm
Krypton	Green	531 nm
	Yellow	568 nm
Dye Laser	Yellow/Green	577 nm
	Red	630 nm
Helium Neon	Red	630 nm
Gold Vapor	Red	630 nm
Krypton	Red	647 nm
Ruby	Deep Red	694 nm
Nd: Yag	Infrared	1064 nm
	Infrared	1318 nm
CO_2	Infrared	10600 nm

PLATE 1.33: Names and types of lasers.

PLATE 1.34: Absorption lengths of different kinds of lasers.

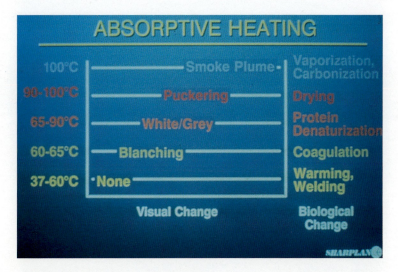

PLATE 1.35: Absorptive heating.

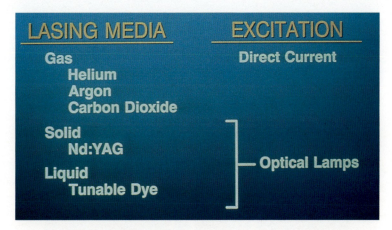

PLATE 1.36: Lasing media.

- Radio Frequency (RF) CO_2 laser operates on a high frequency alternating voltage, with its polarity reversing several tens of megaHertz. This technique was developed by Coherent Laser®.

- Direct Current (DC) CO_2 laser has a constant voltage over time with a positive terminal, or anode, and a negative terminal, or cathode, like in an automobile battery. This technique was developed by Sharplan® (Plates 1.37 and 1.38).

CO_2 laser uses a wavelength of 10,600 nm. It emits in the infrared portion of the spectrum, which is invisible to the human eye. It requires a helium-neon light source to direct the CO_2 laser beam. It is highly absorbed in water, produces no back scatter, and causes flashboiling of intracellular water and ablation of cells (Plates 1.15, 1.39, and 1.40).

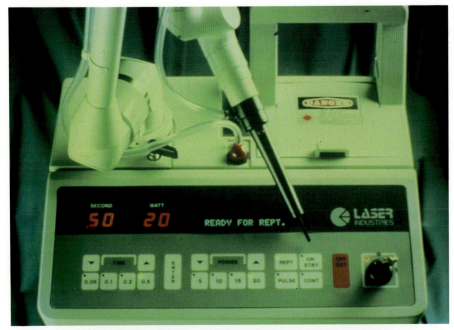

PLATE 1.37: CO_2 laser machine (Sharplan®) showing the laser board.

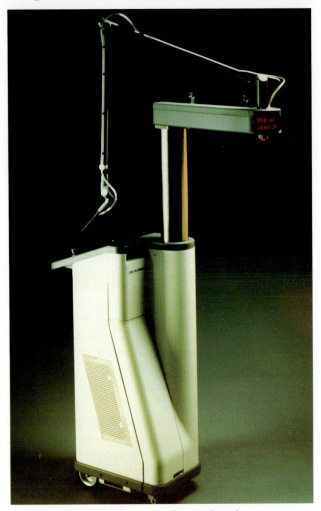

PLATE 1.38: CO_2 laser machine (Sharplan®).

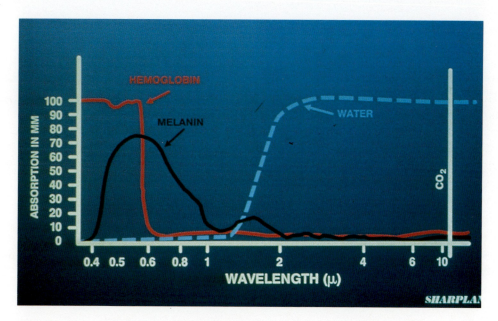

PLATE 1.39: CO_2 laser system: Absorption versus wavelength.

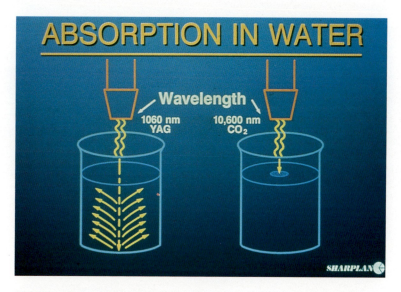

PLATE 1.40: Absorption in water.

By focusing the CO_2 laser beam, the highest energy density is attained and the cutting effect is maximized. In laryngology, the possibility of cutting without contact between the instrument and tissue (up to a distance of 400 mm) through the microscope is an important advantage of this laser technique. It is an aseptic technique. The combination of a slight coagulating effect on small blood vessels without contacting the vocal fold muscle produces minimal tissue damage and maximum precision. Some years ago, the spot size was too large. Today, CO_2 laser techniques allow a tiny spot size of 100 to 200 microns.

Spot size has been one of the parameters to decrease since 1972. The early CO_2 spot size was 600 microns through the microscope. In laryngology, since 1979, we have had an impact of 400 microns on the vocal fold epithelium. The technique used to remove a lesion from the vocal fold was to aim the beam, in the glottic space, tangentially to the free edge of the vocal fold. The disadvantage was a carbonized sample of 400 microns. In 1987 (S. Shapshay) Sharplan® introduced a microspot that is adequate for any laryngeal surgery (Plate 1.41). The latest Acuspot provides a spot size of 150 microns. It uses the standard joystick and is coupled with existing Sharplan® equipment which allows usage of 1 watt of power. In 1991, Ossof reported 50 cases of laryngeal pathology and found a significant clinical advantage to its use for both benign and malignant lesions. Microspot is useful for benign lesions, and the cutting effect is satisfactory with minimal thermal damage. If thermal effects are desired, spot size can be increased by a defocusing ring. Thermal effects are sometimes desirable, for example, when removing a vocal fold or papillomas (Plate 1.25).

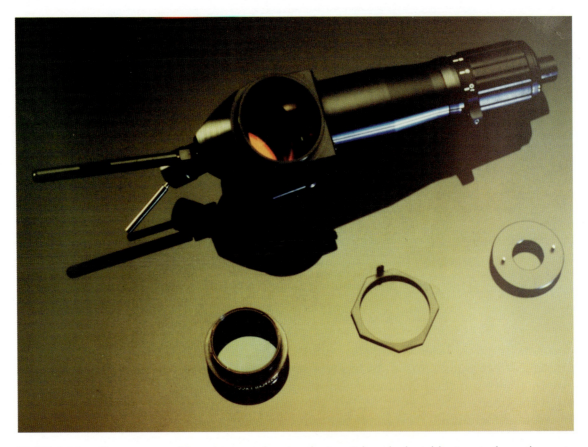

PLATE 1.41: Components of the microspot showing the joystick and adaptable rings to focus the spot.

Two rules must be followed when using the microspot:

1. The tissue to be removed has to be scantily vascularized to avoid bleeding.
2. Laser power must be lowered to 0.8–2 watts from the 7–9 watts used with a normal spot size. There is no charring of tissue on the mucosal edge of the vocal fold.

Parameters are as follows. At a working distance of 400 mm, through the microscope, 1.5 watts of delivered CO_2 energy is used routinely is laryngeal surgery. Less than 100 microns incision width is seen on the sample. For angiomatous polyps, the spot size has to be increased, otherwise the advantage of the laser is lost. For cysts or nodules, on the other hand, the microspot associated with either ultra- or superpulse provides a tremendous advantage in performing very precise surgery with insignificant thermal effects.

In conclusion, CO_2 laser with the microspot and ultra- or superpulse is the most precise laser instrument for soft tissue interaction in direct fire. Surrounding tissue trauma is avoided by using higher energy density. Samples for histological documentation also are more reliable (Plate 1.42).

Wound healing is excellent, and postoperative voice has been better than using traditional techniques. The microspot system permits the microflaps to adhere when lifting the vocal fold for polypoid fold.

Furthermore, CO_2 Laser is the only tool that provides superficial tissue evaporation and minimal destruction of surrounding tissue with a hemostatic effect. The scalpel needs a direct contact and may make the tissue bleed. On

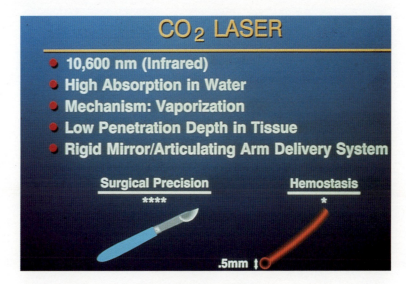

PLATE 1.42: Summary of CO_2 laser systems.

vessels smaller than 0.6 mm, in our experience, the damage looks less extensive after CO_2 Laser use than after the diathermy technique.

In laryngology, its disadvantages are few. It cannot be conducted by a fiberoptic endoscope it is unsuitable for operating in a water medium such as the bladder; and it has a limited ability to coagulate blood vessels larger than 0.6 mm, but it sealed lymphatic vessels (which is very interesting in surgery for early stages of cancer). The advantages of the CO_2 laser for laryngology are numerous: It is absorbed by water, which is the main element in tissue. It has a cutting effect with very little, if any, thermal damage if used with the microspot (Plate 1.43). Using a defocused beam, thermal effects occur which coagulate small vessels without any deep or peripheral effects. Hemostatic capability is limited to microcirculation. A coagulating forceps is necessary to coagulate large vocal fold vessels encountered during cordectomy. CO_2 Laser surgery is a no bleeding, "no tools" surgery: the operating field is dry. The greatest advantage of CO_2 Laser is its precision using the microspot. Using the tangential portion of the beam, we can achieve surgical accuracy of less than 100 microns. It is obvious that it is applicable for any laryngeal tumor from a intracordal cyst to nodules or Reinke's edema. The time required to perform Laser surgery is also shorter than using conventional techniques.

CO_2 laser provides several significant advantages over traditional surgical techniques:

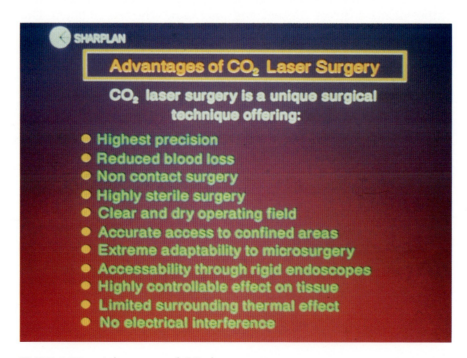

PLATE 1.43: Advantages of CO_2 laser surgery.

- The ability to operate without mechanical movement, thus minimizing the risk of damaging the delicate vocal fold structure (e.g., stripping the vocal fold).
- Less trauma.
- Increased precision.
- Improved hemostasis.
- Sterilization of the excision bed in its path.
- Reduced surgical time.
- Faster healing. Postoperative edema and pain are less (due to lack of contact with the tissues). No postoperative infection is seen.
- A markedly improved success rate of recovering voice with fewer recurrences of benign lesions.
- CO_2 laser vaporizes tissues precisely with minimal to almost no surrounding thermal damage.
- Power ranging from 0.1 to 100 watts. (It is also the least expensive surgical Laser.)

A laser surgeon must be a trained classical surgeon and must know how to perform any kind of micro-instrumental surgery on the larynx in case the laser malfunctions during a surgical procedure.

Argon Laser

The argon laser, introduced in the 1960s, was the pioneering instrument in laser surgery. It is a continuous wave, stable, gaseous laser. Wavelengths range from 488 to 514.5 nm. It is transmitted through clear fluid and structures and emits light in the visible spectrum of blue-green. It can be used through flexible fibers in endoscopy. Spot size is about 100 to 200 microns. It is used in pigmented and vascular lesions and is absorbed by hemoglobin, melanin, and retinal tissue. The average power is 4 to 6 watts, but it can be raised to 30 watts. It has fire coagulation ability and very low cutting effect (Plates 1.44 and 1.45).

Nd-Yag Laser

The Nd-Yag laser has a wavelength of 1060 nm. It is a solid laser: Neodymium-Yttrium Aluminum Garnet Laser. It uses a continuous wave and emits in short infrared wavelengths. It is usable through optical quartz fiber light guides. The ND-Yag laser is transmitted through clear fluids and delivers 10 to 120 watts through a fiberoptic. It produces a high degree of scatter which results in a large spot size, small cutting effect, and substantial charring effect. It coagulates tissue. Thermal effect is important, and it is capable of coagulating vessels up to 2 mm in size. Its tissue penetration ability is 5 to 7

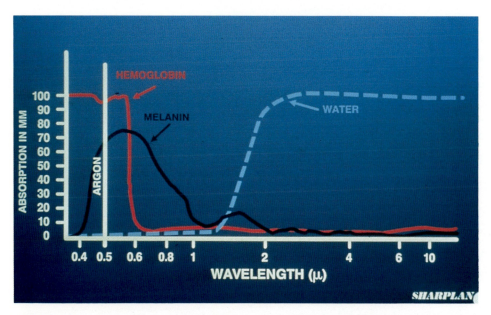

PLATE 1.44: Argon laser system: Absorption versus wavelength.

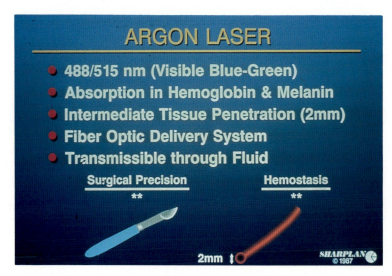

PLATE 1.45: Summary of argon laser systems.

mm. At low powers, it shrinks tissue without any vaporization. Thermal damage is important and could destroy or boil the lamina propria and ruin the voice by a noncontact technique. With a contact tip, the cutting effect is good, but tips must be in contact with the tissue before firing, otherwise the heat will be too high due to the scattering effect (Plates 1.40, 1.46, 1.47, and 1.48). This laser must never be used in the larynx except for malignant lesions. In laryngology, it must not be used alone. It can be coupled with a CO_2 laser through the microscope (Combo Laser) (Plate 1.49). It produces a coaxial,

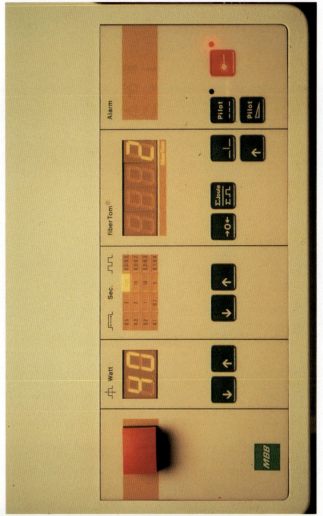

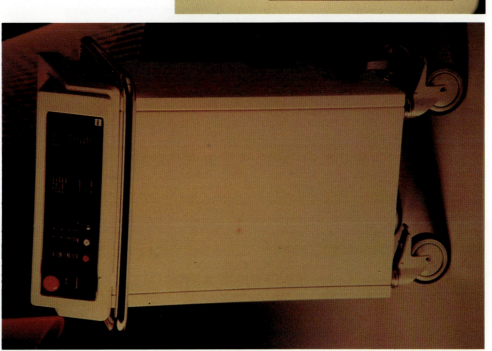

PLATE 1.46: **A.** Nd-Yag laser system (Bernas Medical). **B.** Laser board of the system.

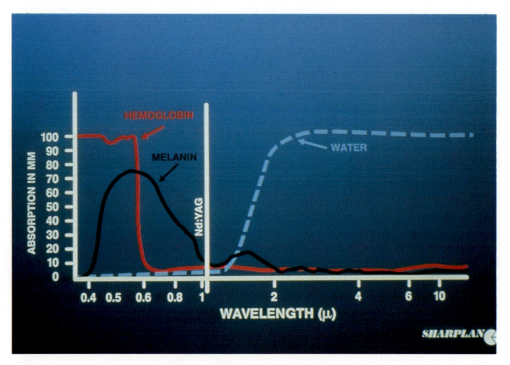

PLATE 1.47: Nd-Yag laser system: Absorption versus wavelength.

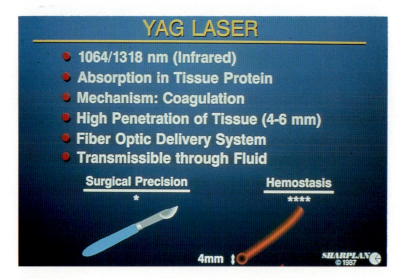

PLATE 1.48: Summary of Nd-Yag laser systems.

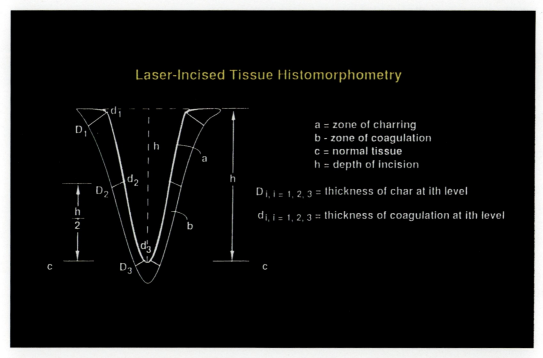

A

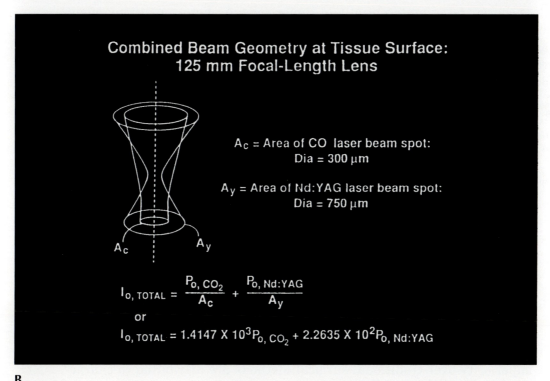

B

PLATE 1.49: Features of the Combo® laser (CO_2 plus Nd-Yag). **A.** Histomorphometry. **B.** Combined beam geometry at the tissue surface.

simultaneous laser beam. Combination laser can be indicated for cases of obstructing laryngeal malignant lesions and carcinoma.

KTP (Potassium, Titanyl, Phosphate) Crystal Lasers

The KTP laser is an Nd-Yag Laser. Recently, its potential for use in surgery was increased with two important improvements: doubling of the frequency of the wavelength and contact surgery. Frequency doubling offers a technique to change the output wavelength from 1060 nm (infrared) to 532 nm (green). It can be done with a special crystal that combines two infrared photons to one green photon. Contact KTP with a conical sapphire which, due to its shape, reflects the laser energy to the tips and heats up to several hundred degrees Celsius on a very focused spot, provides almost a pure cutting effect. KTP laser is transmitted through clear fluids and structures. It does not vaporize well and has a 200 nm spot size when delivered through fibers. Available fibers range from 0.2 to 0.6 mm in diameter. It can be used through the microscope. Perkins originally developed the KTP laser for use in otosclerosis, then it was used in laryngeal surgery.

Photodynamic Therapy

Argon laser or tunable lasers activate Hemato Porphyrin Derivative (HPD) which is concentrated preferentially in tumor cells. A photo-sensitizing agent is administered through an intravenous injection 24 hours before laser activation. Only tumor cells less than 3 mm deep are destroyed. This looks like an interesting technique for carcinoma in situ or T1N0. But, in any case, endoscopic examination and biopsy must be done prior to developing a treatment protocol. Drugs cause photosensitivity. Patients so treated must remain in darkness for 30 days. Twenty-four hours after injection, there is fluorescence of malignant cells only. Laser irradiation destroys the tumor cells. The wavelength of the argon laser is 632 microns. Light dosimetry is calculated based on body surface. It lasts between 20 to 45 minutes. Photo Dynamic Therapy (PDT) is performed under laryngoscopy and general anesthesia. Follow-up appointments are scheduled every week for 2 months and should be made for late in the afternoon to avoid sun irradiation. This technique needs a very early diagnosis for vocal fold carcinoma.

CONCLUSION

The virtues of the laser for surgery have been well described in the literature. Their superiority over traditional surgical methods are attributed to characteristics of the laser that produce minimal thermal effects, precision cutting, very little bleeding, slight postsurgical edema, and fast healing with minimal pain. Several studies (Peak Woo, 1993, Pacific Voice Foundation) have shown laser and cold instruments to have similar results when surgery is performed by an experienced surgeon. In our experience, the surgeon's experience and skill are critical to produce optimal results with laser voice surgery.

The surgeon must look at the vocal folds with the eyes of the laser.

2

Larynx

EMBRYOLOGY

Embryology and Laryngeal Development

Anatomy of the voice cannot be limited to the larynx. Impairment in any of the body's systems can affect the voice. The larynx is, however, the most representative component of voice.

Embryological Development

The larynx, which is the organ of phonation, is anatomically situated in the superior and medial portion of the neck located above the trachea, below the hyoid bone, and in front of the pharyngeal cavity.

Laryngeal mucosa has an endodermic origin and is derived from the cephalic intestine. The upper part of the respiratory tube, which is the anterior bud of the cephalic intestine, will become the future laryngeal cavity.

Cartilages and muscles derive from the mesenchyme. The part of the mesenchyme surrounding the endodermic laryngeal tube, will present the 2nd, 3rd, 4th, and 6th branchial arches. The different structures of the larynx are derived from these four arches:

- **2nd** Smaller cornu of hyoid bone
  Stylohyoid ligament
- **3rd** Greater cornu of hyoid bone
  Pharyngo-epiglottic ligament
  Greater cornu of thyroid cartilage
- **4th** Right and left ala of the thyroid cartilage
  Cricothyroid muscles
- **6th** Supraglottal part of the larynx
  Cricoid and arytenoid cartilages
  Intrinsic muscles of the larynx

The epiglottis originates from the hypobranchial protuberance which buds just in front of the lingual outline, between the anterior part of the 3rd and 4th arches (Plate 2.1).

The constrictor muscles of the pharynx derive from the mesenchyme of the foregut, and the tongue from the mesenchyme of the lateral and medial parts of the foregut (Table 2.1).

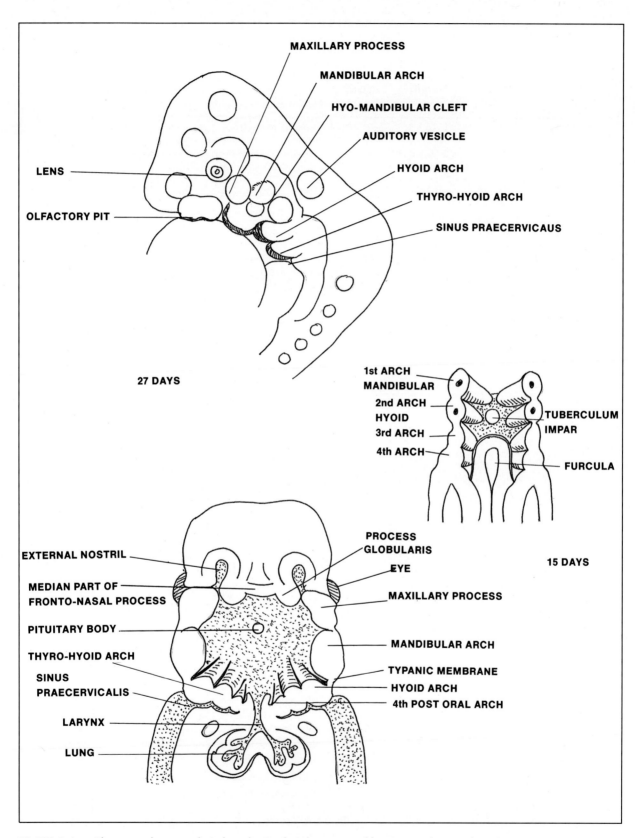

PLATE 2.1: Pharyngo-laryngeal embryologic development of human embryo (after His).

TABLE 2.1. Developmental Stages of the Human Embryo: O'Rahilly and Muller described 23 stages in the embryologic development of the larynx (1984).

Stage	Pairs of Somites	Length (mm)	Age (days)	Features
9	1–3	1.5–2.5	20	Foregut appears.
10	4–12	2.0–3.5	22	Oropharyngeal membrane appears: laryngotracheal sulcus and pulmonary primordium.
11	13–20	2.5–4.5	24	Oropharyngeal membrane rupture.
12	21–29	3.0–5.0	26	Oropharyngeal membrane disappears; lung bud develops.
13	30–?	4.0–6.0	28	Cervical sinus becomes apparent; lung bud separates from digestive tube trachea and esophagus may become recognizable; stomach begins to develop.
14		5.0–7.0	32	Arytenoid swellings and epithelial lamina form in larynx; lung sacs curve dorsally and embrace esophagus.
15		7.0–9.0	33	Pharyngotracheal duct connects digestive and respiratory tubes; lobar buds develop.
16		8.0–11.0	37	Cervical sinus is disappearing; epithelial lamina is complete and separates digestive from respiratory tube; embryonic vestibule of larynx appears; primary palate begins to form.
17		11.0–14.0	41	Vestibule of larynx deepens; skeleton of pharyngeal arches and larynx is dense mesenchyme; segmental bronchial buds develop.
18		13.0–17.0	44	Hyoid chondrification begins; some subsegmental bronchial buds appear.
19		16.0–18.0	47½	Mesenchymal epiglottis and several cartilages appear; infraglottic cavity is expanding.
20		18.0–22.0	50½	Cricoïd lamina develops; ventricle of larynx begins to appear.
21		22.0–24.0	52	Epithelial lamina begins to disintegrate.
22		23.0–28.0	54	Oral cavity is still increasing in width and height; most individual laryngeal muscles are identifiable; secondary (hard) palate is forming; soft palate has not fused; connection occurs between vestibule and infraglottic cavity; large parts of epithelial lamina are still present; ventricle of larynx opens; vocal ligament may appear.

Sources: Arey 1986; Muller et al., 1973; O'Rahilly and Muller, 1984.

At Birth

The birth cry is the first sound a human being makes; it announces the first respiration. Its average frequency is about 500 Hz. It will become an average of about 200 Hz in the adult female and around 120 Hz in males.

Post-Natal Development

- Most characteristics of the larynx develop during the third month of fetal life. At birth, the hyoid bone and thyroid cartilage are fused. They separate slowly. The hyoid bone ossifies at 2 years of age; 20 years later, the thyroid and cricoid cartilages also ossify. The arytenoid cartilages will ossify around age 35, the laryngeal skeleton will complete its ossification in the sixth decade.

- Sexual characteristics: Besides the hormonal receptors found in the epithelium (laryngeal histology), the thyroid cartilage also differentiates the male and female larynx. At birth its angle in males is 110° and in females 120°. The larynx at birth in both males and females is located at level C3 and C4 of cervical vertebrae, at age 6 at C5, and at 20 years between C5 and C7 (Jordan, 1960).

- As the vocal organ descends, the vocal tract grows in length and width.

- The cricothyroid membrane will play a key role for the future voice range in adult life. Its length and flexibility will be one of the characteristics of the voice.

- In childhood, vocal fold length is 6 mm in females and 8 in males. It will increase to 15–19 mm in adult females and 17–23 mm in adult males.

- The vocal ligament appears between ages 1 and 4 years. The ligament is very thin, and no differentiation between the two layers is observed in infants.

- At puberty, the three layers of the lamina propria are identified.

Laryngeal Anatomy

Introduction (Plate 2.2)

The anatomical system and mechanisms leading to phonation involve many body systems. The framework of this complex system includes the:

- Thorax, with the sternum, 12 pairs of ribs, and the lungs;
- Vertebral column;

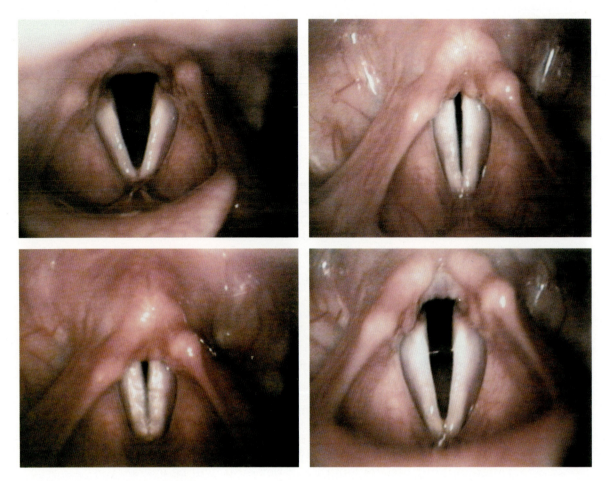

PLATE 2.2: Normal vocal fold.

1	2
3	4

1. During breathing.
2. Starting phonation.
3. End of phonation.
4. Breathing.

- Inspiratory and expiratory muscles; and,
- Abdominal and pelvic diaphragms.

Considering its complexity, one recognizes that many goals for speech and singing are difficult to attain because of the variation in muscular and structural balances within the laryngeal mechanism of each individual.

The larynx is the main organ of voice. According to Negus, voice is an "overlaid function" with its primary functions being respiration and protection of the glottis during swallowing.

Phonatory Anatomy (Plate 2.3)

The larynx may be likened to a valve that connects the respiratory system to the airway passages of the throat, mouth, and nose. The vocal folds vibrate thousands of times each day from the birth cry through a lifetime of speech. Phonation is made possible by the larynx. Two functions of the larynx are essential for speech:

- One is the ability to open to produce about half of the consonants, the half that are voiceless sounds.

- The other function is the ability of the lowest level of the valve (the true vocal folds) to close just enough to vibrate when air pressure pushes against it. These vibrations produce voiced

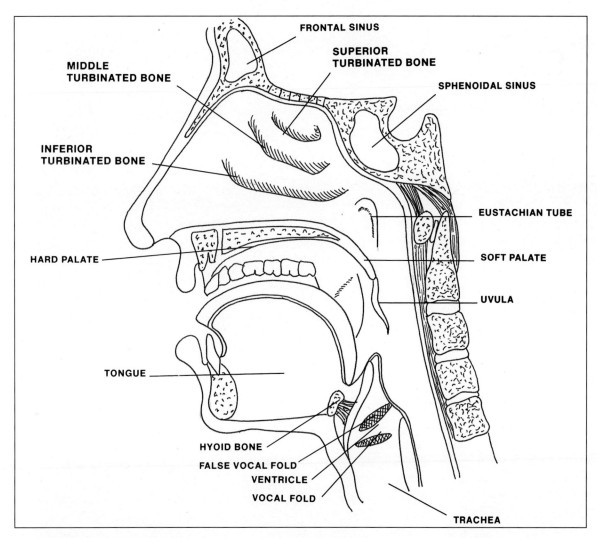

PLATE 2.3: The vocal tract.

sounds, the tones that characterize vowels and semivowels particularly. The ability to control the rate and manner of vibration of this valve accounts for our ability to control pitch, loudness, and, to some extent, quality of the voice.

Laryngeal Anatomy (Plate 2.4)

The larynx is relatively simple in construction. Its framework consists of five relatively large cartilages and about half a dozen pairs of muscles that move these cartilages into different positions. The entire larynx, attached to the top of the trachea, is suspended between the base of the tongue and the sternum. The intricacy of its microstructure and its vast potential for patterns of adjustment and vibration make it well adapted for speech.

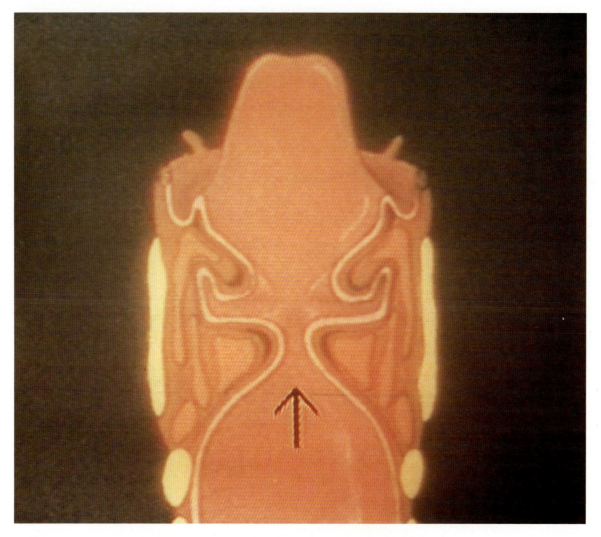

PLATE 2.4: Larynx morphology showing the glottic space. Air = energy.

The larynx is composed of four anatomical units: mucosa, intrinsic muscles, extrinsic muscles, and the skeleton.

Muscles are attached to the different parts of cartilages, and the cartilages are fixed to each other by ligaments and membranes.

MUCOSA

Introduction

There are two different types of epithelium in the larynx:

1. stratified squamous epithelium, and
2. pseudo-stratified ciliated columnar epithelium. (Plate 2.5)

Many transitional areas between these two types of epithelium have been identified. The transitional areas are very fragile and may play a key role in the localization of laryngeal pathologies.

Histology of the larynx

The following structures of the larynx will be described:

- Epiglottis
- False vocal folds and ventricles
- Aryepiglottic folds
- Lower larynx and cricoid cartilage
- Vocal folds
- Particular structures
- Laryngeal histology during lifetime

Epiglottis

- It is situated at the superior portion of the larynx. A central epiglottic cartilage forms its framework.
- The anterior or lingual surface is covered with a stratified squamous epithelium.
- This mucosa also covers the apex and more than half of the posterior or laryngeal surface of epiglottis.
- The stratified squamous epithelium progressively disappears, and a transition is made toward a respiratory epithelium which is a pseudo-stratified, ciliated columnar epithelium.

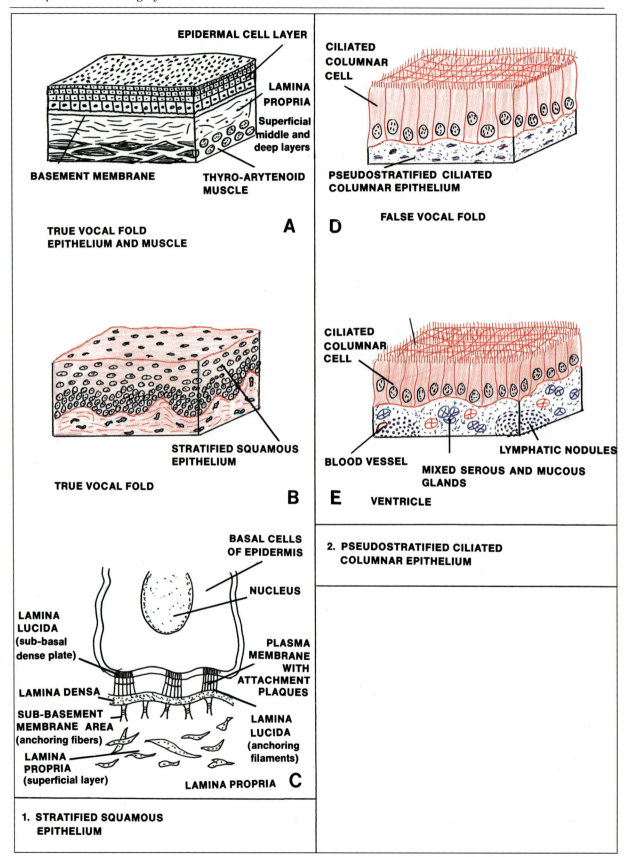

PLATE 2.5: Histology of the larynx: **A.**, **B.**, and **C.** True vocal fold. **D.** False vocal fold. **E.** Ventricle.

- Tubulo-acinous, mucous, serous, or mixed glands are found in the lamina propria. Taste buds are rarely found in the stratified epithelium, but some lymphatic nodules may be present. (Plate 2.6)

False vocal folds and ventricles

- These two structures are covered by a pseudo-stratified, ciliated columnar epithelium. The lamina propria is very rich with mixed glands (mucous and serous acini), lymphatic nodules, adipose tissue, and excretory ducts (Plate 2.5).

- Lymphatic nodules are particularly numerous in the external wall of the ventricles.

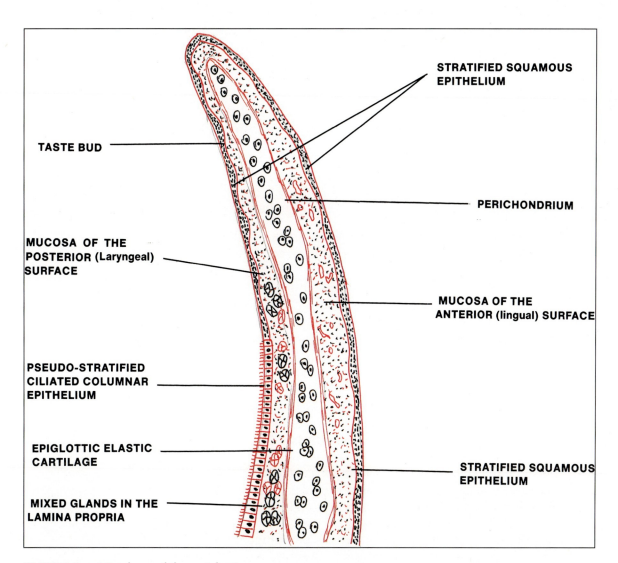

PLATE 2.6: Histology of the epiglottis.

Aryepilglottic folds

- They are covered by a stratified squamous epithelium, as are the vocal folds.

Lower larynx and cricoid cartilage

- They are covered with a respiratory epithelium (pseudo-stratified, ciliated columnar epithelium).

- Mixed glands and lymphatic nodules are found in the lamina propria.

Vocal folds

- The most complex and important structure of the larynx is a "four dimensional structure" formed by the three space dimensions: length, width, and height plus a fourth one which is the "vibratory dimension."

- The vocal fold consists of the lamina propria and the epithelium and, in our concept, is composed of two specific masses.

    Both are supported by the thyroid cartilage.
    1. The vibratory mass complex
    2. The muscle mass complex (Plate 2.7) consists of the vocalis muscle

- The vibratory mass complex consists of the epithelium and the lamina propria. The vocal fold has a layered structure.

The **epithelium** is a noncornified, stratified squamous epithelium. It can be considered as a thin, stiff capsule that maintains the shape of the vocal folds.

- The basement membrane of the stratified squamous epithelium shows microridges on the outer surface of epithelial cells which increase the cell surface area. (see Plate 2.5)

- Desmosomes, located at the junction of two cells, decrease when approaching the vocal fold surface and almost disappear by the time the squamous cells migrate into the last few layers. (Plate 2.7)

- Between the epithelium and the superficial layer of the lamina propria, there is the basement membrane zone responsible for securing the two layers. Different types of proteins have been identified:

    1. In Lamina Lucida: laminin bullous pemphigoid antigen which is involved in the attachment between the epithelium of the dermis.

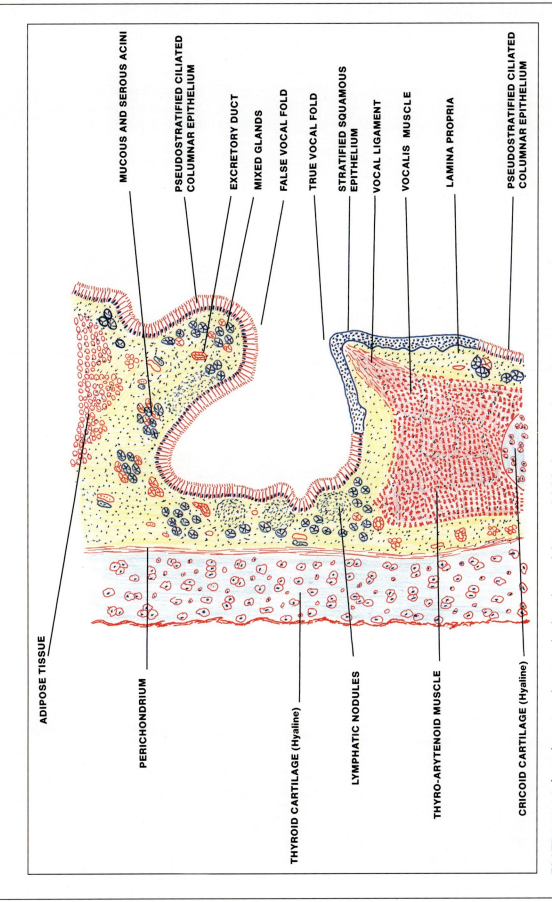

PLATE 2.7: A frontal section showing the histology of the vocal fold, the ventricle, and the false vocal fold.

2. In Lamina Densa: a type IV collagen, proteoglycan, and KF-l antigen. This KF-l antigen plays a role in the integrity and strength of the basement membrane zone located under the epithelium. This antigen also plays a role in binding the basal cell layer to the basement membrane zone. The concentration and integrity of this antigen might help to explain some vocal fold diseases.
3. The sub-Lamina Densa zone contains type VII collagen and AF-l and EBA antigens.

The **lamina propria** is composed of three different layers, each layer having a specific mechanical property:

1. The superficial layer of the lamina propria is composed of an amorphous substance and is the main location of vibrations during phonation. It can be regarded as somewhat like a mass of soft gelatin. The superficial layer is referred to as Reinke's space. It is pliable with an adaptive characteristic. It is composed of an amorphous substance and is the location of vibrations during phonation.
2. The intermediate layer of the lamina propria consists chiefly of elastic fibers and can be likened to a bundle of soft rubber bands.
3. The deep layer of the lamina propria, which primarily consists of collagenous fibers, is something like a bundle of cotton thread.

The portion that consists of the intermediate and deep layers of the lamina propria is known as the vocal ligament. Situated at the apex of the vocal fold, it consists of dense elastic fibers that spread out across those two layers, and then into the skeletal vocalis muscle.

Any impairment of the lamina propria will lead to dysphonia.

There are no glands, no lymphatic nodules, and few blood vessels in the three layers of the lamina propria of the vocal fold. Glands located in adjacent structures (ventricle, false vocal fold, lower larynx) are responsible for humidification of the vocal folds. They play a key role in cooling and lubricating the vibratory mass. (Dryness after radiation therapy causes a hoarse voice.)

Capillaries run roughly parallel to the free edge of the vocal fold. Rarely vessels enter into the mucosa, emerging from the muscle. These blood vessels help to maintain the vocal fold's temperature and oxygenate the cells as well. They can also, if necessary, increase the vocal liquid mass. These blood vessels can also be expanded by inflammation or by hormonal effects. This phenomenon may be responsible for dysphonia.

Aberrations of the basement membrane zone have been identified in the formation of nodules (Gray, 1991).

Different types of collagen comprise the lamina propria, which is a network of collagen type III and elastic fibers (Gray & Titze, 1988). The structure of the lamina propria is composed of fluids, interstitial matrix, fibroblasts responsible for the synthesis of collagen, elastic fibers, and ground substances.

Elastic fibers are very particular: they can be stretched to twice their length and then return to their original size.

- The **vocalis muscle** constitutes the body of the vocal fold. It can be likened to a bundle of rather stiff rubber bands. The structure of this muscle is basically the same as the other skeletal muscles of the body. Muscular fibers are long, cylindrical, and composed of myofibrils.

From a mechanical point of view, the five layers of the vocal fold can be reclassified into three sections:

1. The cover
   a. Epithelium
   b. Superficial layer of the lamina propria
2. The transition
   c. Intermediate layer
   d. Deep layer of the lamina propria
3. The body
   e. Vocalis muscle

Each layer has its own mechanical properties.

The mechanical properties of the four outer layers (mucous membrane) are controlled passively. The mechanical properties of the innermost layer (vocalis muscle) are regulated by receptors, blood vessels, and neurological factors.

Particular structures: Mitochondria

- Mitochondria supply the energy of the cells. Their size and configuration may vary according to the nutritional status and function of the organ. For example, the mitochondria of a normal skeletal muscle, such as the biceps, may have mitochondria of 0.7 µm in length. In vocal fold muscles, their size may be doubled: 1.4 µm. (Plate 2.8)

- The most important role of mitochondria is the formation of energy-producing ATP (adenosine triphosphate) from phosphorus and ADP (adenosine diphosphate).

- Mitochondria contain their own DNA and RNA which are independent of nuclear DNA. The existence of an independent mitochondrial genetic system suggests that cellular function, and possibility configuration, depends on the interaction of at least two genetic systems: nuclear and mitochondrial (Wagner, 1969). Are voice quality and strength congenital or acquired?

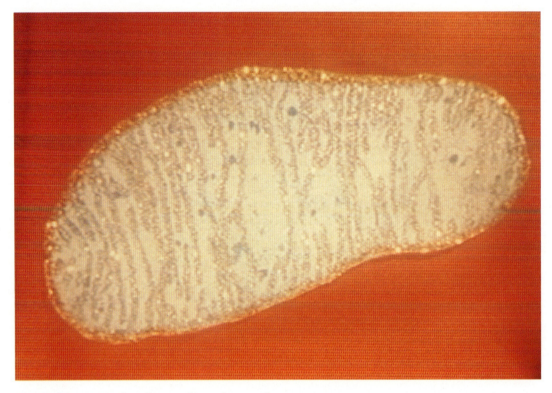

PLATE 2.8: Mitochondria as shown by an electron microscope.

- Accumulation of fat and proteins may be observed in the immediate vicinity of the mitochondria. Fat inclusions are six times more numerous in the vocal fold muscle than in other muscles of the body. This occurs because of their role in energy production.

STRUCTURES IN CHILDREN

Between 1 and 4 years of age, the vocal ligament appears. The lamina propria has two layers; the elastic fibers and collagenous fibers are in the same layer. After puberty, the structure of the lamina propria with three layers is defined. The composition of the two layers of the lamina propria is the main histological difference between the newborn and adult larynx. (Plate 2.9)

STRUCTURE IN GERIATRICS

The lamina propria of the aged vocal fold reveals a decrease in glandular cells and less fluid in vocal folds. The epithelium of the vocal fold is thinner in the intermediate layer and less pliable. Elastic and collagenous fibers decrease and become atrophied as do muscle fibers. Histologic changes are more pronounced in men than in women. Voice training appears to forestall or lessen these age-related changes.

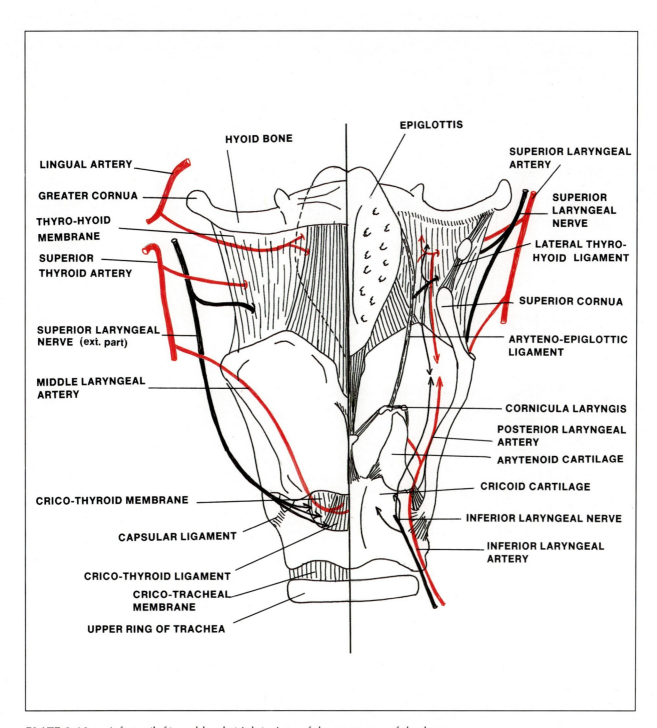

PLATE 2.10: A front (left) and back (right) view of the anatomy of the larynx.

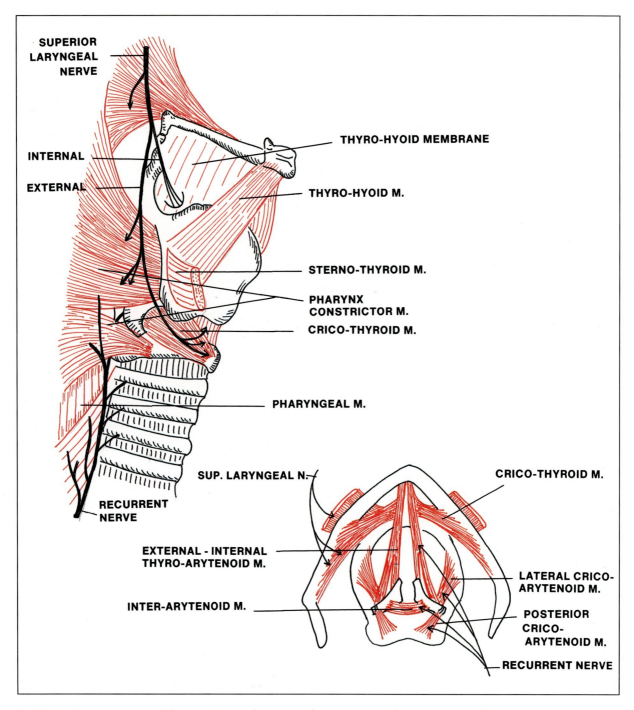

PLATE 2.11: Anatomy of the intrinsic and extrinsic laryngeal muscles. (M. = muscle, N. = nerve)

One is innervated by the superior laryngeal nerve:

1. Cricothyroid muscle

Thyroarytenoid Muscles

The muscles set into vibration to produce sound are part of the thyroarytenoids. This large muscle consists of two parts:

- The **internal thyroarytenoids** (or vocalis muscle) which are the vocal folds. Its origin is the angle of the thyroid cartilage and its insertion site is the vocal process of the arytenoid cartilage. Fibers of the vocalis muscle are attached to the inferior and lateral surfaces of the vocal ligament.

- The **external thyroarytenoids**, which are located lateral to the vocal folds. The external thyroarytenoids also originate in the angle of the thyroid cartilage and insert in the base and anterior surface of the arytenoid cartilage. Laterally, they attach to the inner wall of the thyroid cartilage.

The action of the thyroarytenoid muscles may relax and shorten the vocal ligament for the singing of low pitches, draw the vocal processes of the arytenoids downward and inward to approximate the vocal folds, pull the vocal folds apart by a lateral contraction, stabilize the vocal folds throughout their entire length, vary both the length and thickness of the vibrating segment, and render a portion of the vocal fold tense while the remainder is relaxed. (Elliptic opening of the vocal folds is maintained for producing higher pitches.) The contraction of vocalis muscle stiffens the vocal folds. This stiffening action is independent of vocal fold length.

Posterior Cricoarytenoid Muscles

The posterior cricoarytenoids are flat muscles arising from the back wall of the cricoid cartilage and inserting into the muscular processes of the arytenoid cartilage. They are the major muscles responsible for translating and gliding the arytenoids apart. They play a major role in abduction of the vocal folds (which opens the glottis vocalis).

Lateral Cricoarytenoid Muscles

The lateral cricoarytenoid muscles arise from the upper and lateral borders of the cricoid cartilage and insert into the muscular processes of the arytenoid cartilage. They have an opposite effect from the posterior cricoarytenoids: They adduct the arytenoids and can also squeeze the anterior tips of the vocal processes tightly together in a condition of a medial compression. This action moves the vocal processes inward, closing the glottis vocalis.

Interarytenoid Muscles

The **transverse arytenoid** muscle originates on the posterior and outer surface of each arytenoid. It inserts on the outer border of each arytenoid. It draws the arytenoid cartilages together and closes glottis respiratoria between arytenoids.

The **oblique arytenoid** muscles originate on the base of the posterior surface of one arytenoid cartilage and insert on the apex of the posterior surface of the opposite cartilage. Fibers of each muscle cross to form an ×. They stabilize the arytenoids by drawing the arytenoid tips together and aid in closing the glottis.

Cricothyroid Muscles

Oblique fibers:

The cricothyroid muscles originate from the anterior border of the cricoid cartilage and insert into the lower lamina and inferior cornu of the thyroid cartilage. Their contraction pulls the two cartilages together, thereby approximating, lengthening, and stiffening the vocal folds, rendering them tense in preparation for phonation.

Anterior fibers:

These fibers of the cricothyroid muscles originate from the front and superior surface of the cricoid cartilage. They insert on the anterior border and lower lamina of the thyroid cartilage. They depress the thyroid cartilage and elevate the arch of the cricoid cartilage, or draw the thyroid downward and forward. This combined action increases the distance between the vocal processes of the arytenoid and the lamina of the thyroid. It elongates the vocal folds and provides tension. This action gives stability to the phonated sound and permits intensity to increase as the pitch is maintained. The degree of thyroid tilt affects the pitch, intensity, and quality of the vocal sound.

The Extrinsic Muscles:

There are eight:

Four are located below the hyoid bone:

1. Thyrohyoid muscle
2. Sternothyroid muscle
3. Sternohyoid muscle
4. Omohyoid muscle

Four are located above the hyoid bone:

1. Digastric
2. Mylohyoid
3. Geniohyoid
4. Stylohyoid

They will not be described in this chapter.

Function of the laryngeal muscles:

The laryngeal muscles are of great importance in regulating the mechanical properties of the vocal folds, as described by Hirano (1981). They control the position, shape, elasticity, and the viscosity of each layer of the vocal fold. Table 2.2 shows the functions of the five major intrinsic laryngeal muscles.

TABLE 2.2. Functions of the five major intrinsic laryngeal muscles.

	Cricothyoid Muscle	Vocalis Muscle	Lateral Cricoarytenoid Muscle	Interarytenoid Muscle	Posterior Cricoarytenoid Muscle
Position	Paramed++	Adduct+++	Adduct+++	Adduct+++	Abduct+++
Level	Lower++	Lower++	Lower+++	0	Elevate+++
Length	Elongate+++	Shorten+++	Elongate++	Shorten+	Elongate+++
Thickness	Thin+++	Thicken+++	Thin++	Thicken+	Thin++
Edge	Sharpen+++	Round+++	Sharpen++	0	Round++
Muscle (body)	Stiffen+++	Stiffen+++	Stiffen++	Slacken+	Stiffen++
Mucosa (cover and transition)	Stiffen+++	Slacken+++	Stiffen++	Slacken+	Stiffen++
S.L.N.	+	0	0	0	0
R.L.N.	0	+	+	+	+
S.T.A.	+	+	+	0	0
I.T.A.	0	0	0	+	+

Note: 0 = No Effect, + = Slight Effect, ++ = Moderate Effect, and +++ = Marked Effect. S.L.N.: superior laryngeal nerve; R.L.N.: recurrent laryngeal nerve; S.T.A.: superior thyroid artery; I.T.A.: inferior thyroid artery

Laryngeal Membranes and Ligaments

The cartilages of the larynx are attached to joints, are held together by ligaments, and are covered with membranes (see Plates 2.12 and 2.13). Those ligaments and membranes are:

Hyothyroid Ligament:
  Connects the hyoid bone and the thyroid cartilage and extends from cornu of hyoid bone to cornu of thyroid.

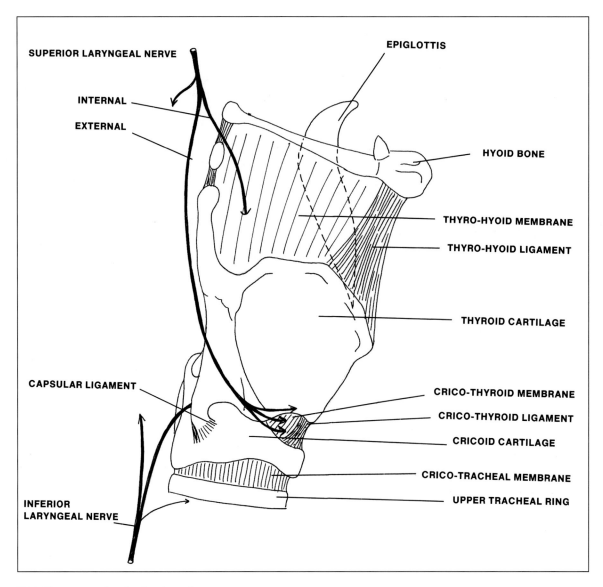

PLATE 2.12: The "voice box."

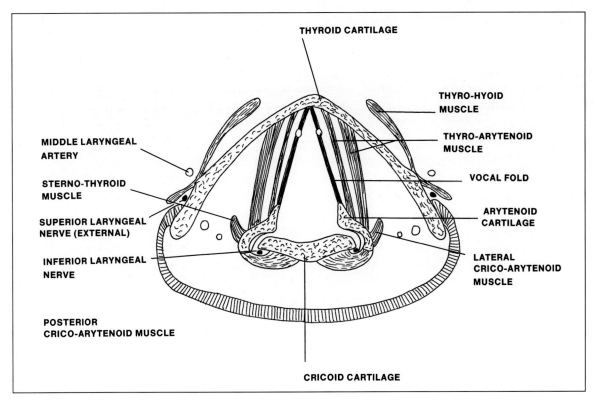

PLATE 2.13: The glottic space illustrated in a horizontal section.

Cricotracheal Ligament:
Connects the cricoid cartilage and the trachea.

Thyroepiglottic Ligament:
Connects the epiglottis and the thyroid cartilage.

Cricothyroid Ligament (medial):
Connects the cricoid and the thyroid cartilage at its anterior position.

Cricothyroid Ligament (lateral):
Connects the cricoid and the thyroid cartilage at its inferior cornu and the posterior surface of the cricoid.

Cricothyroid Ligament (posterior):
Connects the cricoid and the thyroid cartilage at its inferior cornu and the posterior surface of the cricoid.

Cricoarytenoid Ligament:
Connects the arytenoids and the cricoid cartilage.

Corniculate Pharyngeal Ligament:
Connects corniculate cartilage with the cricoid cartilage at the pharyngeal wall.

Vocal Ligament:
Paired thickened strips that originate at the inner surface of the angle of the thyroid cartilage and extend posteriorly to the vocal process of each arytenoid cartilage. The vocal ligament is an integral part of the mucosal cover of the vocalis muscle called the lamina propria. The cover consists of an almost gelatinous superficial layer that provides a loose connection between the outer epithelial covering of the glottal edge and the intermediate and deep layers of the lamina propria (transition layer) that attach to the vocalis muscle. The intermediate layer, which contains elastic fibers, blends into the deep layer containing collagenous fibers. Together, these two layers form the vocal ligament. This arrangement permits the mucosal membrane to vibrate more or less independently of the vocalis muscle, which vibrates synchronously but not as vigorously. This explains why the vocal folds, when seen vibrating in ultra-slow motion, appear like a flag flapping in the breeze.

Aryepiglottic Fold:
From the epiglottis, the two aryepiglottic folds pass backward to the tips of the corniculate cartilages and form the lateral boundaries of the vestibule, which contains the corniculate and the cuneiform cartilages. Their function is to draw the opening of the vestibule together.

Conus Elasticus and Cricothyroid Membrane:
The conus elasticus is a short cone-shaped tube which hangs between the thyroid and arytenoid cartilages. It is the framework on which the muscular function of the vocal folds is based. The anterior portion of the cone forms the cricothyroid membrane. As the thyroarytenoid muscle contracts, the conus become firm. It has three points of attachment: the lower border of the thyroid cartilage, the upper surface of the cricoid cartilage, and the inferior surface of the vocal process of each arytenoid.

Cartilages of the Larynx (Plate 2.14)

The cuneiform cartilages, the epiglottis, and the apices of the arytenoids are composed of yellow fibrocartilage, which shows little tendency to calcification; whereas the thyroid, the cricoid, and the greater part of the arytenoids consist of hyaline cartilage and become more or less ossified as age advances. Ossification starts about age 25 in the thyroid cartilage, somewhat later in the cricoid and the arytenoid cartilages. By age 65, these cartilages may be completely converted into bone. The cornicula laryngis consists of white fibrocartilage, which becomes osseous about age 70.

The **cricoid cartilage** is a complete cartilage ring. It is the foundation of the larynx to which the other cartilages attach. It differs from the other tracheal rings, which are all incomplete circles.

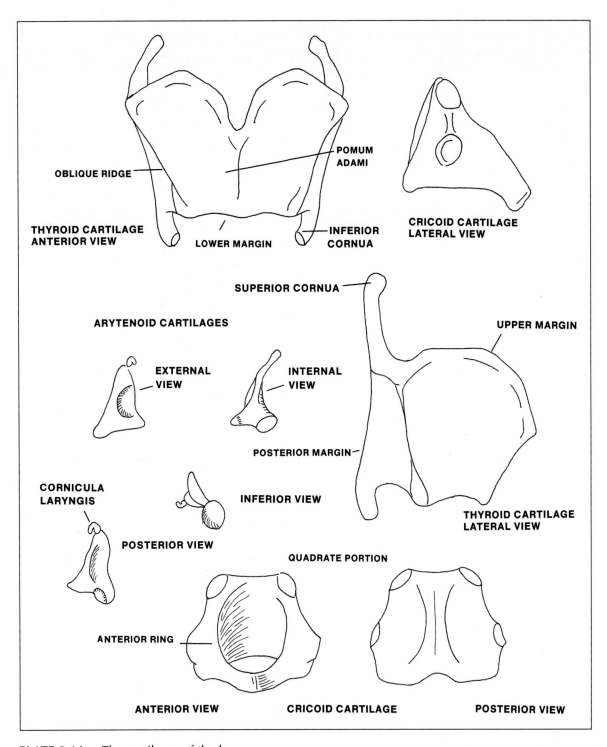

PLATE 2.14: The cartilages of the larynx.

The **thyroid cartilage** is like a wing-shaped shield and has an anterior prominence called the Adam's apple. It has two horns, the lower providing a pivotal attachment to the cricoid which permits these two cartilages to rock back and forth in relationship to each other. This ability to tilt the thyroid forward and the cricoid backward is the basis for changing the length of the vocal folds in pitch adjustments.

The **arytenoids**, a pair of small pyramidal cartilages, are mounted opposite each other on the rim of the signet portion of the cricoid cartilage. The arytenoids have two different motions: translation and gliding, which occur together. By translating or gliding, the vocal folds can be abducted (opened) for voiceless sounds (or breathing) or adducted (closed) to a variety of phonatory positions. Each arytenoid has three projections: one, located anteriorly, is the vocal process to which the vocal folds attach; another, located laterally, is the muscular process, to which several of the muscles responsible for translation and gliding attach. The upward projection is called the apex.

The **epiglottis** is a leaf-shaped flap that provides the anterior wall of the tube leading from the vocal folds to the throat.

All of these structures, as described, will delimit in the vicinity of the vocal fold. Certain structures play a major role in phonation.

Other Structures (Plate 2.15)

Glottis

The glottis is a space (and not a structure) situated between the vocal folds. It is said to be closed when the glottal edges of the vocal folds make contact when adducted. The glottis is open in abduction.

Supraglottal Cavity

The tube that extends upward from the level of the glottis through which the airstream from the larynx enters the throat is the aditus or supraglottal cavity. The cavity is formed anteriorly by the epiglottis, posteriorly by the arytenoids, and laterally by the aryepiglottic folds. The contraction of the aryepiglottic muscle tends to tilt the arytenoids toward the epiglottis and to pull the epiglottis down, assisted by a push of the base of the tongue.

False Vocal Folds

Also called ventricular folds, the false vocal folds are situated above the true vocal folds. They consist of thick folds of mucous membrane that protrude into the airway, but not as far as the true vocal folds. They originate just below the attachment of the epiglottis and insert into the lateral edges of the arytenoids below the apex. They are soft and passive structures.

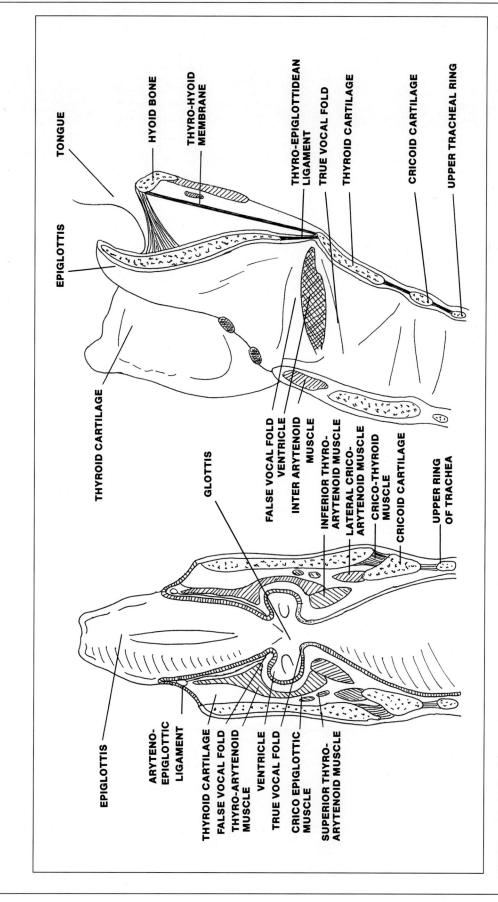

PLATE 2.15: The larynx shown in a coronal section (left) and in profile (right).

Laryngeal Ventricles

Between the false vocal folds above and the true vocal folds below, is a deep indentation of the mucosal wall of the larynx, the laryngeal ventricle or ventricle of Morgagni. It extends almost the full length of the vocal fold and is bound laterally by the external thyroarytenoid muscle. Within the ventricle, mucous glands provide lubrication of the true folds. The ventricles also serve as spaces into which the folds can move when vibrating.

ANATOMY AND PHYSIOLOGY

Laryngeal Physiology

There are three components of speech: exhalation, phonation, and articulation. Exhalation of the lungs produces a subglottal air flow (direct current) which is interrupted (alternating current) by the glottis when closed and when vocal folds vibrate. (Plate 2.16)

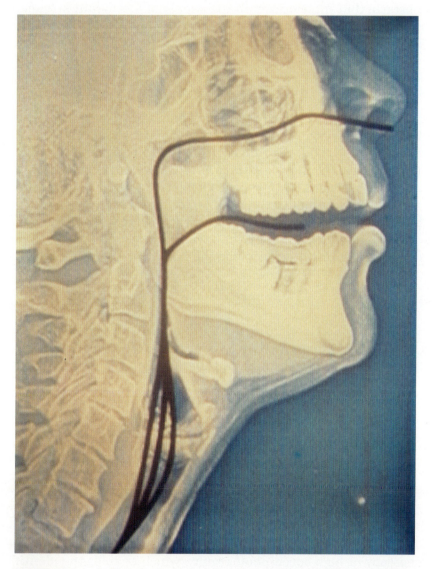

PLATE 2.16: Airflow in the larynx showing resonance of the vocal tract.

The larynx is involved in many other functions: breathing, swallowing, coughing, and sneezing. The sound produced at the level of the glottis is the primary laryngeal tone or glottal sound, also called source. This sound is then modified by the resonance organs of the vocal tract by attenuation or amplification of some frequency components. The last step involves the tongue, palate, and lips. The glottal sound is finally modulated into speech.

Lungs (Plate 2.17)

The lungs are responsible for exhalation, which is the energy source of the voice. The respiratory pattern can affect voice directly (disorders due to central nervous system or reduced vital capacity) or indirectly (via muscle contraction). Any obstacle that interferes with the supply of a constant stream of air from the lungs across the glottis (e.g., tracheostomy, bronchial or laryngeal web) will modify voice characteristics.

Resonance of the Vocal Tract (Plate 2.18)

The vocal tract functions as a tube closed at one end and open at the other. Resonant frequencies vary with the length and the shape of this tube. If the inside wall of a resonator is rigid, the range within which the sound amplified is narrow. Because the wall of the vocal tract is soft, the range of the human vocal tract is wide. The resonant frequency of a subject is directly bound to the volume of the resonator. The smaller the volume, the higher the resonant frequency (Holmholtz resonator). The human vocal tract has many resonant frequencies. The vocal sound is modified by the vocal tract resonators which act as acoustic filters that augument or decrease the amplitude. (Plate 2.19)

Articulation

Articulation involves the lips, teeth, tongue, hard and soft palate, and uvula. They are used in different combinations to produce plosive, fricative, or nasal consonants. However, vocal fold vibration is generally not disturbed by resonance at any fundamental frequency.

Vocal Folds

Closure of the glottis, associated with airflow due to exhalation, generates vocal fold vibrations. Two antagonistic forces are necessary to maintain this vibration: the opening force due to subglottal pressure and the closing force due to elasticity of the vocal fold associated to the Bernoulli effect (think of a thin shower curtain being drawn toward the jet of water during a shower). The vibration of the vocal fold during phonation is very rapid, and it can be studied by stroboscopy or high speed-photography, which enables the identification of nine stages in the glottal cycle.

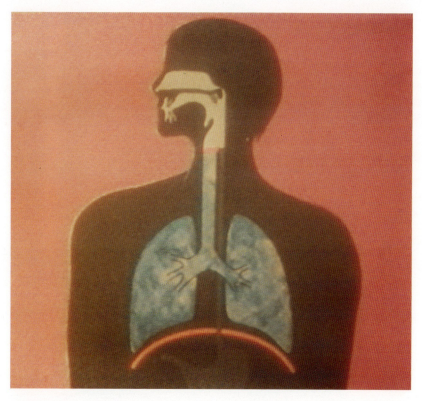

PLATE 2.17: Diagram of the larynx, lungs, and diaphragm, the energy source of sounds.

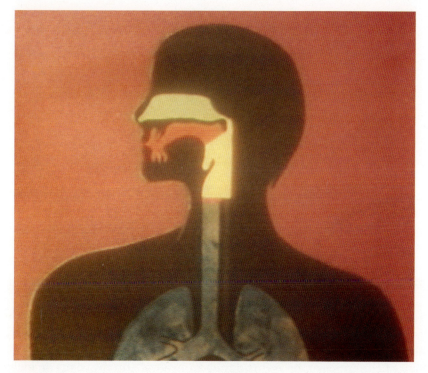

PLATE 2.18: Resonance of the vocal tract.

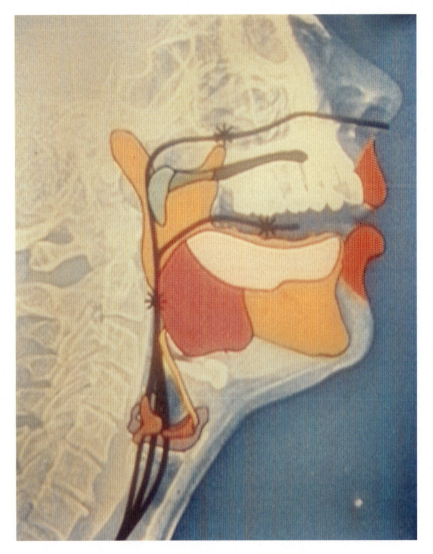

PLATE 2.19: Resonators used for voice production.

We will see later that this movement can also be recorded by electroglottography (EGG). The subglottal pressure overpowers the vocal fold resistance just enough to start the first slight opening phase. Air flow then continues during the opening phase, until the escape of air decreases subglottal pressure, which leads to the closing phase. The more compliant the vocal folds are, the more they can absorb the impact of the air below and the longer they remain closed.

When air passes through a narrow glottis, the negative pressure pulls the vocal folds apart (via the Bernoulli effect). This movement depends on the mobility of the vocal fold mucosa. If mucosa loses its mobility (submucosal tissue connection, rheology of the mucosa, or redundancy in area of the mucosa) or loses its lubrication (excessive dryness of the vocal fold), the quality of the vocal fold vibrations decreases, the vocal mass loses its adaptability, and voice is altered.

This cycle of opening and closing of the glottis is permanent. The ratio of the duration of one period of openness to the duration of the entire cycle is termed the opening quotient (OQ). Vocal folds open from bottom to top and also close from bottom to top in the vertical phase. In the horizontal phase, the folds open from the middle toward the front and back and spread out simultaneously anteriorly and posteriorly. The point of highest pressure is located in the middle third where most vocal fold pathology occurs.

Sound and Speech

Sound can be classified as tone and noise.

- Tone is periodic, unique or multiple, and consists of a sinusoidal wave.
- Tones are produced by the vibrations of the vocal folds.

A tone consisting of a single sinusoidal wave is a pure tone (tuning fork). Most tones are composed of many sinusoidal waves: they are complex tones. The frequency components of a complex tone are called partial fundamentals. The lowest natural frequency is F_0 or fundamental frequency. If partials are integral multiples of F_0, they are named harmonics. F_0 equals the first harmonic and multiples are called F_1, F_2, F_3 and so forth ($F_n = F_0 \times n$).

- Noise is aperiodic. It contains no harmonics. It occurs when sound is distributed randomly over a frequency range so that there is no pattern among the frequencies at which vibrations occur. Noise is generated by turbulences of air in the resonant cavities during phonation and emission of formants.
- Quality of voice. The quality of voice (timbre) depends on the wave shape of the glottal sound (its periodicity, the amount of noise it contains). Glottal opening and closing affects the timbre of the voice, and serves as a factor in voice identification.

Intensity of Voice: Intensity is regulated by three factors: power, glottal efficiency, and resonance. In most cases, the best way to increase vocal intensity is to increase the effort of exhalation. Changing the shape of resonator cavities can also increase the intensity of voice. Air density slightly affects the voice.

Fundamental Frequency: F_0 is the frequency at which the vocal folds vibrate. The mean range for men during speech is 120 to 180 Hz, for women 220 to 250 Hz.

Pitch is expressed in Hertz (Hz). It is mainly regulated by tension, mass, viscosity, and length of the vocal folds. The pitch is elevated by stretching the vocal folds (i.e., by increasing the stiffness). The cricothyroid muscles play a major role in this process.

Modifications of mass tend to lower the vocal pitch. Two types of vocal mass may be distinguished: a static vocal mass, which is the thyroarytenoid muscle. It does not vibrate. It plays a major role in the vocal fold tension. There is also a dynamic vocal mass, which is the cover of the vocal fold (the epithelium the basal membrane, and the lamina propria). It vibrates at the pitch frequency. Thickening of the vocal folds due to administration of anabolic steroids or male hormones tends to lower vocal pitch in women, creating a condition known as androphonia.

The vocal folds in men are longer and thicker than those in women and children.

Conditions for normal phonation:

1. Initial glottal area
2. Subglottal pressure
3. Stiffness of the vocal folds
4. Mobility of the vocal fold mucosa

Normal speech production is diagrammed in Plate 2.20.

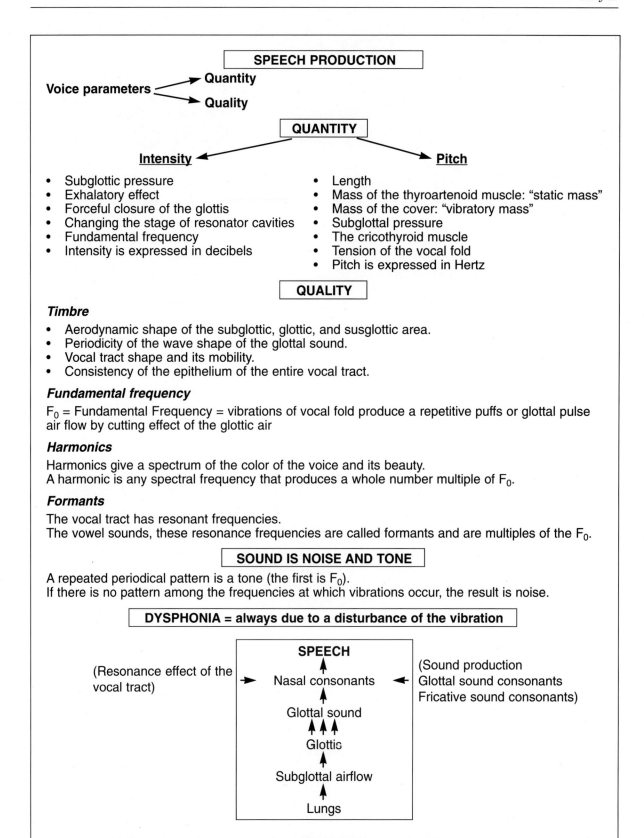

PLATE 2.20: The dynamics of normal speech production.

EXPLORATION OF NORMAL VOICE

History

The ability to look at the voice in action was a mystery first solved by Manuel Garcia in 1854. At Place de l'Odeon in Paris, in a cottage that belonged to his sister, a Diva, Manuel Garcia had the idea to look at the vocal folds by a complex mirror system using sunlight. It was the birth of laryngology. In 1861, Charles Bataille wrote the first book on phonation. In 1877, Edison invented the phonograph.

We then had to wait until 1939 when Jean Tarneaud wrote the first book on vocal fold vibrations. Paul Moore and Hans von Leden were pioneers in vocal fold cinematography with the ultra high speed technique. In the early 1970s in Japan, Sato, Isshiki, and Hirano developed the fiberscopic examination. In the early 1980s, Gould, Feder, Brewer, Colton, Sataloff, and others lectured extensively at the Voice Foundation and elsewhere on that subject.

We developed Dynamic Vocal Exploration in 1981. The origin of this technique is the association of five techniques in perfect synchronization. It was published in "Larynx Imprint," a videotape available through the Voice Foundation.

Dynamic voice evaluation includes five techniques of video documentation: (1) the patient's posture (position of the neck, thorax, etc.), (2) electroglottography, (3) flexible and telescopic laryngoscopy, (4) stroboscopy, and (5) recording the acoustic signal by microphone (Plates 2.21 and 2.22). Voice evaluation using various techniques, particularly fiberoptic laryngoscopy, has changed the standard of otolaryngologic evaluation of voice patients. Similar techniques have been used by this author, Lawrence, von Leden, Gould, Sataloff, and others to recognize previously overlooked effects of pathology and to diagnose pathologic conditions previously missed. Evaluations are performed not only during easy vocal tasks, but also under stress. This unmasks dysfunction in the voice, just as stress testing uncovers heart dysfunction in cardiology. With the technology available today, the evaluation of voice function can be performed applying technology to voice users in a manner similar to that used in the evaluation of athletes by sports medicine specialists.

Procedures

A wide range of diagnostic procedures for the study of voice disorders has become available over the past 10 years. Microlaryngoscopy is no longer used as a diagnostic tool but only for a therapeutic goal. These invasive procedures

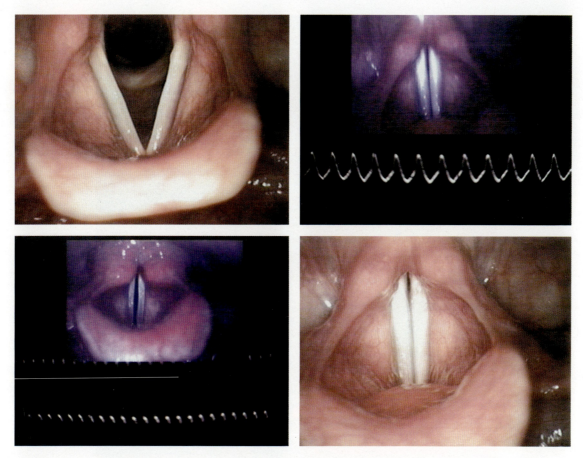

PLATE 2.21: Exploration of normal voice with telescope and EGG before and during phonation.

are justified when histopathology is needed and to remove benign and early malignant lesions.

Testing voice performance can be carried out through multiple techniques. Each of them adds to our understanding of voice pathology and normal voice production.

In the past decade, the field of voice has introduced new procedures including:

- Televideoscopy
- Fiberscopy
- Stroboscopy
- Electroglottography
- Spectrography

In some cases, functional respiratory exploration and invasive procedures, such as electromyography and smear testing, also are used.

Atlas of Laser Voice Surgery

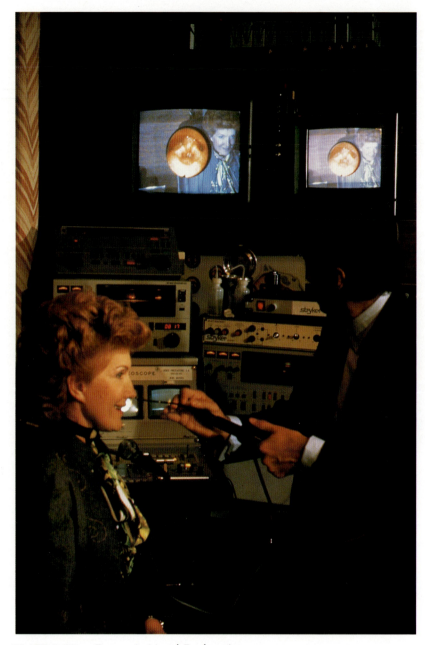

PLATE 2.22: Dynamic Vocal Exploration.

Indirect Laryngoscopy

Indirect laryngoscopy is the main laryngeal examination. The larynx is visualized through the use of a laryngeal mirror, instead of sunlight as used by Manuel Garcia in 1854. (Plate 2.23)

The tongue must be pulled forward, the mirror introduced into the oropharynx, and the patient asked to produce a high pitched "ee" sound. The "ee" vowel enhances visualization of the vocal folds by removing the tongue and epiglottis from the larynx area.

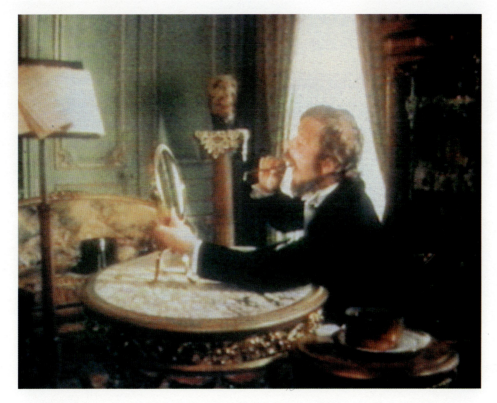

PLATE 2.23: Manuel Garcia developed the first method of indirect laryngoscopy in 1854.

This examination provides assessment of the real color of the mucosa and gives more information in three dimensions but cannot provide information about natural voice production.

Laryngeal Televideoscope

Laryngeal televideoscopic examination allows accurate assessment of laryngeal pathologies. This technique provides a wide angle objective and a sharp image with a focus from almost nil to infinity. Some telescopes have a fixed focus and need a zoom lens which is adjusted by a ring. (Plates 2.24, 2.25, and 2.26)

We use the same technique for observing vocal folds that is used in indirect laryngoscopy. This instrument is a rigid tube that allows observation of the vocal folds during respiration and pronunciation of the vowel "ee." The main advantage is that it increases and magnifies the true and false vocal folds. Very small lesions can be diagnosed during stroboscopy by this technique, for example, varicosities, soft nodules, or slight edema.

Fiberscope

The flexible fiberoptic laryngoscope is a bundle of flexible fibers used for two purposes:

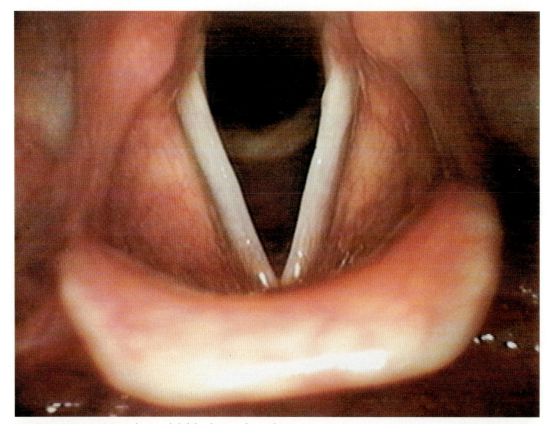

PLATE 2.24: Normal vocal folds during breathing.

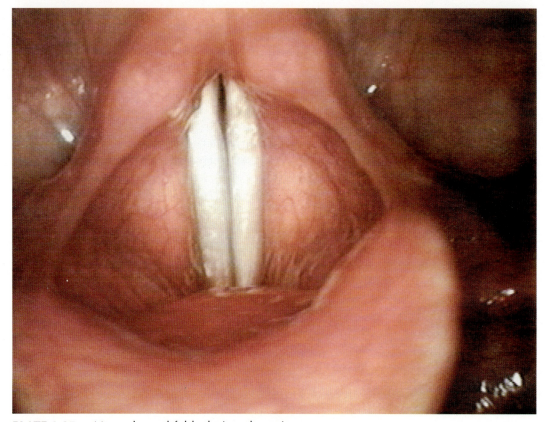

PLATE 2.25: Normal vocal folds during phonation.

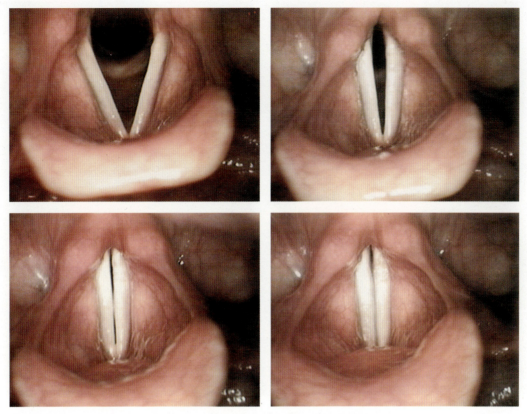

PLATE 2.26: Exploration of normal voice with tele-videoscopy.

- to carry light to the larynx
- to bring the image to the eye or to a video camera and to record the patterns. (Plate 2.26)

This flexible instrument has a diameter of 2.7 to 4.2 mm. Resolution has improved greatly since 1990. Assessment by laryngo-fiberscopy does not require anesthesia. The laryngoscope is introduced into the right or the left nasal fossa depending on the septum, running along the floor of the nasal fossa, then above the soft palate, and arriving over the pharynx. It is slowly pushed along on the base of the tongue and the epiglottis, toward the larynx and the glottis. Its movable lens tip is adjustable and can be rotated to observe the full larynx. Usually, the fiberscope, positioned vertically, is stopped near the epiglottis to observe voice production. It can be moved closer to the vocal folds during breathing and slowly into the glottic space for a more detailed visualization. By video fiberoptic laryngoscopy, pharyngeal and laryngeal mechanisms become easier to understand. (Plates 2.22, 2.27, and 2.28)

This method is particularly helpful when specific anatomical conditions, such as hyperactive gag reflexes, a thick tongue base, or an overhanging epiglottis, are present and in the examination of children. The examination is fully videotaped for careful review and to share the results and observations with

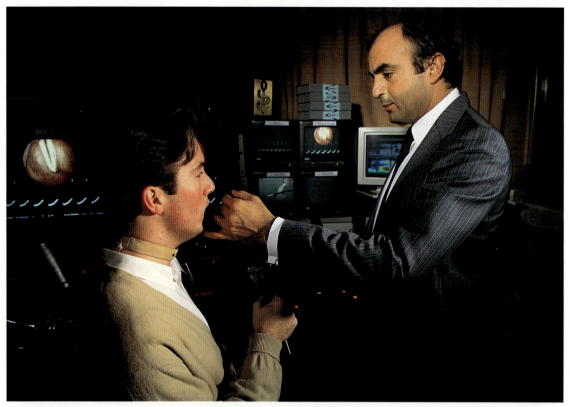
PLATE 2.27: Dynamic Vocal Exploration of the vocal folds with EGG.

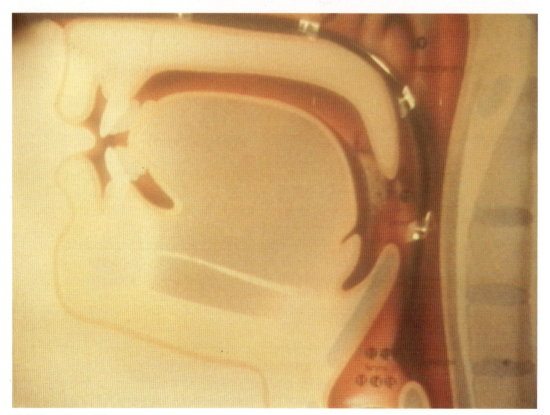
PLATE 2.28: Fiberscopy.

colleagues and patients. The advantages of videofiberscopy are that the patient has normal voice production during an examination for speaking and singing, but also normal breathing production for whistling or playing a wind instrument. The disadvantages are inherent in the fiberscope structure:

- There is a lens distortion effect on the border area of the image
- The use of a zoom diminishes definition of the picture because of the fiber bundles which are all surrounded by a specific structure (honeycomb). (Plates 2.22 and 2.27)

Stroboscopy

Stroboscopy has been used in laryngology for more than a century. It was first developed by Oertel in 1878 in Munich on the human larynx. Light flux was periodically released and interrupted through a rotating perforated disk (the vocal fold vibrates). Muschold, in 1898 in Berlin, made the first photographic picture. Many names are closely connected with the development of laryngostroboscopy; for example, Seeman in 1921 and Tarneaud in 1939 to whom stroboscopy owes its decisive breakthrough into practical laryngology. (Plate 2.29)

The stroboscopic effect is based on an optical illusion that arises from the persistence of vision. According to Talbot's law, every light admission to the retina leaves a positive after image for 0.2 seconds. A sequence of individual frames presented at intervals shorter than 0.2 second appears as a continuously moving picture. Vocal fold vibrations that cannot be resolved by the human eye will become visible for these reasons. When the frequency of the flash coincides exactly with the frequency of vibrations of the vocal fold, the vocal fold seems motionless. If the frequency of the flash is slightly different from the vibration's frequency, the vocal folds will be illuminated in each passage but not exactly at the same moment and the entire vibratory cycle can be seen in "slow motion." (Plates 2.30 and 2.31)

Clinical Process of Stroboscopy

The stroboscopic examination is more precise through a tele-video-endoscope. To obtain stroboscopic frames, we need:

- a microphone placed on the patient's neck near the thyroid cartilage
- emission of a fundamental frequency to light the stroboscopic lamp
- a telescope introduced in the mouth, or fiberscope through the nose, and an activated foot pedal to control the light ignition.

The patient substains the vowel "ee" for at least 2 seconds, and various pitches are performed.

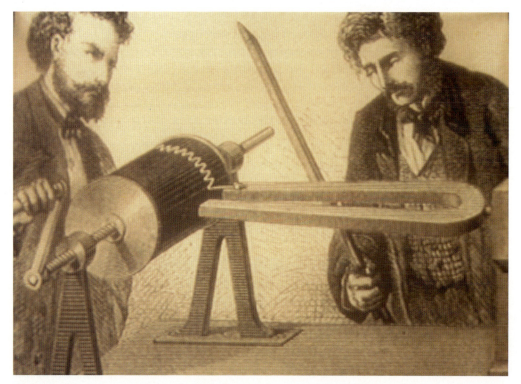

PLATE 2.29: The stroboscopic effect is based on the optical illusion that arises from the persistence of vision.

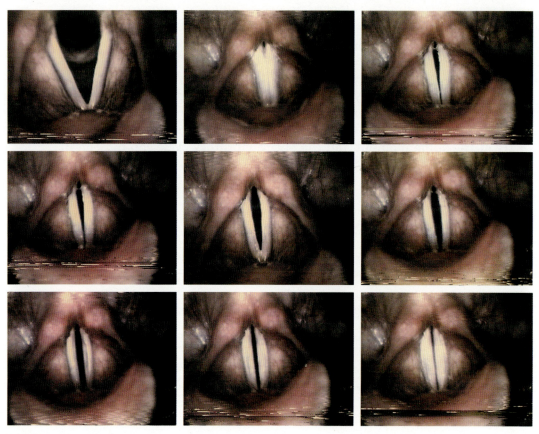

PLATE 2.30: Stroboscopy.

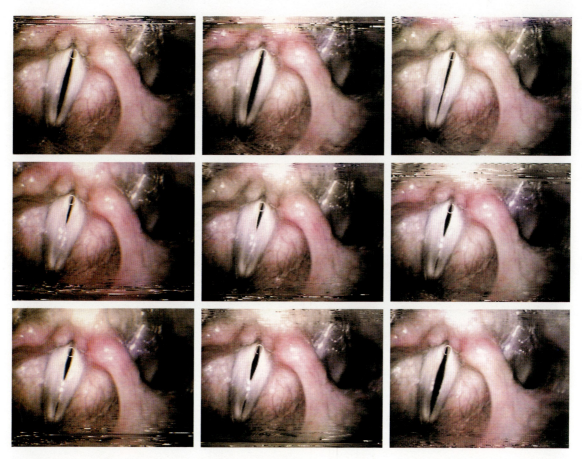

PLATE 2.31: Soft nodules as shown by stroboscopy.

Stroboscopy has provided patterns in laryngology and phoniatrics. Early diagnosis of vocal fold lesions such as soft nodules (Plate 2.32), vascular pathologies, and premalignant lesions can be enhanced. For example, early premalignant tumors look like a surfboard on a wave.

Stroboscopy is an indispensable part of a laryngeal examination. It provides information during phonation about symmetry, regularity, periodicity, and amplitude of the glottal closure and the integrity of the epithelium. (Plate 2.30)

Electroglottography (EGG)

Electroglottography is an electrical impedance method used to observe vocal fold vibratory contact during phonation. It was developed by Fabre in 1957. (Plate 2.33)

Two measuring electrodes are placed superficially on either side of the thyroid cartilage. Each electrode is 1.5 inches in diameter. Electrode A has a 4 MHz transmitting voltage applied between the central conductor and the guard ring. Electrode B serves as a current pick-up. The power is usually 30 mW.

Atlas of Laser Voice Surgery

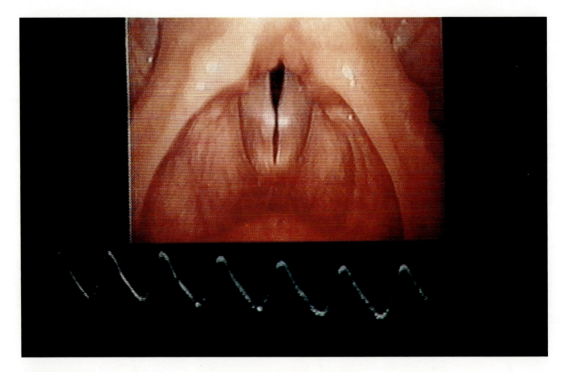

PLATE 2.32: A kissing nodule shown by telescope and EGG.

The electric output is connected to an oscillograph, and a hard copy of the electroglottograph can be printed.

In dynamic vocal evaluation, this pattern is associated and synchronized with the laryngeal videoscopy. (Plate 2.34)

During breathing the wave is flat, and during glottic closure without phonation, the wave is also flat. (Plates 2.35, 2.36, and 2.37)

During phonation, the electroglottographic recording is periodic or aperiodic. (Plate 2.38)

When the vocal fold contact area increases during vibration, the current flow increases and vice versa. To facilitate the analysis of the mucosal wave, we have outlined six different steps. (Plates 2.39 and 2.40)

Periodicity is one of the most important values. It assesses the stability of the vibrations and the impedance of the vibratory mass. If the impedance is important, the wave is wide and vice versa. Normal voice is regular and periodic, abnormal or pathological voice shows disturbed waves. Pathologically, the most important feature is obtained at the closure phase. (Plates 2.41, 2.42, 2.43, and 2.44)

The electrolaryngogramm or E.G.G. waveform provides information about vocal fold vibration behavior. As illustrated below, the upward slope of the E.G.G. waveform corresponds to closing of the folds and the downward slope corresponds to opening of the fold. The peak indicates maximum vocal fold contact.

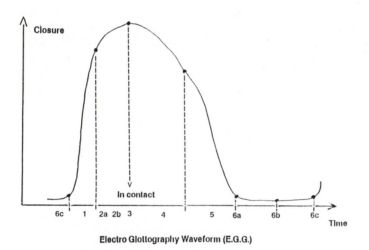

Electro Glottography Waveform (E.G.G.)

NOTE :

1. Normal vocal fold vibration produces a periodic E.G.G. waveform in which closing / opening phases are regular and constant.

2. E.G.G. means something only if there is vibration of the vocal folds. If the two vocal folds do not vibrate but they are in contact, the waveform is flat as if the glottic space is open.

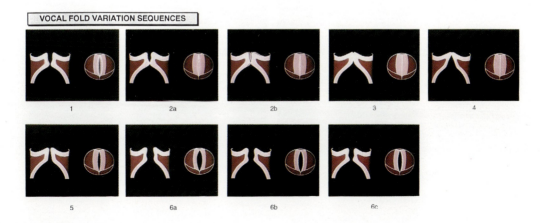

PLATE 2.33: Nine sequences of vocal fold vibrations shown by EGG.

Atlas of Laser Voice Surgery

Sources of error include

- Movements of the head
- Thickness of the fat tissue of the neck and short necked patients
- Vertical movements of the larynx (which increase the electrical resistance)
- Nasal sounds are more effective than vowels
- Dryness of the larynx (e.g., from radiotherapy)

Spectrography

Abnormality of the voice is often described as "hoarseness." Dynamic Vocal Exploration gives a precise description of vocal fold lesions and functions and seems indispensable before treatment. However, analysis of acoustic data was still poor before spectrography and computerized analysis.

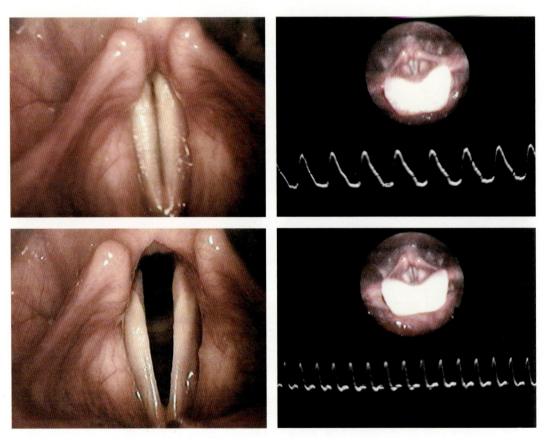

PLATE 2.34: Exploration of the voice.

1	2
3	4

1. Medium pitch.
2. Low pitch.
3. Breathing.
4. High pitch.

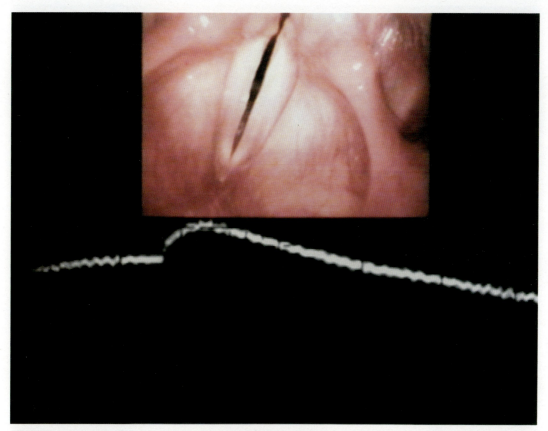

PLATE 2.35: Attack: waveform of EEG started.

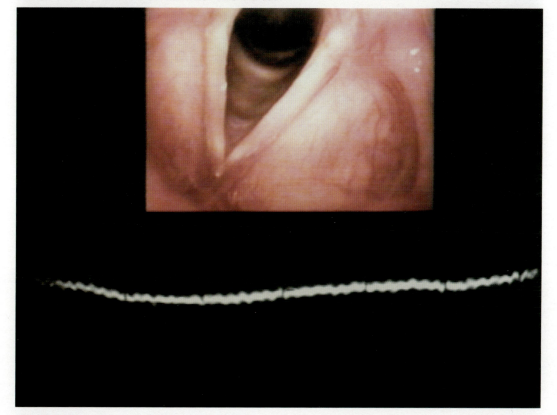

PLATE 2.36: No sound during breathing.

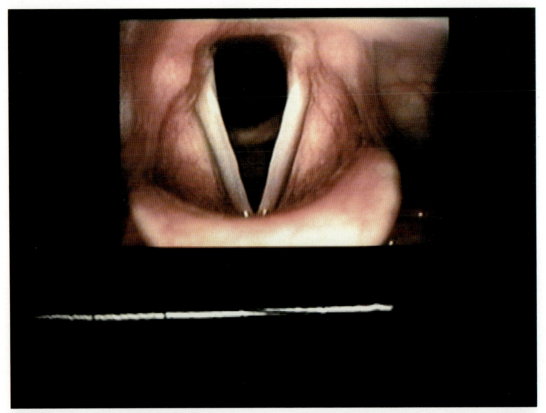

PLATE 2.37: Exploration of the normal voice.

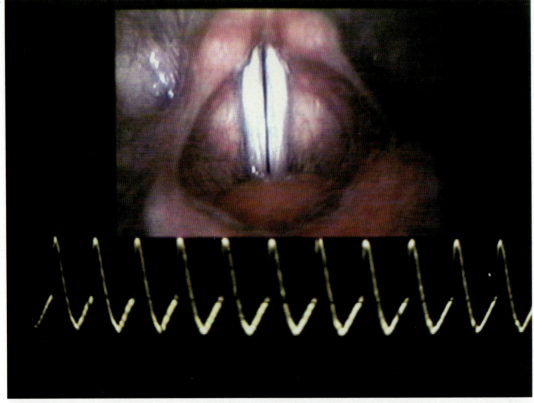

PLATE 2.38: Normal vocal folds closed. The electroglottographic waveform shows the different steps of the joining of the free edges of the vocal folds during phonation.

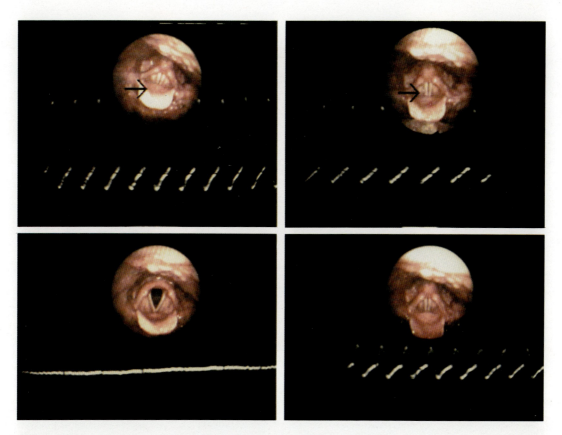

PLATE 2.39: Exploration of the normal voice.

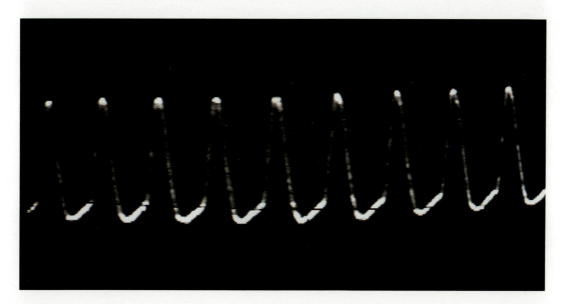

PLATE 2.40: Electroglottographic recording: normal voice.

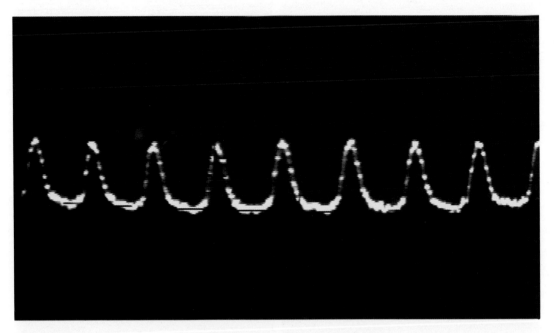

PLATE 2.41: Exploration of the pathology of voice: mini nodules.

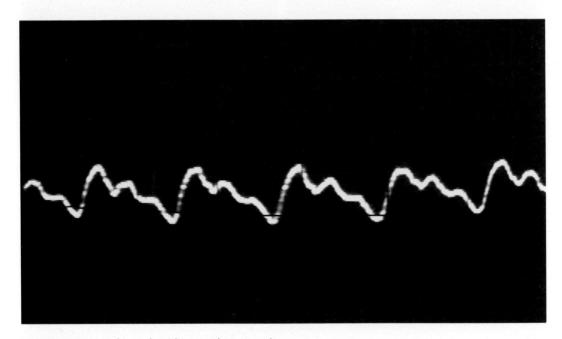

PLATE 2.42: Sulcus glottidis or sulcus vocalis.

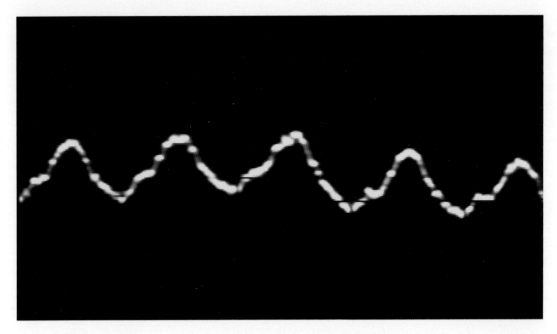

PLATE 2.43: Exploration of the pathologic voice: kissing nodules.

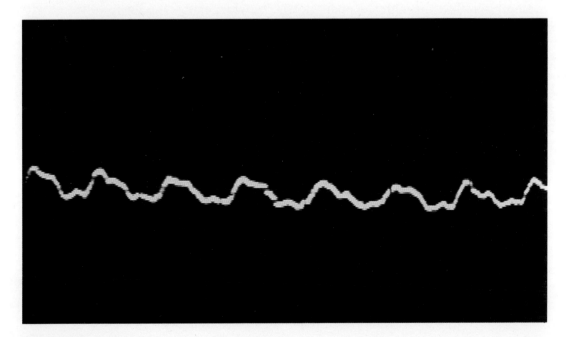

PLATE 2.44: Edematous polyp with microvarix.

From an acoustic point of view, voice is recorded on a video and/or audio tape recorder. In phonosurgery the audio portion is rarely analyzed as it is before otosclerosis surgery. Most otolaryngologists subjectively rate degrees of hoarseness to evaluate the voice disorders and to assess the results of laryngeal therapies. We now have an objective anatomical image of the larynx before and after treatment from Dynamic Vocal Exploration, but we rarely have an objective imprint of the voice by sonograms. Spectrographic classification of the degree of hoarseness may be undertaken. Signal-to-noise or harmonic-to-noise ratios must be evaluated, including the fundamental frequency, the formants, and the noise or turbulence. During recording, the distance between mouth and microphone must always remain constant.

Speech is generated by three structures:

1. One structure consists of those that enclose the air passage below the larynx. Through control of the muscles and through forces generated by the elastic recoil of the lungs, pressure builds up below the larynx. Air pressure provides energy for the speech signal.
2. The second structure, located above the trachea, is the larynx. The vocal folds can be positioned in many ways. Air flow proceeds through the glottic space with or without setting the vocal folds into vibration. The degree of the airflow leakage during phonation will produce "noise." In both phonation and aspiration, sound is generated as a random frequency distribution and may properly be called noise. Aspiration noise arises from turbulence developing in flow through the open glottis. In whispering, the basic vowel sound is generated in this fashion. In normal speech, "h" is an example of an aspirated sound. In phonation, sound is produced by a mechanical interaction between expired air and the vocal folds. The latter are alternately pushed apart by an increasing subglottal pressure and drawn together by Bernoulli forces combined with elastic recoil. To analyze the vocal folds sounds with spectrograms, the isolated vowel sounds yield the best data. Basic vowel sounds are produced by phonation. The pitch of a phonated sound is determined by the length, mass, and tension of the vocal folds and the density and pressure of the expired air. When the vocal folds are set into vibration, the expired air flow through the glottic space is periodically interrupted, creating the modulation effect and producing the "signal." The signal-to-noise ratio (S/N) provides a useful representation of voice quality. It is related to the vertical striations on the spectrogram.
3. The third structure includes the resonators and their components: the pharynx, tongue, teeth, jaw, velum, sinus, nasal fossa, nostrils, and lips which participate in producing the formants. By changing the configuration of the vocal tract, one can shape the detailed characteristics of the sounds being produced. Loudness, however, depends on the subglottal pressure.

The area of the glottal opening during vibrations and the configuration of the cavities of the upper airway act as resonators. On the spectrographic scale from red to black, intensity or loudness is the red color.

The speech signal, as recorded by a microphone, reflects sound pressure as a function of time. The process of determining the components of a speech wave is called Fourier analysis. It is a dissection technique whereby a complex vibration is split into its component simple harmonic vibrations. The spectrogram is produced by computing the short-time Fourier transformation of the speech signal. The speech spectrogram is a three-dimensional display: the x-axis represents time (2 sec.), the y-axis represents frequency (0 to 4,000 Hz), and the z-axis (black to red of the marking) the intensity (0–50 decibels). The appearance of the spectrogram depends on the characteristics of way the sound was filtered, or "the window function." Two kinds of windows are used: narrow band is 58.6 Hz, wide band is 300 Hz. The display in the upper part is the harmonics; the display of the lower part of a sonogram is the formants.

From the wide band sonograms, we observe that the quasi-periodic sounds have vertical striations and correspond to the onset of periodic excitation. Broad bars correspond to the resonant frequencies of the acoustic cavities, and turbulent sounds are characterized by noisy spectra with primarily high-frequency energy. Silence is an absence of acoustic energy at all frequencies (black on the print).

Because we wanted a possible international analysis we performed the sonograms on "A." A given spoken language is made up of a finite number of basics sound units (Plate 2.45)

Vowels are produced with no constrictions in the vocal tract (in English there are 16 vowels: beat, bit, bait, bet, bat, bought, boat, but, buht, burt, boyt, bott, butt, boot, bite, beaut), and a neutral second vowel with or without /r/ coloration as in butt*er*, *r*oses, *a*bbot).

Fricatives are produced with a constriction in the vocal tract, narrow enough to produce turbulence. (There are eight fricatives in English: *s*ue, *z*oo, *s*ure, lei*s*ure, *f*an, *v*an, *th*in, *th*is).

Stops are produced by first making a complete closure in the vocal tract and allowing the pressure to build up behind the constriction. This is followed by a sudden release of the constriction, characterized by the generation of the turbulent noise. (There are six stops in English: bee, pea, dee, tea, geese, key).

In English there are also two consonants produced as a combination of a stop and frication (chop, job).

Nasals are produced by closing off the vocal cavity while lowering the velum, a soft piece of tissue connecting the vocal cavity to the nasal cavity, thus allowing airflow through the nasal tract. (There are three nasal consonants in English: *S*am, *s*un, *s*ing.)

Liquids or **glides** are produced by some constrictions in the vocal tract. (There are four liquids in English: wet, yet, let, red.)

Atlas of Laser Voice Surgery

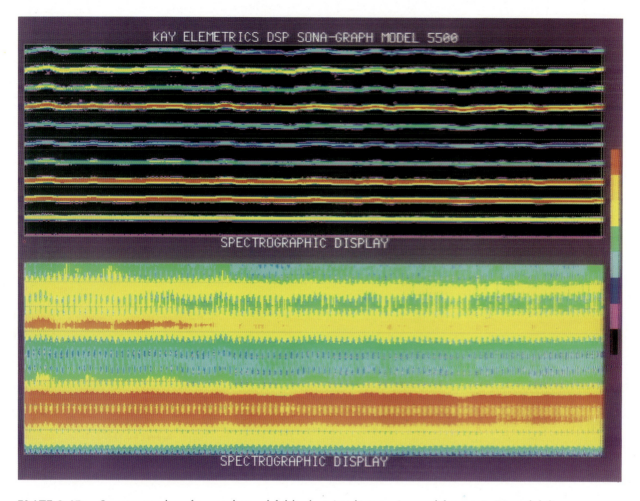

PLATE 2.45: Spectrography of normal vocal folds showing harmonics and formants (Vowel /a/).

There are two principle kinds of sources:

1. **Turbulence noise**, present in fricatives, must not exist in vowel production. Turbulence occurs by producing rapid airflow at a constriction and consists of fluctuations in the velocity and the control of the airflow. *When the constriction is at the glottis, the noise is called aspiration.* The spectrum is rather flat, and it tends to have a broad peak in the vicinity of 2,000 Hz. *When the constriction is above the glottis, the noise is called frication.* The spectrum is flat, with a broad peak at around 4,000 Hz.
2. **Vocal fold vibration** is present in the production of vowels and nasals. The glottal waveform is almost periodic. The inverse of the period of replication is called the fundamental frequency or F_0. We typically observe the following frequencies:

	F_0 Average	F_0 Minimum	F_0 Maximum
Men	120 Hz	80 Hz	200 Hz
Women	220 Hz	150 Hz	350 Hz
Children	300 Hz	200 Hz	500 Hz

The spectrum of the glottal excitation is a line spectrum with energy at multiples of the fundamental frequency F_0.

Procedures

Dynamic Vocal Exploration is performed on each patient. Laryngeal images are recorded on videotape for review, storage, and repetitive studies.

For the acoustic signal, the sound is stored. A hard copy is made directly from the screen of a Kay Elemetrics Sona-Graph which digitizes the signal. The signal-to-noise ratio is excellent.

A Kay DSP Sona-Graph 5500 was used to analyze the signals. The sonagraph stores the signal digitally. Digital storage of the signal results in considerably less noise than magnetic recording. The analyzing filter bandwidths are 300 Hz and 58.5 Hz. Using a 300 Hz filter during recording, the duration of the window is 6 msec. When we know that the male fundamental period is around 10 msec and the fundamental period of women is 7 msec, time spaces of the glottic vibrations can be stored, and the display shows the vertical striations. With a 58.5 Hz narrow filter, the duration of the window is 25 msec; the vertical striations of the glottal vibrations cannot be stored, but we observed horizontal bars, the harmonics. They have been labeled F_1, F_2, and so on [$F_n = F_o \times n$]). The movement of the several formant bars is a consequence of the change in shape of the vocal tract as it moves from one vowel to the other. If a 300 Hz bandwidth is used with a fundamental of 100 Hz, the individual harmonics are too close to each other to be resolved. They are merged into wide bars of energy. These bars represent the frequency components emphasized by the vocal tract formants. The position of the formant bars chiefly tells us the vocal tract resonances. The 58.5 Hz bandwidth is narrow enough to resolve the individual harmonics in the vocal signal. The harmonics are more intense in the region of the formants than elsewhere. (Plate 2.46)

Outside of the formant regions, harmonics are very weak and tend to disappear from the screen. From bottom to top, the horizontal bars represent ((harmonics)) F_1, F_2, and so forth. Fricative sounds are characterized by airflow through a tight constriction in the vocal tract. The spectra of fricatives contain a strong continuous spectrum component extending over a frequency range

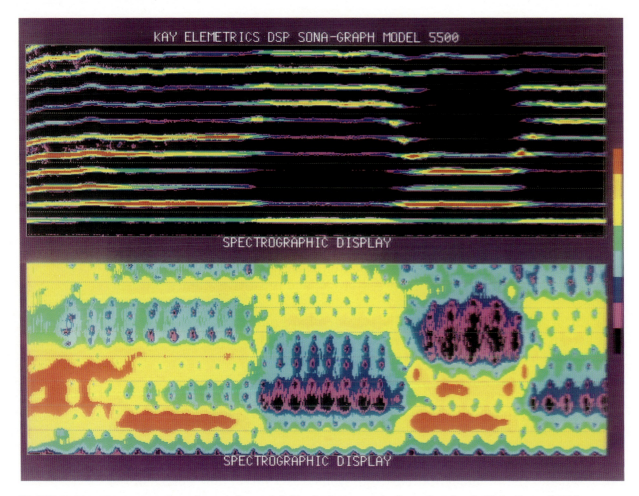

PLATE 2.46: Spectrography of normal vocal folds during vowel phonation for A, E, I, O, and OU.

that is broad, but limited. Vowels are characterized by pulsed glottal airflow that remains laminar as it goes through the supraglottic space. Beside /i/, we used a French phrase to illustrate the spectrogram: "Le Petit Caillou de Fillou" and an English sentence "two plus seven is less than ten." (Plate 2.47)

Electromyography (EMG)

Electromyography is an invasive procedure. Electrodes are inserted into the intrinsic or the extrinsic laryngeal muscles to measure their electrical activity. Laryngeal EMG was formerly used primarily to differentiate between vocal fold paralysis and arytenoid dislocation or fixation. However, in the last few years, diagnostic electromyography has been found to be of a great deal more value in a variety of patients with subtle neurolaryngological problems (Spiegel, Mandel, & Sataloff, 1994).

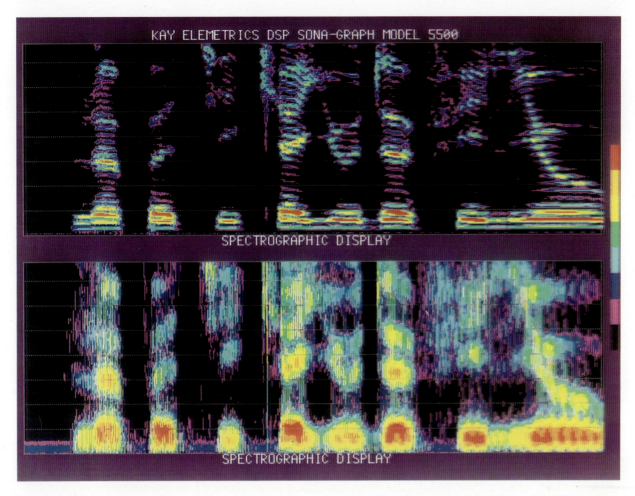

PLATE 2.47: Spectrography of normal vocal folds during phonation of the French phrase, "Le Petit Caillou de Filliou."

Aerodynamic and Respiratory Studies

Speech requires air volume, flow, and pressure. The respiratory system can provide considerably more air volume, flow, or pressure than is required for speech and singing. Only a small portion of the total available volume is normally used for speaking.

Air Volumes and Capacities:

Clinicians do not agree on the importance of the analysis of a patient's respiratory system, which measures lung volume, vital capacity, residual capacity, and phonation volume. The air volume, pressure, and flow needed for speech can also be measured.

Measurement of airflow includes four parameters that vary during one vibratory cycle according to the opening or the closing of the glottis:

- subglottal pressure
- supraglottal pressure
- glottal impedance
- velocity of the air flow at the glottis.

A spirometer is used to measure the respiratory function. Two major parameters are evaluated:

- **Mean Airflow Rate (MFR)**

    The mean flow rate (MFR) of a sustained vowel is a practical way to assess phonatory function. It is obtained by dividing the total volume of air used during phonation by the duration of phonation. The average value of the MFR is 90 to 140 ml/sec with males producing higher flows than females. It appears reasonable to consider values under 40 and over 200 ml/sec as abnormal.

    The magnitude of air pressure in the subglottic space is important in producing vibration and in determing the intensity of sound. The mean range is between 2 to 20 cm H_2O pressure depending on the intensity. (5 cm H_2O) for conversational speech). Variability of airflow may be important in vocal pathology.

- **Maximum Phonation Time**

    Objective measures of phonatory function are numerous, but one of the most important is the maxium phonation time. It is measured with a stopwatch on vowel /a/. Following a deep inspiration the patient sustains the vowel as long as possible at a comfortable pitch and intensity. The test is repeated three times, and the greatest value is recorded. Normal values are 22 to 30 seconds for males and 17 to 22 seconds for females.

- **Phonation Quotient (PQ)**

    The phonation quotient is the value obtained when the vital capacity is divided by the maximum phonation time (MPT). The average value is between 120 and 190 ml/sec. Recurrent laryngeal nerve paralysis, nodules, polyps, or neoplasms can increase PQ. The same results are obtained for the MFR. The phonation quotient is the value obtained when the vital capacity is divided by the maximum phonation time (MPT).

Respiratory Movements:

Control of respiratory movements is important for speech, and essential for singers. Assessment of the movement of thorax and abdomen during speech may provide important information about the control exerted by a voice patient.

Radiography

Radiotomography and xerography of the larynx can be interesting in the observation of the vocal proces and the ventricles. (Plates 2.48 and 2.49)

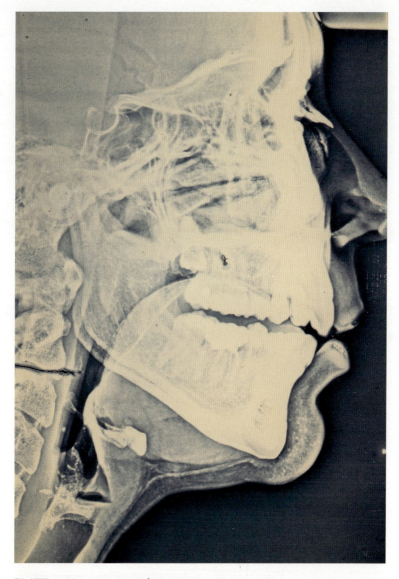

PLATE 2.48: Xerography.

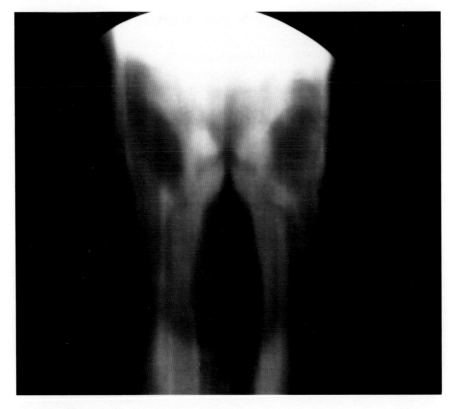

PLATE 2.49: Tomography of the larynx.

The angles of the subglottic space and the larynx tomography (frontal view) show air penetration angle through the glottic area during phonation and breathing.

This exploration provides a dynamic view of the "airflow" vibration. It also allows a view of the bone structure (cervical vertebrae and cartilages of the larynx), as well as the sinuses of the larynx.

A computed tomography (CT) scan or magnetic resonance imaging (MRI) is prescribed if carcinoma is diagnosed or suspected. They also provide interesting tools for voice research.

Smear Test of Vocal Folds

Smear tests of the vocal fold by direct laryngoscopy were first performed by Perello and Comas on five patients in 1959. Since 1983, we have developed an easier, more effective technique. Through the inlet of the fiberscope, which has an operating channel, a micro-brush is introduced and a brush of the vocal epithelium is done.

This invasive test is interesting in the study of voice performers who have voice disorders before menstruation but particularly to diagnose early cancer and fungus infections. (Figures 2.50 and 2.51)

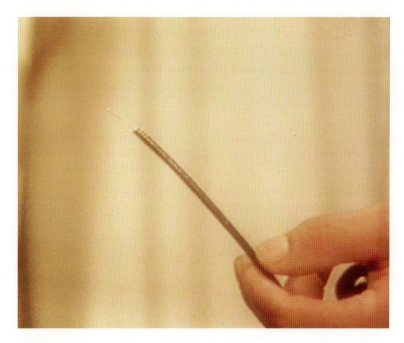

PLATE 2.50: Smear-test: The micro-brush goes toward the channel to perform the vocal fold smear test.

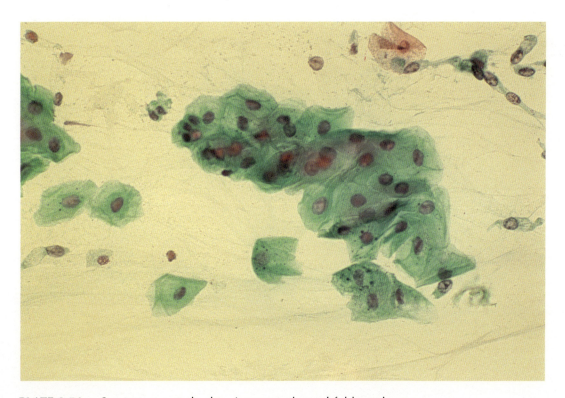

PLATE 2.51: Smear-test sample showing normal vocal fold cytology.

Audiology

Hearing tests are a vital part of every otolaryngologic examination and are systematically included in our clinical procedure. Audiometric tests include tuning fork tests, audiologic evaluation with testing of pure tones by air- and bone-conduction, speech audiometry, impedance testing, and stapedial reflexes.

To complete this evaluation, a high frequency air-conduction audiometry is necessary for vocal performers.

Normal hearing is necessary to get good feedback in the audiophonatory loop, which includes pitch, intensity, and timbre.

> These patterns may demonstrate the importance of good audition to voice quality.
>
> During the adult life, normal hearing is necessary to maintain an accurate pitch.

Audiometry is a very useful parameter to analyze the effects of hearing accuracy of patients who have dysfunctional voice disorders.

Micro-Laryngoscopy

INDICATIONS AND PREOPERATIVE PROCEDURES

- After many years of experience, except for suspicious lesions, large polyps, cysts, or papillomas, I have seen organic lesions such as nodules or microvarix cured by voice therapy; and other lesions, such as small spindle-shaped edemas remain intact and justify phonosurgery. There is no rule for benign lesions except one:

  "Don't touch the vocal fold if the patient does not ask for it."

- The most difficult lesions to cure are not big polyps or huge Reinke's edemas, but tiny lesions such as sulcus vocalis or scarred vocal folds following a laryngeal trauma. The epithelium of the vocal fold and the lamina propria can be damaged, and the web between the vocal vibratory mass and the muscle will destroy the perfect glide surface that leads to voice by the vocal fold vibrations.

Removing the roots of a lesion is more important than removing the lesion itself. Extirpation of a polyp with a tiny root on the vocal fold will be an easy laser surgery; however, removal of a nodule with a large root will be hard to perform. Slight edema with rheological laryngeal changes may cause more dysphonia than a nodule. If the mechanical properties are damaged, voice production will be disturbed. Pathologies are numerous, ranging from epithelial inflammation or glottic leakage to excessive tensing of the vocal folds.

Voice therapy must always be performed before and after laser phonosurgery, except for voluminous lesions which have to be removed first. Voice therapy will synchronize airflow, air pressure, closure of the vocal folds, and head and cervical vertebra positions.

When Is Phonosurgery Indicated?

There is no debate for premalignant and malignant lesions, nor for benign lesions in which a secondary reaction on the opposite vocal fold (pits, inflammatory edema, or contact lesion) appears. Some patients can benefit from treatment with antibiotics and antacids in the preoperative period.

Phonosurgery must be avoided during the menstrual period and the two days before, because of the modifications of the rheological aspect of the vocal fold. The advice of the voice therapist is helpful in the management of small benign lesions.

The surgeon is responsible for deciding when to operate or not to operate. In voice and communication surgery, the risk of modifying, touching, changing, or restoring the pitch must be kept in mind before proceeding.

After having decided to undergo surgery, patients should be told that their voices may require several weeks before recovering after sugery and sometimes require the help of voice therapy.

For voice performers, we can never certify the liability of surgery of the voice —any scar can be worse than a nodule.

If the surgical procedure depends on the surgeon, the capability of healing depends on the patient.

SURGICAL INSTRUMENTS AND PROCEDURES

Laser Phonosurgery Instruments

In the 1960s, Oskar Kleinsasser and Karl Storz pioneered the instrumentation needed for phonosurgery. If a good position of the patient and a good exposure of the larynx are the main requirements for a satisfactory laryngoscopy, adapted instruments permit good surgical craftsmanship.

Laser phonosurgery requires few instruments. Our set consists of 12 instruments including adult and pediatric laryngoscopes (manufactured by Micro-France®). All instruments are matted to prevent reflection of the laser beam and light (see Plate 3.1). We generally use four kinds of laryngoscopes (Plate 3.2), depending on the patient morphology and the pathology we have to treat:

Rarely Used

The pediatric laryngoscope is suitable for children, some women, and patients with restricted access to the larynx (jaw pathology, retrognathism).

The laryngoscope with a long spatula (Micro-France®) is used for patients with long necks.

Frequently Used

The A-Laryngoscope has a spatula including one lateral channel for light and one lateral channel for suction. It is used for pathologies of the entire vocal fold and the anterior commissure (Abitbol spatula).

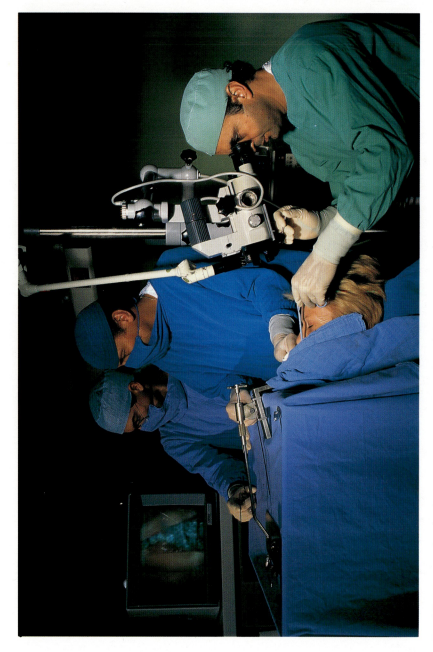

PLATE 3.1: Setup for laser microsurgery showing instruments.

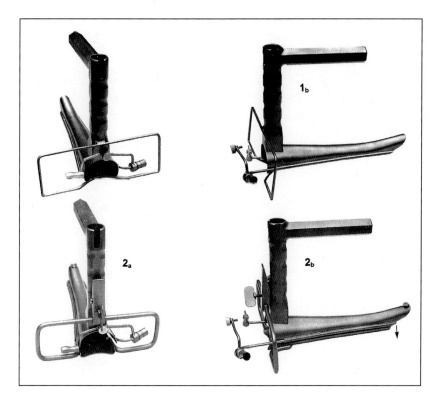

PLATE 3.2: Laryngoscopes. **1.** A-spatula (Abitbol spatula for usual laryngoscopy). **2.** P-spatula (Abitbol-Boutmy spatula for posterior commissure).

The P-Laryngoscope includes a spatula with a lower articulated valve with an adjustable aperture. A tube guide, shaped as a half-ring, is fixed on the superior surface of the upper valve (Abitbol-Boutmy spatula). It is indicated for lesions of the posterior commissure and the arytenoid.

All of these laryngoscopes have a broad and flat surface, which is necessary to spread the pressure over the upper jaw teeth, protected by the dental plate. Distal illumination is provided by a glass fiber with a 250 watt cold light. Excellent illumination must be achieved all the way to the anterior commissure.

The laryngoscope support, easy to install, is fixed to the table. To straighten the neck, a supple shaft is necessary, such as the one we have on the Micro-France® spatula.

The Zeiss or Wild operating microscopes, using an electrical-driven zoom, are fitted with 400 mm lenses.

We use few instruments because the laser will do most of the difficult work to "micro-cut" the lesion.

We work with small suctions and forceps 22 cm long. All of our forceps (see Plate 3.3) have suction for smoke removal and a unipolar coagulating system. If arteries are more than 0.6 mm in diameter, we use the laser to treat the bleed-

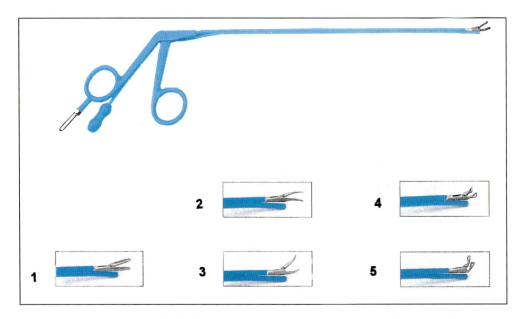

PLATE 3.3: Forcep used in laser voice surgery. Suction and unipolar coagulating forceps: **1.** fenestrated jaws, atraumatic. **2.** serrated jaws, curved right. **3.** serrated jaws, curved left. **4.** heart-shaped forceps curved left. **5.** heart-shaped forceps, curved right.

ing. Scissors are not used, but we recommend having them ready and, more importantly, knowing how to use them, because if the laser stops working, the surgeon must be prepared to proceed with traditional surgery with cold instruments.

The 12 instruments used are:

1. A fenestrated jaws forceps, atraumatic;
2. A triangle-shaped forceps curved to the right;
3. A triangle-shaped forceps curved to the left;
4. A serrated jaws forceps curved to the right;
5. A serrated jaws forceps curved to the left;

All of these forceps have a suction device and a unipolar coagulating system.

6. A thin suction tube, with an easy finger contact device (see Plate 3.4);
7. A thick suction tube, with an easy finger contact device;
8. A pair of microscissors;
9. A pediatric laryngoscope;
10. A long spatula laryngoscope;
11. An A-Laryngoscope;
12. A P-Laryngoscope.

There must not be any medical, anesthetic, or technical contraindication for operating on these patients, even in the case of suspicious lesions.

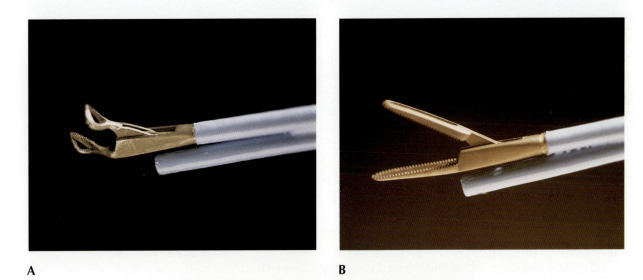

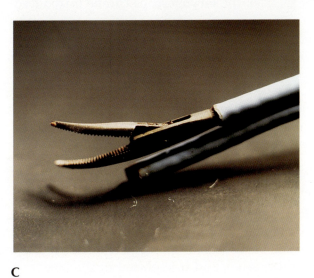

PLATE 3.4: Laser phonosurgery instruments.

These contraindications include:

- **Medical and anesthetic:** cardiac, respiratory, or metabolic disease.
- **Technical:** Microlaryngoscopy can be impossible because of cervical spine disease, arthrosis, ankylosis, short neck, prognathism, or obesity.

By using cytology with the help of a fiberscope and brush, we can diagnose a fungus infection instead of a malignant tumor and eventually may avoid a general anesthesia.

Microlaryngoscopy Procedures

The secret of a good microlaryngoscopy is good positioning of the patient which allows an optimal introduction of the laryngoscope.

Suspension laryngoscopy is possible with many head positions: elevated, extended, or flexed, but to provide a satisfactory view of the vocal folds, some rules must be followed:

The patient must lie flat on the operating table, head in extension, with a ring under occiput to avoid rotation during the operation.

A disposable dental plate is placed when anesthesia is induced. The pediatric endotracheal tube with a cuff is put in place; and when the respiratory pressure is quiet and positive, all monitors are controlled, and the mouth, tongue, and pharyngeal muscles are relaxed, the laryngoscope can be introduced slowly.

The endotracheal tube is behind the lower lip of the laryngoscope valve. The tongue is above the superior lip of the laryngoscope valve. The spatula is then advanced after having raised the epiglottis, through the subglottic space.

- If the laryngoscope is pushed too far (see Plate 3.5), the anterior commissure cannot be seen, nor can the anterior third of the vocal folds and the entire length of the false vocal folds.

- If the laryngoscope is not in far enough (see Plate 3.5), the false vocal folds will obscure the true vocal folds.

- When the laryngoscope is in place, the anterior commissure is well seen, as is the entire vocal fold. The A-spatula support can then be fixed to the bridge table. The endotracheal tube is small (it is a pediatric-size tube), and it is placed in the posterior commissure between both arytenoids. The operating field is now clear, and a moist and icy green gauze is placed under the vocal folds. It will protect the cuff, and will lift and add slight tension to the vocal fold process.

In this position, any lesion of the anterior third of the vocal fold (superior surface or free edge) can be removed, from a nodule or Reinke's edema to a complete cordectomy for a vocal fold cancer.

- Using the posterior spatula, the endotracheal tube is placed on the upper half-ring located on the superior valve of the spatula. The laryngoscope is pushed slowly. The tube is placed in the anterior commissure and the green gauze is pushed in the posterior subglottic space. The articulated valve is slowly opened. Surgery can then be carried out for posterior lesions, such as granuloma or arytenoidectomy.

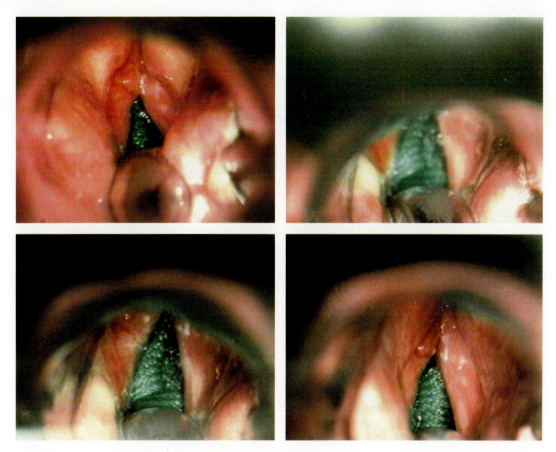

PLATE 3.5: Microlaryngoscopic technique showing how to place the laryngoscope.

1	2
3	4

1. The tip of the laryngoscope is not introduced far enough.
2. The tip of the laryngoscope is too far, through the glottis.
3. The tip of the laryngoscope is too far again. The vocal folds are stretched too much.
4. This is the optimal adjustment of the laryngoscope. The anterior commissure is well visualized, as are the false vocal folds in relief.

At that moment, the surgeon, through the microscope, examines the entire larynx and then focuses on the lesion. Green gauze in place, a checklist is done to confirm that suction, laser, and coagulation are ready to work. A joystick allows the surgeon the control of the laser beam. A ring controls the focus, from 100 to 500 microns.

A first spot is fired to control the parallelism between the Helium Neon laser and CO_2 laser with a power of 1 watt on the superior surface of the false vocal fold.

Now, laser phonosurgery can begin.

Vocal fold epithelium is fragile, and the vibratory mass must be preserved as much as possible. We avoid direct suction on the vocal fold mucosa; suction is performed through moist icy cottonoid placed over the mucosa.

Irregular scars can easily cause webs between the vibratory mass and the vocal muscle. They are very hard to cure.

The goal of this surgery is to restore voice. If we leave scarred tissue, the voice will remain disturbed, and our goal is lost. Surgical experience is very important in this procedure, and a soft movement of the laser beam is fundamental. Firing on the borderline of the free edge of the vocal fold must be direct and frank; firing for polyps, nodules, or granulomas must be tangential to the epithelium; and firing for other lesions must remain on the superior surface of the vocal fold.

When operating, one hand holds the joystick that drives the laser beam, and the other holds the suction-coagulating-forceps.

Phonosurgical Procedures

After having visualized the laryngeal field, as well as testing of the laser focused on the lesion, the suction, and the coagulation devices, laser microsurgery is ready to start.

Dissection will require adaptable forceps, and if no thermic effect is required, the Microspot CO_2 laser with a power of 1.5 watts is used. We have used this kind of spot for many years, in coordination with Bernas Medical and Sharplan®. Progress is significant for the cure of tiny lesions and cysts.

- The trianglar forceps will help to grasp nodules or polyps.
- The serrated jaws forceps is used to grasp the epithelium in laryngitis when the vocal fold needs to be "decorticated" by laser.
- The fenestrated jaws forceps, atraumatic, grasps the false vocal fold, the vocal fold, or the arytenoid that needs to be removed, using a classical CO_2 spot (250 to 500 microns) with a power of 7 to 10 watts.

For removal of benign lesions with a CO_2 laser, we use the normal spot. One of the main rules is that the angle of shooting on the lesion must be 90° (perpendicular to the vocal fold). Generally, bleeding is not observed. Using the microspot for the same lesions (polyps, for example), light bleeding can be observed. In this case, we have to increase the spot size to 3 on a scale of 10 and fire with 7 watts power. Before that, a moist icy cotton will control, with light pressure, the slight bleeding.

Laser generally must be used on clean mucosa. During cordectomy or arytenoidectomy, coagulation with the forceps that we have developed appears very useful, mainly in the case of the posterior arytenoid artery bleeding. Its diameter is 0.6 mm.

In our experience, after many years of using our suction and coagulating forceps, we never had to ligate the superior laryngeal artery.

Laser phonosurgery restores voice. Surgeons must be aware of the complex anatomical structures of the vocal folds, and of the vocal fold vibratory mass, composed of the epithelium and the lamina propria, sites where phonosurgical acts are mainly performed!

As Kleinsasser (1990) said in his book, *Microscopy and Endolaryngeal Microsurgery*, "If laser is used, it should be employed as a scissor or scalpel in dissection, and not for vaporization of the tissues." This is the only way to perform phonosurgery. We vaporize with a precision of 100 microns on the free edge of the vocal fold, at the insertion of the lesion. The cutting effect is satisfactory and the spot size precise. Preservation of the Reinke's space is possible and necessary. Otherwise, the vibratory complex adheres to the vocal muscle, leading to a hoarse voice.

Some examples will now be described:

Nodules and polyps are attached on the superficial epithelium and vibrate with it. The laser beam must be tangential to the vocal fold, vaporizing the insertion, and skimming the free edge. Frozen section examination can be performed, as well as histological examination.

Papillomas and premalignant or malignant lesions are always rich in blood vessels. In these cases, CO_2 laser is used with the spot size of 300 microns.

Laser surgery for Reinke's edema is simple: it consists of a microsuction with a lifting of the vocal fold epithelium. The vocal fold epithelium is open on its superior surface by a CO_2 laser incision; the under epithelial fibrin glue is suctioned, and the excess epithelium is removed, if necessary, by a second laser incision. We use CO_2 laser surgery on one vocal fold if both of them need to be operated on, except when the anterior commissure is involved. Otherwise, the second side is operated on 6 months later. Sometimes, after this first step, the patient does not need a second operation. After having stopped smoking and after serious voice therapy, the patient, generally a woman, likes her new voice, and does not want to change it anymore.

In chronic laryngitis, CO_2 laser will decorticate the vocal ligament as deeply, and widely, as necessary. Frozen section and histological examination are then carried out.

COMPLICATIONS OF LARYNGOSCOPY

Complications of laryngoscopy are rare; but they occur, in three different areas:

- **Pharyngeal tissue:** Besides general complications, laryngoscopy can involve injuries. Tonsillar hematomas and lesions of the basal tongue are difficult to prevent, because these structures cannot be seen during the surgery. They are caused by the spatula pressure, and only a preventative approach, consisting of a soft introduction of spatula, will help to avoid these complications.

- **Teeth:** These incidents are easy to prevent. A patient suffering from periodontal disease must be informed that teeth could be accidentally extracted during laryngoscopy. The surgeon and the anesthesist must always check the patient's teeth and tell him what the risks are.

- **Neurologically**, taste disturbances can last from 6 weeks to 6 months after surgery, as well as a partial paralysis of the tongue.

Complications of laser phonosurgery inherent to the surgeon include hemostasis incident (we have never had one) and injuries of the lip caused directly by the spatula. They can be avoided as can scarring of the epithelium related to a improper use of the laser beam. Complications inherent to the patient are granulomas and recurrences, both of which are very rare.

Patients usually stay 2 days in the hospital; voice rest is necessary during the 8 days following the surgery. We systematically prescribe antibiotics, anti-inflammatory, anti-coughing, and anti-reflux drugs for 8 days in association with vitamins and magnesium for 1 month.

The enemies of phonosurgery are coughing, throat clearing, sneezing, and reflux laryngitis. Voice therapy is helpful after most cases of phonosurgery.

ANESTHETIC TECHNIQUES

Anesthesia for laryngeal laser surgery has three major goals:

1. To ensure good ventilation for the patient;
2. To obtain muscle relaxation that prevents any motion of the vocal folds, thus increasing the surgeon's comfort;

3. To choose anesthetic drugs with a rapid turnover that allow a good recovery of pharyngeal and laryngeal reflexes postoperatively.

Numerous anesthetic techniques have been developed specifically for laser phonosurgery: endotracheal tubes protected by metallic taping or coating, jet (high- or low-frequency) ventilation, and neuroleptic analgesia. The aim of the laser phonosurgery is to remove lesions with minimal damage to the surrounding normal tissue such as vocal ligaments or the anterior commissure. We will first analyze the ventilation techniques and then the problem of drug administration.

Ventilation

Spontaneous ventilation may not be acceptable for laser phonosurgery because of the lack of immobility of vocal folds with this procedure in our experience. Other techniques currently used are described.

Orotracheal Intubation

We reject metallic tubes, indeed a perfect protection against laser beams, but responsible for a number of scratches on the vocal folds, as well as "laser shields" that cause glottic trauma. An exception may be the Oswal-Hunton tube which is flexible.

We perform a classical orotracheal intubation with small diameter, lubricated cuffed tubes (see Plate 3.6). These tubes may be coated with adhesive aluminum foil over the 10 cm before the cuff. Once intubated, chest auscultation is performed. The patient's ventilation is then manually assisted using an anesthetic mask connected to a flow meter. A mixture of air and 30% oxygen, carefully excluding nitrous oxide, avoids tube ignition.

Jet Ventilation

Jet ventilation is an intermittent positive-pressure ventilation that works according to the Venturi effect. The jetted gas leaves a narrow cannula and, when entering the trachea, entrains outside air *inside* the lungs because of the depression created in the larger tracheal volume. This causes the gases to move forward. Two techniques are described.

> **Manual Jet Ventilation or Low-Frequency Jet Ventilation:**
>
> Initally described by Saunders in 1967 for patients undergoing bronchoscopy, it includes an injector connected to a gas reservoir (air and/or oxygen), a flow interrupter with a manual trigger, and a large bore catheter placed distal or proximal to the vocal folds. It allows a relatively low-frequency ventilation with 10 to 16 insufflations per minute and a time of insufflation of 1 to 3 seconds.

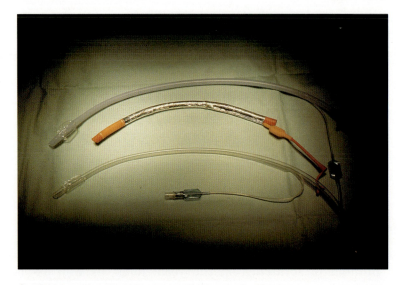

A

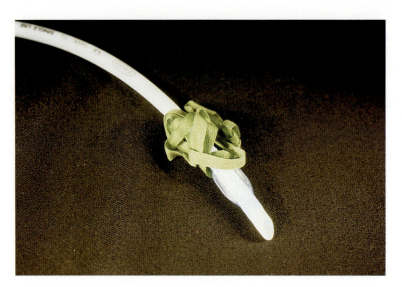

B

PLATE 3.6: Orotracheal intubation. **A.** The tubes. **B.** The tube with the green gauze that protects the cuff.

High-Frequency Jet Ventilation:

Air and oxygen (30% FiO_2) are delivered at a frequency of 100 to 300 insufflations/min., under a pressure of 3 bars. A Venturi effect is produced at the distal end of the injector, imposing an additional air circuit with a flow of 10 to 20 l/min. The sum of the two volumes (ventilation system plus displaced gas) equals the patient's tidal volume (i.e., 5ml/kg). We rarely use this technique in our patients, who often present with chronic obstructive pulmonary diseases, distention, and asthma, all the more dangerous because it predisposes the patient to alveolar hypoventilation and pneumothorax. Moreover, it causes the vocal folds to vibrate, disturbing laser sharp-shooting, particularly on 0.5 to 1 mm nodules.

Transtracheal Ventilation

Used in cases of difficult or nonfeasible intubation and emergency or maxillofacial trauma, this method allows a proper access to the airway through either tracheotomy or a 14-gauge needle inserted into the trachea through the cricothyroid membrane. Except for a few contraindications (e.g., goiter, subglottic tumors), this technique uses jet ventilation.

General Anesthesia Without Intubation

We never use this technique because of its various drawbacks and dangers. Successive intubation, extubation, and reintubation may jeopardize the mucosa and lead to bleeding or regurgitation; smoke exhalation prevents the surgeon from adjusting the laser beam.

Anesthetic Agents

The success of laser surgery in otorhinolaryngology depends on the skills and cohesion of the whole surgical team. Duration of the procedure is generally short, ranging from 10 minutes to a maximum of 1 hour. Drugs, therefore, have to induce a rapid and deep anesthesia and, at the same time, allow a fast recovery of pharyngeal and laryngeal reflexes.

Preoperative Procedures

Besides the history and physical examination, routine preoperative evaluation includes screening for any previous intubation problem and dysmorphic features, or maxillofacial trauma resulting in limited mandibular or cervical vertebrae mobility. Pre-existing dental pathology is also assessed. We currently use a standardized checklist for these criteria. A test battery includes examinations such as chest x-ray, electrocardiogram (ECG), and laboratory blood tests. Pulmonary function tests are recommended for patients with a history of lung disease.

Premedication is limited to Hydroxyzine (100 mg orally) and Atropine (0.5 to 1 mg intramuscularly). In the operating room, a large intravenous line (14 to 18 gauge) and noninvasive monitoring are established.

Gas exchanges are monitored using PO_2, SaO_2, FiO_2, and PCO_2, as well as ventilation curves and analyses of volumes, pressures, and flows. Cardiovascular function is monitored via automatic pressure-measuring systems, transcutaneous oximetry, and cardioscope (with variable position of lead II and CM5) to detect dysrhythmia or myocardial ischemia.

Anesthetic Procedures

We do not use neuroleptic analgesia or Benzodiazepine anesthesia because of their prolonged postoperative effects. Indeed our method is simple, using induction drugs that have a rapid onset of action and a short half-life, such as Thiopental (Pentothal®, Nesdonal®) or Propofol (Diprivan®), 2mg/kg intravenously. The use of analgesic morphine-like substances such as Alfentanyl, 5 to 15 µg (Alfenta®) are particularly well-suited to the average duration of the procedure (10 to 45 minutes). Anesthesia is maintained with reinjections of Thiopental or Propofol administered via an infusion pump at the rate of 6 to 12 mg/kg/hr.

Muscle relaxation is obtained with short-acting potent drugs like Suxamethonium (1 mg/kg at intubation) and maintained by continuous infusion (2 to 15 mg/kg/hr). Anaphylaxis or dual block may rarely be encountered with these drugs.

Once the straight laryngoscope is suspended, the surgeon covers the endotracheal tube and cuff with a swab soaked with a 2% Lidocaine-Epinephrine iced solution. This prevents tube ignition and potential damage to the surrounding tissue. Wet compresses placed on the patient's face, after careful eye closure, protect him from the laser beam. On the A-spatula there is a special arch to fit the wet drapes. At the end of the procedure, Dexamethasone (4 mg) is injected intravenously.

Conclusion

Laser surgery endangers the otolaryngologic patient because of a number of problems the anesthesiologist will have to deal with, forcing him to choose a technique that ensures good ventilation and complete muscle relaxation to bring as much comfort as possible to the surgeon.

COMPLICATIONS OF CO_2 LASER SURGERY

Complications due to CO_2 laser surgery rarely occur if safety rules are carefully respected. There are many potential complications, concerning the entire respiratory tract, ranging from facial burns to endotracheal blasts of variable gravity.

Ventilation-Related Accidents

Nonspecific

Hypoventilation, laryngeal obstruction from blood aspiration, and regurgitation may occur.

Specific

With jet ventilation, pressure trauma in the mediastinum or subcutaneous emphysema may occur, as well as respiratory alkalosis and rejection of a catheter or tube.

Specific to these procedures, other incidents like hypertension with tachycardia, due not to hypercapnia but to hypoanalgesia, may occur. (The richly innervated oral, pharyngeal, and laryngeal areas are exposed to very strong nociceptive stimuli.)

A sinus bradycardia, with regular, normal P waves and without modification of PR interval or QRS complex, may appear during laryngoscope suspension, either because of inadequate analgesia or cervical hyperextension. Flexion of the neck will usually correct this situation if the primary stimulation was reflex bradycardia from carotid sinus compression.

Laser-Related Accidents

Cutaneous and mucosal burns of the face, tongue, lips, and eyes can be avoided by efficient protection with moist compresses on the face of a patient and the use of the A-spatula. Protective eyeglasses must be worn by the entire surgical team. The most serious accident is the tracheal burn due to a mixture of oxygen and nitrous oxide, which contraindicates its use. Finally, laryngeal complications specific to this surgery, such as stenosis or synechiae, can occur.

To avoid these potential hazards, we subject ourselves to strict protocol control, use of a checklist before each procedure, from which, in no case, do we deviate. The occurrence of these complications represents, in our experience, an infrequent and often minor event, which, however, can be serious if not remedied immediately. Potential hazards are detected by close clinical supervision and adequate monitoring of the patient.

This does not allow us to conclude that our anesthetic techniques are absolute. However, our techniques have been well modified to minimize the complications that we have faced and after 15 years of experience allow us to use simple and efficient therapeutic solutions.

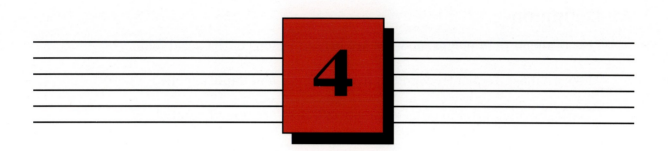

Laryngeal Pathologies

NODULES

A. Definition

Less common than polyps, nodules are benign lesions of the vocal fold.

They are most frequently found in male children and adult females.

Classically bilateral and often symmetrical, they are due to vocal abuse.

B. Location

- Nodules usually occur in the superficial layer of the lamina propria of the vocal fold.
- They are located typically on the upper lip of the free edge of the vocal fold, near the junction between the anterior and the middle third, close to the point called "nodular point."
- In contrast to polyps, nodules are rarely unilateral and may result from a contralateral lesion. When unilateral, the growth is generally a small cyst or a polyp classified as a secondary lesion.

C. Etiology and Histopathogeny

1. Etiology

Nodules occur as a result of repetitive vocal abuse.

They appear mainly in male children and adult females.

They are caused by several factors including a tissue reaction to the constant stress in the weak point of the vocal fold (Luslinger & Arnold, 1965) induced by frequent hard oppositional movement and high flow rate exhalation pressure.

2. Pathogenesis

Vocal fold nodules in children are very frequent in boys and are found especially from the fourth year until puberty. In adults, they are almost exclusively found in adult women.

Patients with nodules may have an airflow slightly higher than normal. Tanaka and Gould (1985) reported a mean value of 275 ml/sec; the average value for normal subjects is close to 125 ml/sec. Woo and Al (1987) reported a mean flow rate of 265 ml/sec in nodules.

Voice mutation during sexual maturation is well known. We have noticed in our patients that the mass of the nodules located in the middle third of the free edge of the vocal fold increases 1 week before menstruation.

3. Macroscopic Aspect

We can distinguish two main types of nodules:

- **Soft Nodules** are due to a localized edema associated with vocal abuse and voice fatigue. Nodules are pearly white in color, and the consistency is soft, the surface friable. They also occur in women before menstruation without any vocal abuse. They may be edematous with a slightly inflamed larynx.

- **Hard Nodules** are due to a vocal abuse and may be seen in voice professionals. They occur most often in women and boys. These lesions are white, thick, hyalinized, and fibrotic.

4. Histology

Nodules present initially as a simple, localized fusiform thickening of the mucosa of the vocal fold. In the course of development, the lesion thickens, and its base extends along the free edge of the vocal fold. Nodules are epithelial lesions, and consist of acanthotic hyperplasia with or without keratinization. They lie on a thickened basal membrane (lamina propria). Slight edema of the corium and minimal inflammatory reaction may be found. No vascular changes occur. Reinke's space, the vocal ligament, and muscle are not affected by nodules, but their mechanical properties may be modified.

D. Clinical Approach

1. Primary Symptoms

- ☐ Voice fatigue
- ☐ Hoarseness
- ☐ Breathiness and sore throat
- ☐ Loss of high pitch
- ☐ Reduced vocal range and register
- ☐ Increasing of spectral voice and lowering of the maximum phonation time.
- ☐ Dysphonia depends on the location (more anterior, less voice), the type, and the volume of the nodule.

2. ***Tele-Video-Naso-Fiberscope and Telescope*** show a pseudo-tumor located on the free edge of the vocal fold. The location is most often at the junction of the anterior third and the posterior two thirds of the vocal fold. During phonation, we can observe the hourglass shape.

3. ***Stroboscopy*** shows a subnormal symmetry of vibrations and periodicity and a reduced amplitude at the nodule site with an incomplete glottic closure. In hard nodules, vibration waves are slightly asymmetrical and glottic closure is incomplete with an anterior and posterior chink. Nodules are most often located on the upper lip of the free edge of the vocal fold.

4. ***Electroglottography (EGG)*** shows a decreased closing time and irregular spikes. Patterns are irregular.

5. ***Spectrography***
   - ☐ Fundamental frequencies are modified in hard nodules, lowering pitch.
   - ☐ The spectral energy distribution is aperiodic.
   - ☐ Harmonics are always decreased on high frequencies and can sometimes disappear.
   - ☐ Formants are less individualized.
   - ☐ The signal-to-noise ratio is increased.

E. Conclusion

Female voice professionals and children are the populations in which we find nodules. Many amateur or professional singers are afraid of the word "nodules." In all cases, voice therapy must be the first step of the treatment, with institution of vocal hygiene.

Nodules must never be removed for a "plastic" anatomic vocal surgery or in any case where voice does not please the otolaryngologist but is pleasing to the patient. Nodules can be a "vocal imprint" of the voice personality. Surgery must be decided after the failure of at least 1 year of voice therapy. In fact, small nodules can disappear spontaneously or after voice therapy, but even for large nodules that require surgical removal, voice therapy is necessary.

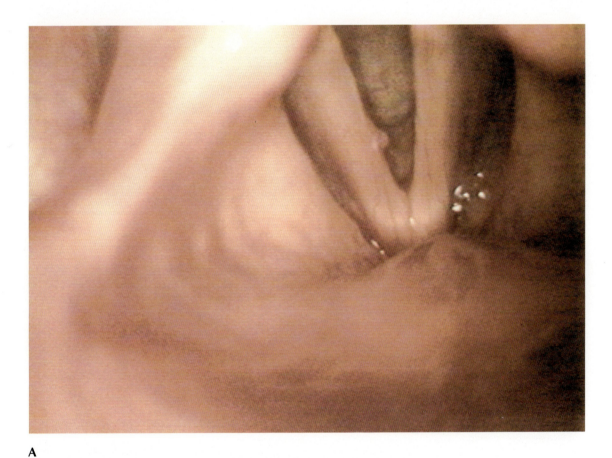

A

PLATE 4.1: **A.** Unilateral nodule of the right vocal fold. Tele-videoscope during breathing.

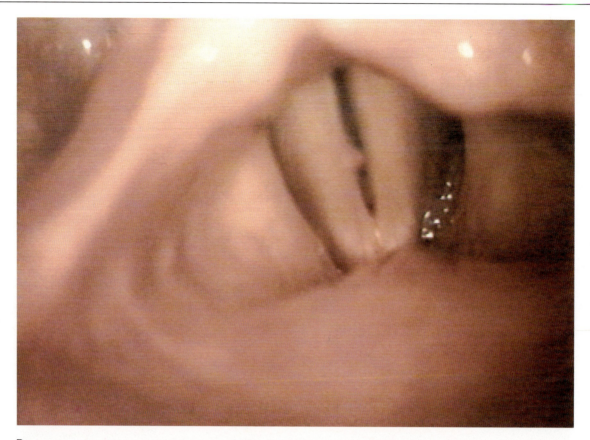

B

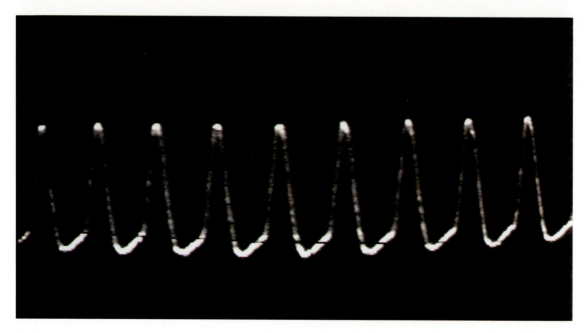

C

B. During phonation. The closure is almost normal; parallel free edges can be observed. **C.** EGG is perfect with a normal open/closure phase. **D.** Spectography is normal. Harmonics are all found with high harmonics at 3800 Hz. The formant display is synchronized.

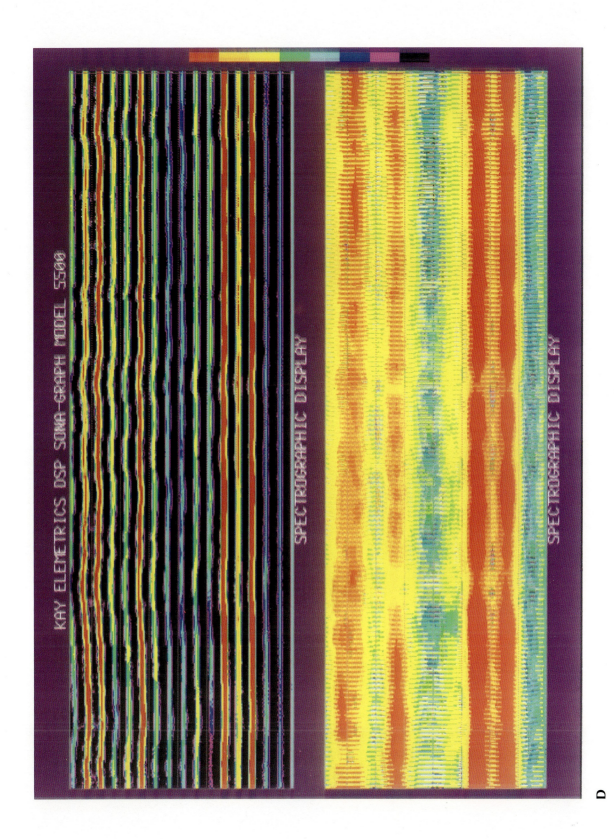

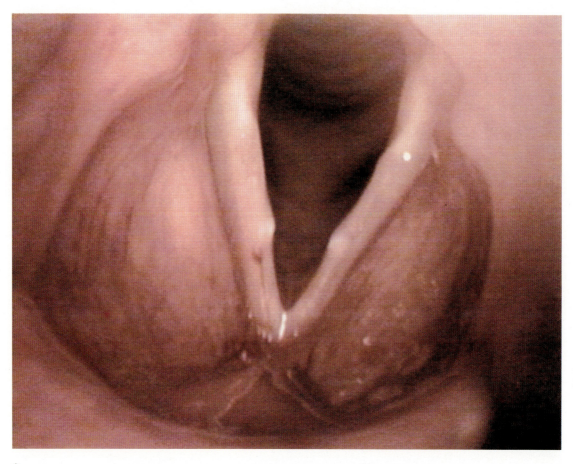

A

PLATE 4.2: **A.** Bilateral soft nodules with microvarice on the right vocal fold during breathing with tele-videoscope. **B.** During phonation showing an "hourglass" shape.

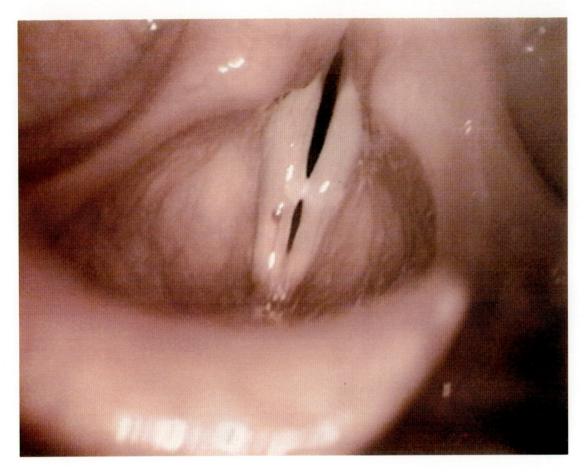

B

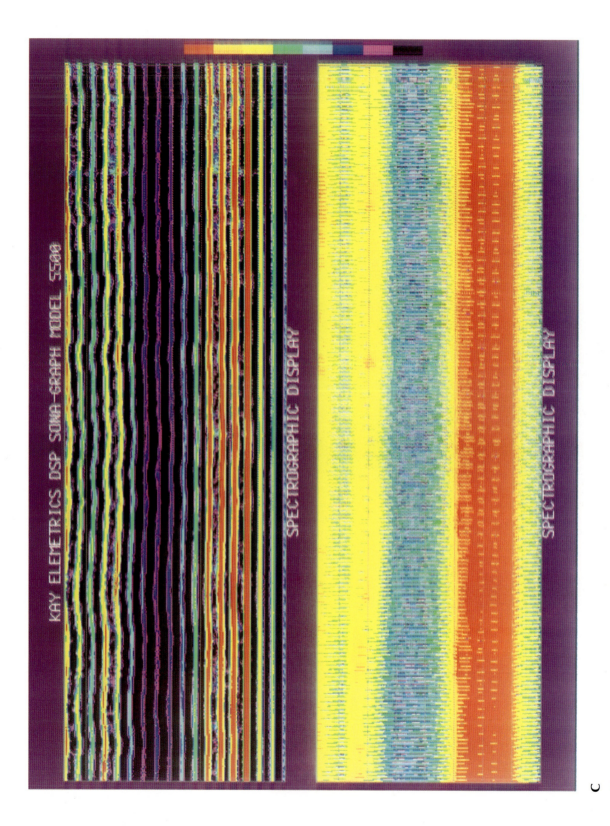

C. Spectography is normal with strong partial harmonics on high and low pitches as well as formants.

Laryngeal Pathologies: NODULES

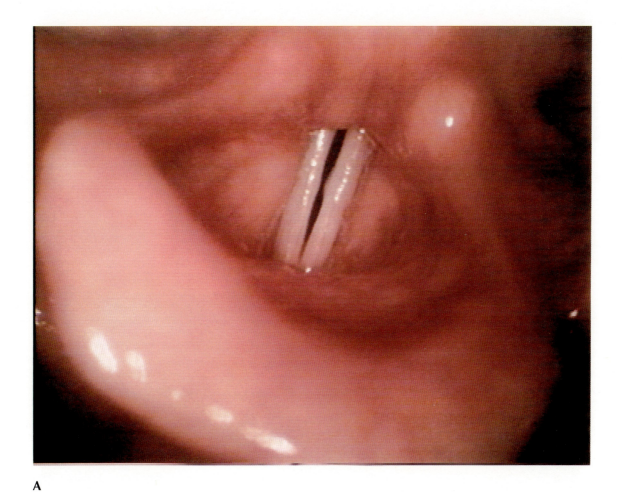

A

PLATE 4.3: **A.** Soft nodule during phonation seen with tele-videoscope. We can see a very soft epithelium.

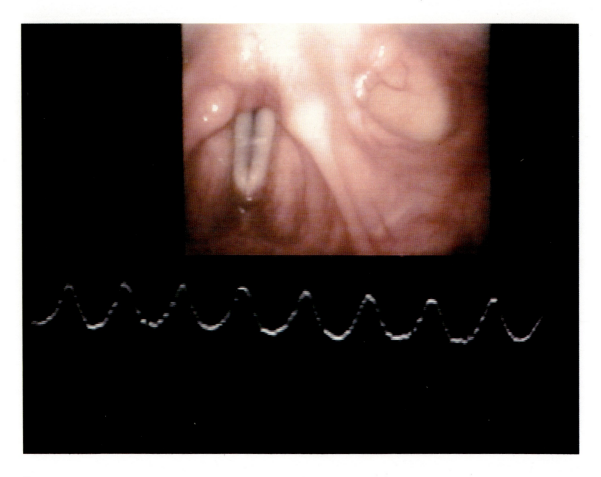

B. Soft nodule with normal EGG. The closure of the vocal folds is almost normal during phonation.

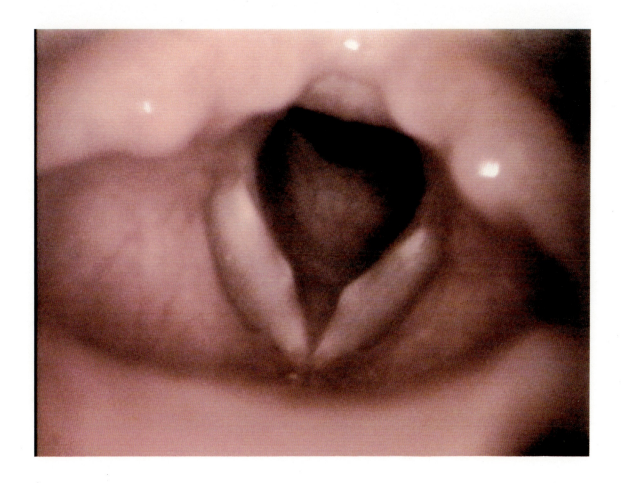

A

PLATE 4.4: **A.** Bilateral hard nodules in male child, 7 years of age. Tele-videoscopy during breathing.

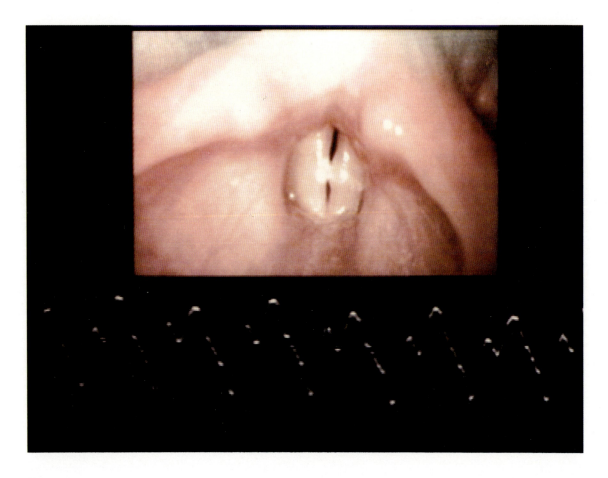

B

B. During phonation with EGG: EGG has a double wave on the display. **C.** Spectography shows the low harmonics with high intensities. The higher harmonics have low intensities, and register is slightly reduced. The formants are almost normal.

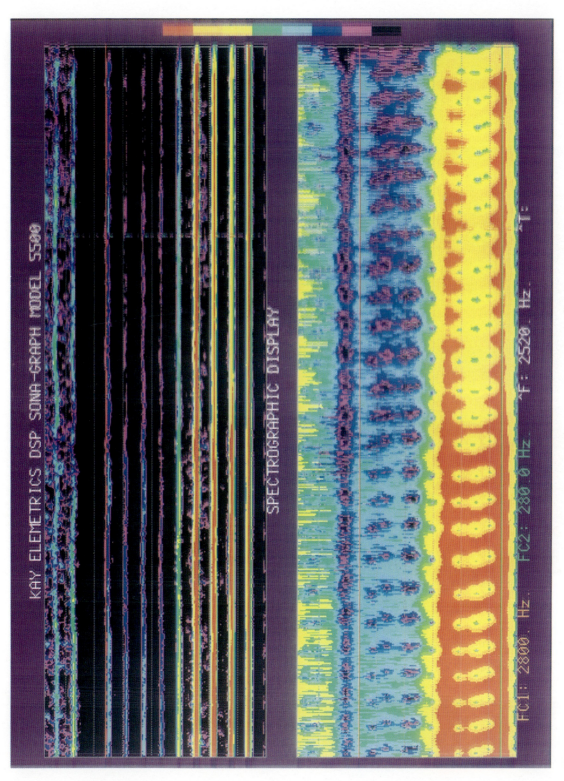

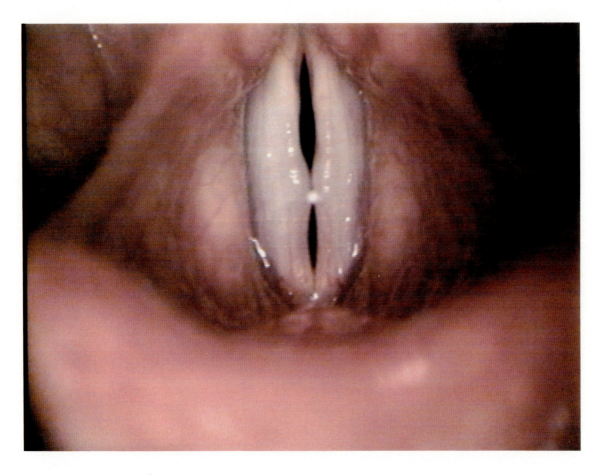

A

PLATE 4.5: **A.** Bilateral hard nodules during phonation. Tele-videoscopy. "Hourglass" frame is seen with slight edema on both vocal folds.

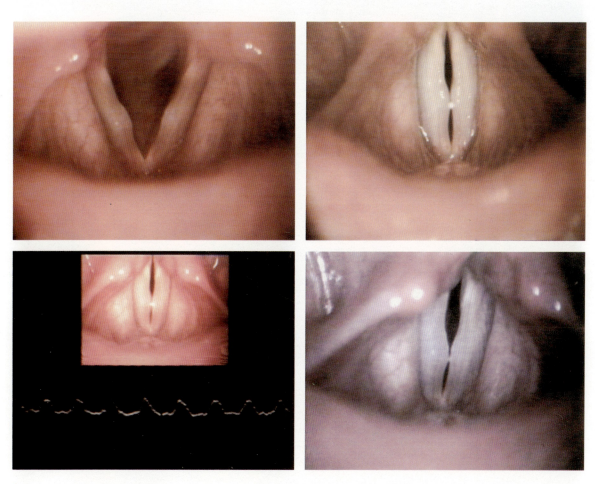

B

B. Bilateral hard nodules:

1	2
3	4

1. During breathing,
2. During phonation,
3. With EGG: long open phase,
4. During stroboscopy.

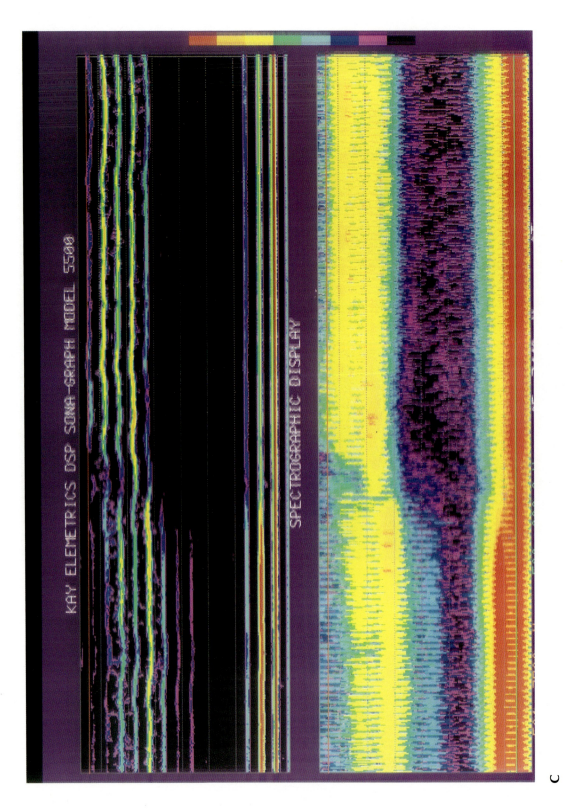

C. Spectrographic display of bilateral hard nodules shows a reduced range. Few harmonics are present, and noise level is low.

Laryngeal Pathologies: NODULES

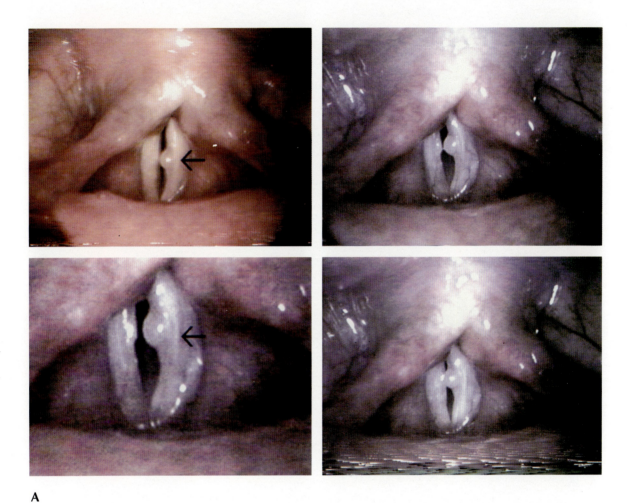

A

PLATE 4.6: A. Hard nodule with secondary lesion on the left vocal fold. Tele-videoscopy during stroboscopy. Four main steps are observed: Closure of the glottis is incomplete. Leakage is important. This hard nodule can be discussed as a cyst.

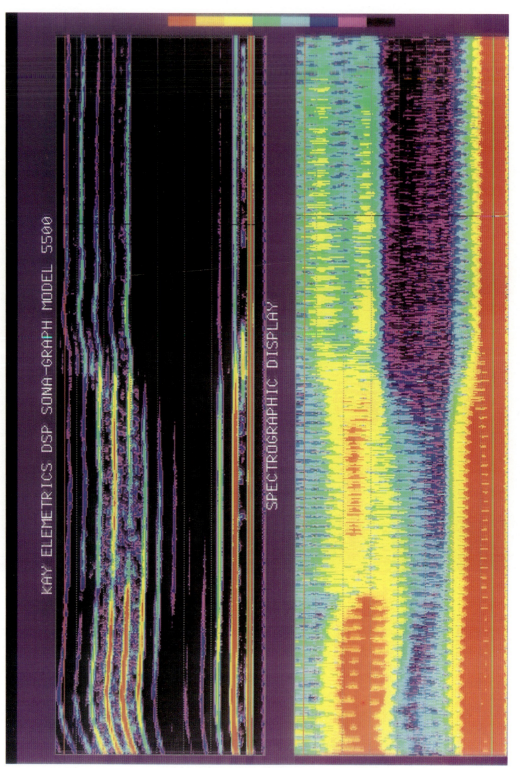

B. Spectrography before surgery. Spectrographic display is very reduced with only three low harmonics. Formants are reduced.

Laryngeal Pathologies: NODULES

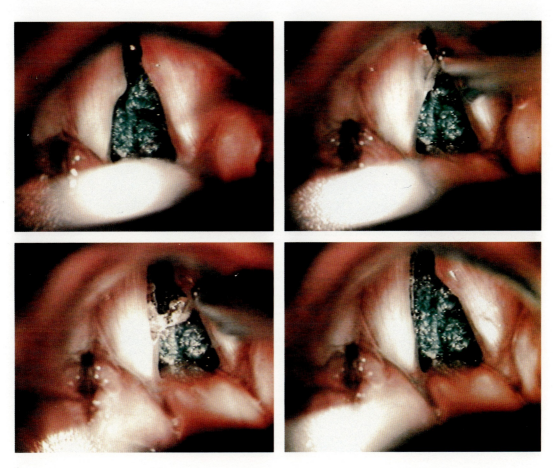

A

PLATE 4.7: **A.** Hard nodule of left vocal fold with secondary lesion. Laser microsurgery.

1	2
3	4

1. Larynx exposure.
2. Hard nodule of the left vocal fold is grasped with the A-forceps, removed by the laser.
3. Sample is collected for histopathology.
4. The excision bed is smoothly cleansed with an icy gauze.

(continued)

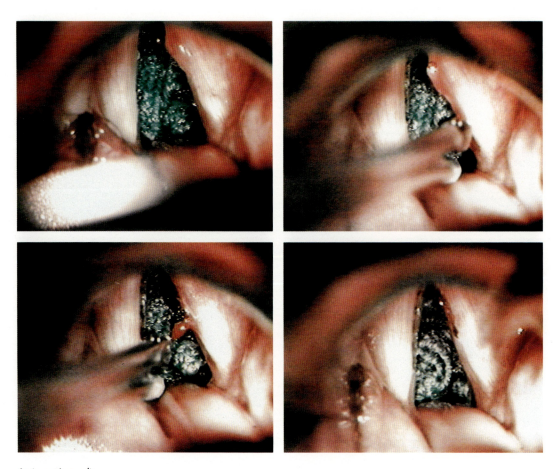

A *(continued)*

5	6
7	8

5. The right nodule is now going to be removed.
6. The first laser spot coagulates the small blood vessel running on the surface of the fold.
7. Then the A-forceps grasps it and removes it, using the laser beam (7 watts, continuous fire).
8. End of surgery.

Laryngeal Pathologies: NODULES

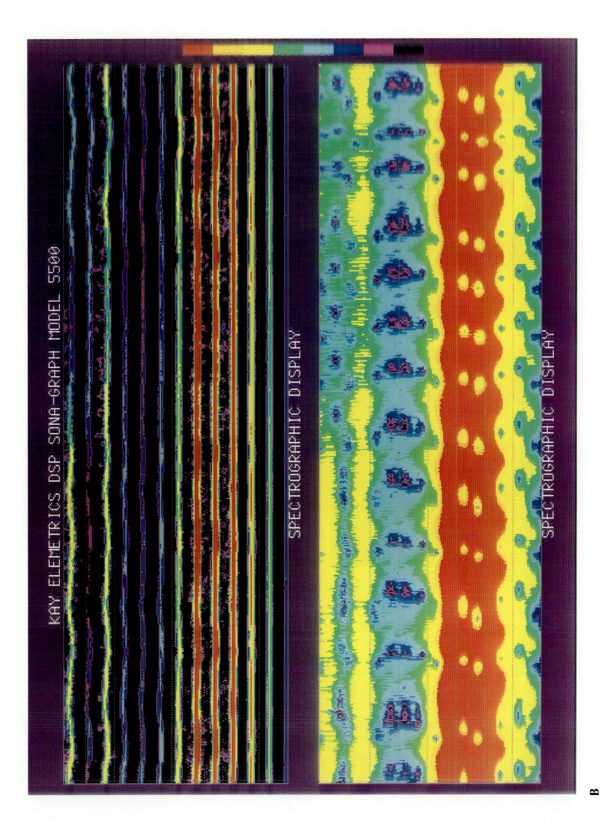

B. Spectography 4 weeks after surgery is almost normal.

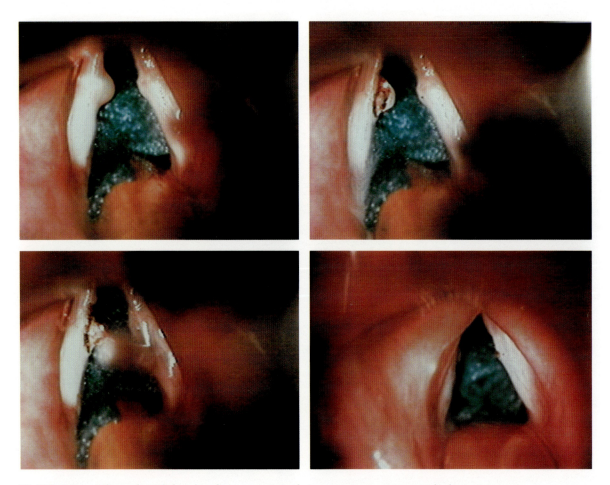

PLATE 4.8: Bilateral nodules: hard, asymmetrical. Laser microsurgery with the microspot.

1	2
3	4

1. Exposure of the larynx: a voluminous hard nodule is seen on the left vocal fold, a small one is seen on the right vocal fold.
2. Microspot laser is performed without grasping the nodule to avoid notch: continuous power, 1.5 watts.
3. Removal of the nodule with the A-forceps and with the laser.
4. The right nodule is vaporized tangentially to the free edge. End of surgery.

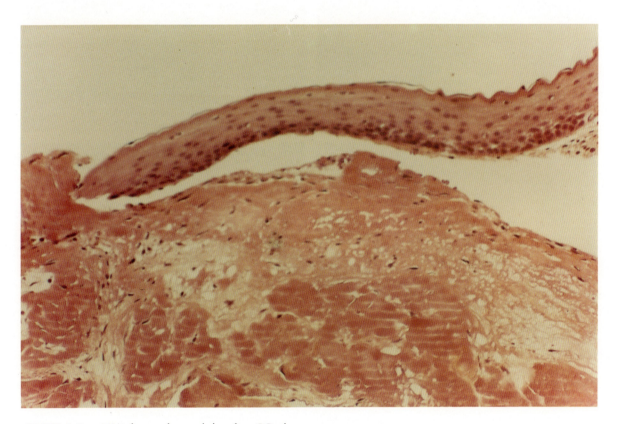

PLATE 4.9: Histology of a nodule after CO_2 laser surgery.

Atlas of Laser Voice Surgery

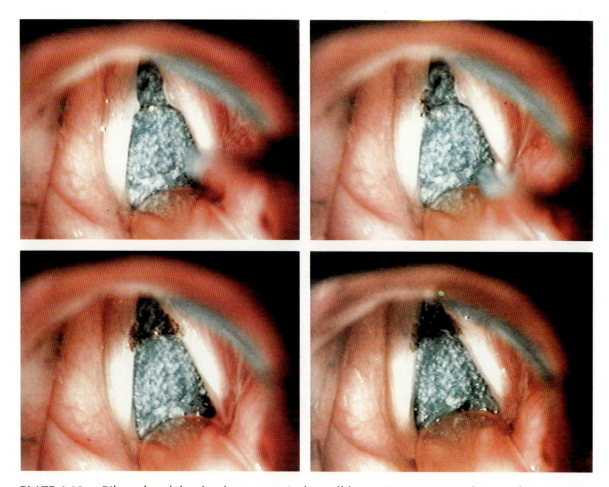

PLATE 4.10: Bilateral nodules: hard, asymmetrical, small laser microsurgery with normal spot, power of 7 watts, continuous mode. The nodules are vaporized tangentially to the free edge. No sample.

1	2
3	4

1. Exposure of the larynx with nodules.
2. Left nodule is vaporized.
3. Right nodule is vaporized.
4. Iced cottonoid is used to remove charred tissue.

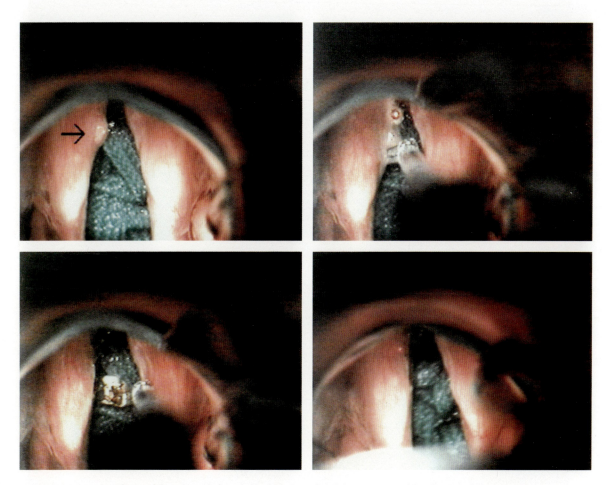

PLATE 4.11: Unilateral hard nodule of the left vocal fold is removed by laser microsurgery.

1	2
3	4

1. Exposure of the larynx.
2. Microspot shot is well seen, tangential to the free edge, with almost no thermic effect.
3. The sample is removed.
4. The glottal anatomy is restored.

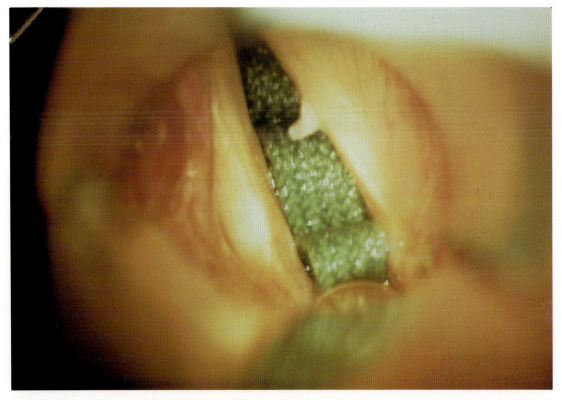

A

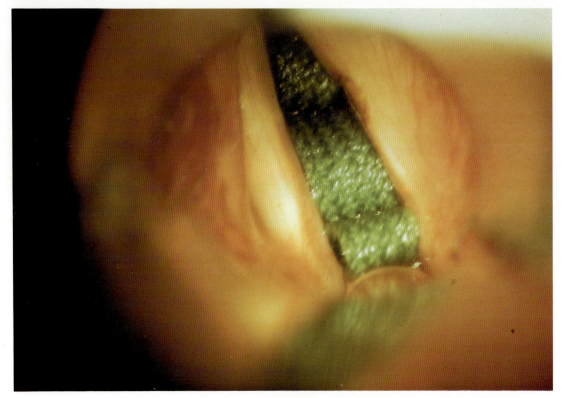

B

PLATE 4.12: **A.** Unilateral pseudo-nodule, spikelet-like, of the right vocal fold: laser microsurgery larynx exposure. **B.** After laser surgery.

Laryngeal Pathologies: NODULES

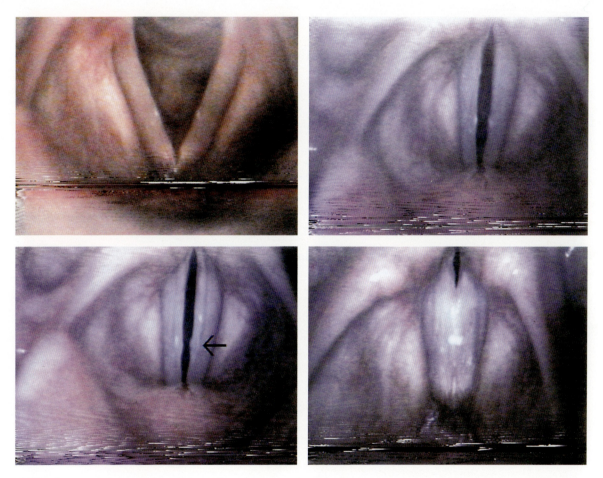

PLATE 4.13: Ephemeral nodules. They appear 2 days before menstruation and disappear 3 days after. Medical treatment is performed only.

1	2
3	4

1. During breathing
2, 3, and 4. During stroboscopy.

POLYPS

A. Definition

Polyps are benign lesions of the vocal fold.

They are common in adults, and rare in children.

Classically unilateral, they can be sessile or pediculated, edematous or angiomatous.

B. Location

- Polyps usually occur in the superficial layer of the lamina propria of the vocal fold.
- They are usually located on the middle third, rarely on the anterior or posterior third of the free edge of the vocal fold. Polyp implantation on the inferior or superior surface of the vocal fold is even more rare.
- In opposition to nodules, polyps are classically unilateral, rarely bilateral or multiple.

C. Etiology and Histopathogeny

1. Etiology

Polyps are caused by several factors, including excessive vocal abuse or traumatic incidents such as yelling during a football game.

They frequently increase in size in women during menstruation, after vocal abuse.

2. Pathogenesis

The pathogenesis of polyps is not well known, although it is evident that vocal abuse plays a major role as does excessive vascular fragility.

3. Macroscopic Aspect

We can distinguish two main types of polyps:

- Sessile polyps
- Pediculated polyps

Both can be edematous or angiomatous, but they are mostly pale, translucent, and edematous.

- Polyps are rounded, mono- or multilobulated masses and rarely are ulcerated. Their size, appearance, color, and consistency can vary.
- Sessile polyps will have more effect on vibration of the vocal fold and consequently greater voice impact than a pediculated polyp. This difference can be seen on spectrography.
- Size, softness, and location of the polyp will increase voice fatigue, breathiness, and laryngeal discomfort.

4. Histology

- Polyps are pseudo-tumors characterized by degenerative and exsudative local inflammatory processes located in the superficial epithelial layer of the lamina propria.
- The main histological changes occur in the corium.
- The different features of polyps can be explained by the age of the lesion, and explain endoscopic polymorphism, but histological changes (vascular abnormalities, angiomatous tissue, constant edema with fibrin exsudation, or hemorrhage) are constant. Inflammatory infiltration remains discrete.
- Amyloid deposits and fibrosis may be found in old lesions.
- The epithelium is often normal, but in the course of development, it can become thinned or hyperplasic with a variable degree of acanthosis and keratosis.

D. Clinical Approach

1. Primary symptoms

- ☐ Voice fatigue
- ☐ Hoarseness
- ☐ Low pitch
- ☐ Flat voice
- ☐ Reduced vocal range and register
- ☐ Lowered maximum phonation time
- ☐ Increased spectral noise

2. ***Video-Naso-Fiberscope and Telescope*** show a pseudo-tumor often located on the middle third of the free edge of the vocal fold, unilateral, partially or totally obscuring the glottis. Hoarseness and breathiness depend on the polyp's size and location on the vocal fold (anterior more than posterior).

3. ***Stroboscopy*** shows an incomplete glottal closure, during phonation, with anterior and posterior air leakage (more important for sessile polyps). Asymmetry of vibration of the vocal folds is noted. The pattern of mucosal waves depends on the type of the polyp (hemorrhagic, fibrous, or edematous) and its location.

4. ***Electroglottography (EGG)***

   The display shows decreased closing time and double or irregular spikes. The patterns are irregular.

5. ***Spectrography***
   - ☐ Fundamental frequency is slightly modified.
   - ☐ Spectral Energy Distribution (aperiodic vibration).
   - ☐ Harmonics are decreased on high frequencies.
   - ☐ Formants are less individualized.
   - ☐ Signal-to-noise ratio is increased.

E. Conclusion

Polyps are benign lesions found mostly in adults after vocal abuse. The specific way in which they occur is not well known. Glottal attack, capillary fragility, inappropriate pitch level, and excessive vocal trauma may induce this type of lesion. Voice therapy will help to avoid recurrences. Most polyps, except small angiomatous polyps, require surgery.

The aim of laser phonosurgery is to:

- Remove the distended epithelium
- Respect the vocal ligament
- Control excision of the lesion and preserve normal epithelium along the superior and inferior borders of the free edge of the vocal fold
- Avoid the anterior commissure
- Control and focus the laser spot

Voice rest is necessary for 8 days. After 3 weeks, the patient has a satisfactory voice.

Laryngeal Pathologies: POLYPS

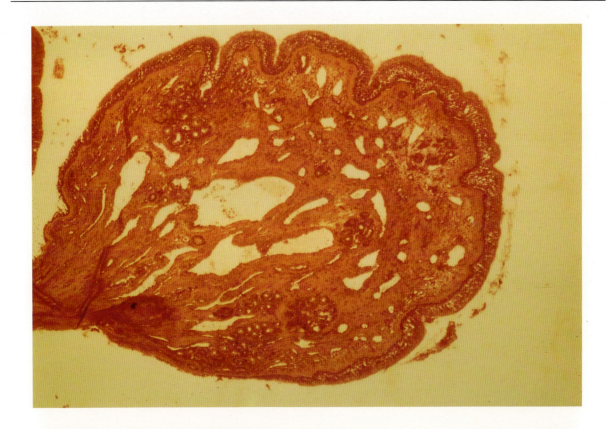

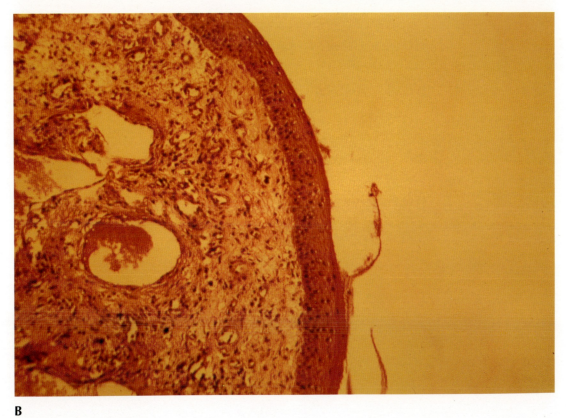

B

PLATE 4.14: Sessile polyp after laser surgery. **A.** Cross-section showing histology. **B.** Magnified view.

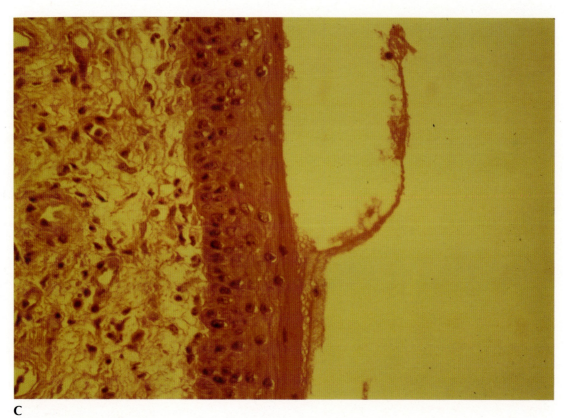
C. Increased magnification.

Laryngeal Pathologies: POLYPS

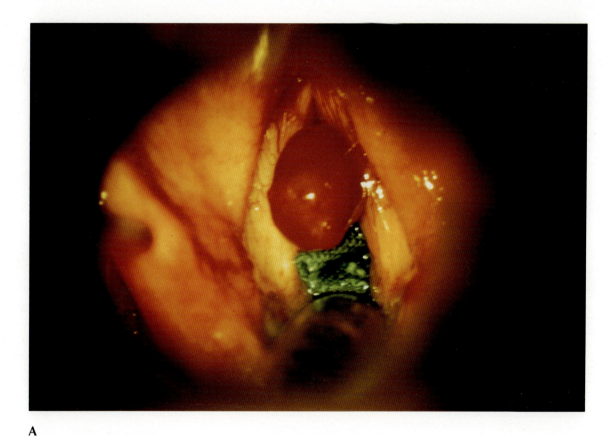

A

PLATE 4.15: A. Voluminous angiomatous polyp after hemorrhage. Laser microsurgical procedure: larynx exposure. The roots of the polyp must be well identified before shooting.

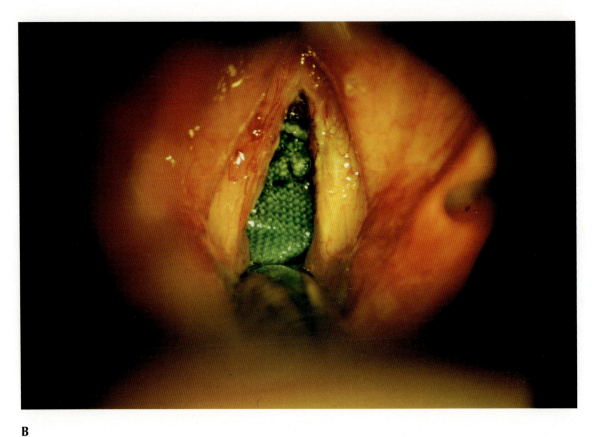

B

B. After laser surgery: Bloodless because the vessels were first vaporized at 4 watts, discontinuous fire, 0.1 second, normal spot size. Then the polyp was removed at 7 watts, continuous fire.

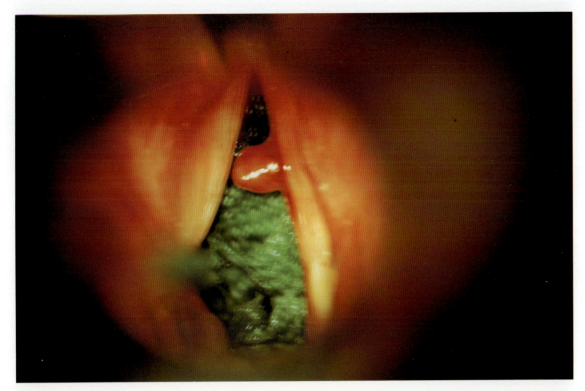

A

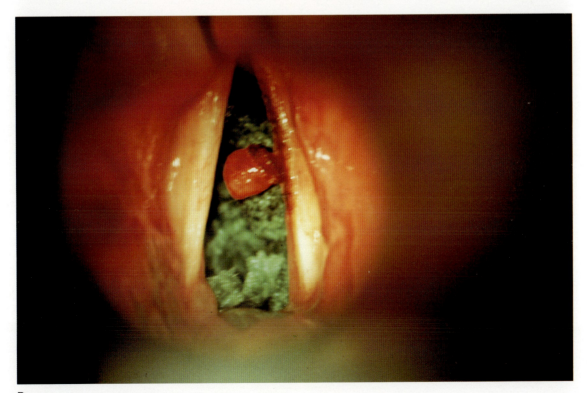

B
PLATE 4.16: **A.** Angiomatous polyp after hemorrhage. Laser microsurgery procedure: larynx exposure. **B.** During laser microsurgery: the first laser impact was in front of the polyp, then back of the polyp, then removal of the polyp.

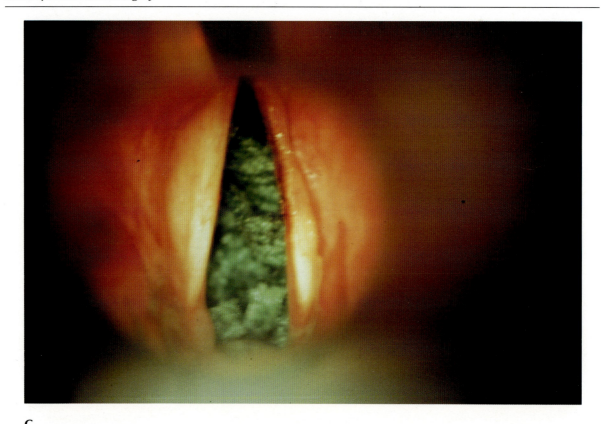

C

C. End of the procedure.

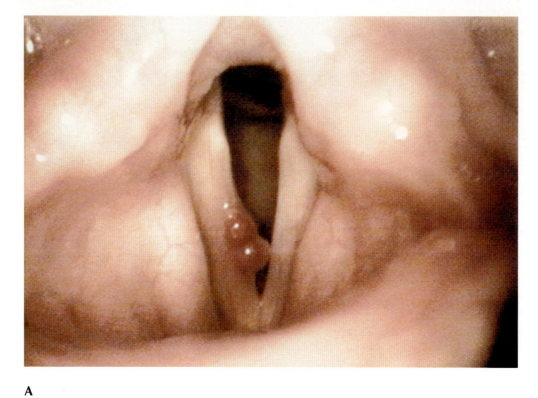

A

PLATE 4.17: **A.** Bilobular angiomatous polyp on the right vocal fold.

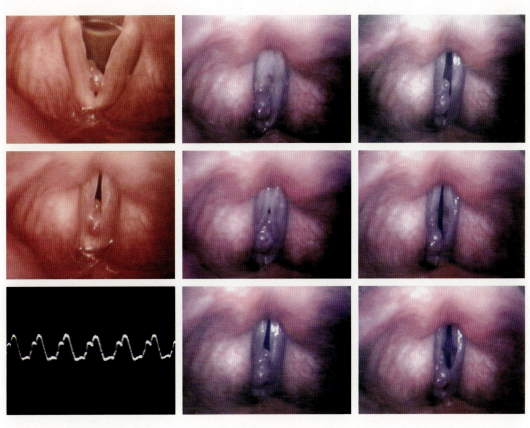

B. Bilobular angiomatous polyp on the right vocal fold: stroboscopy and EGG.

1	2	3
4	5	6
7	8	9

1. During breathing.
2,3,4,5,6,8,9. Stroboscopy.
7. EGG: double waveform.

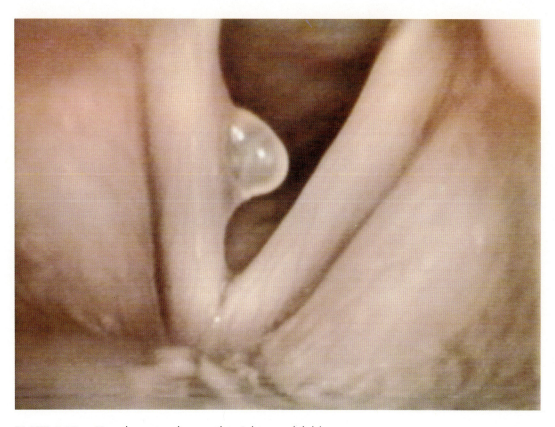

PLATE 4.18: Translucent polyp on the right vocal fold.

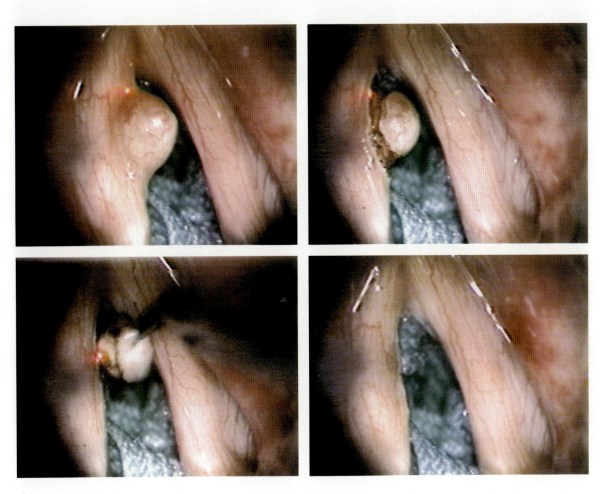

A

PLATE 4.19: **A.** Sessile polyp of the left vocal fold.

1	2
3	4

1. Exposure of the polyp: fibromatous, thick, sessile polyp of the middle third of the left vocal fold.
2. Laser impact: 8 Watts, continuous fire from front to back of the implantation of the polyp.
3. The polyp is removed for histological examination.
4. The excision bed is smoothly cleansed.

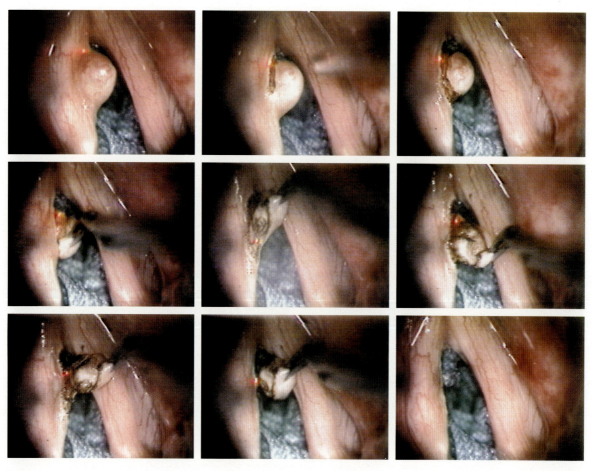

B

B. Sessile polyp of the left vocal fold.

1	2	3
4	5	6
7	8	9

1. Exposure of the polyp: fibromatous, thick, sessile polyp of the middle third of the left vocal fold.
2. Fire with 8 watts, continuous CO_2 laser, from front to back without grasping the polyp.
3. Impact on the implantation base of the polyp.
4. A-forcep grasps polyp. Fire on the anterior third of base of implantation of the polyp.
5. Fire on the posterior third of the vocal fold.
6. Fire on the middle third: discontinuous 0.10 second.
7. Removing the base.
8. The polyp is removed for histological examination.
9. The excision bed is smoothly cleansed.

Laryngeal Pathologies: POLYPS

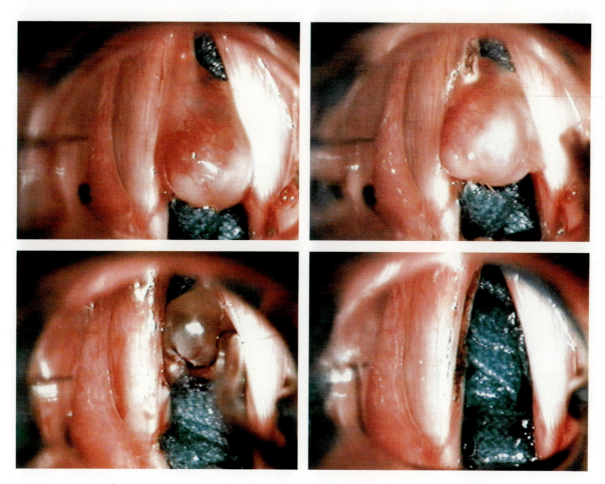

PLATE 4.20: Voluminous sessile polyp of the anterior two thirds of the left vocal fold.

1	2
3	4

1. Exposure of the lesion.
2. Incision of the implantation of the polyp from front to back.
3. Ablation of the polyp held by the forceps.
4. Regularization of the free edge of the vocal fold at the end of the intervention.

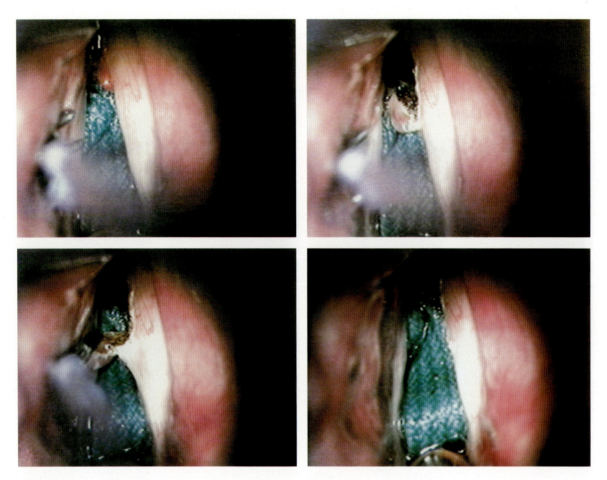

PLATE 4.21: Mini-angiomatous thick sessile polyp of the right vocal fold.

1	2
3	4

1. Exposure of the polyp: mini-angiomatous thick polyp of the anterior border third of the right vocal fold.
2. Impact on the anterior border of the implantation base of the polyp: 9 watts, continuous fire.
3. Polyp is grasped by the A-forceps. The specimen is removed for histological examination.
4. The excision bed is smoothly cleansed with icy cottonoid.

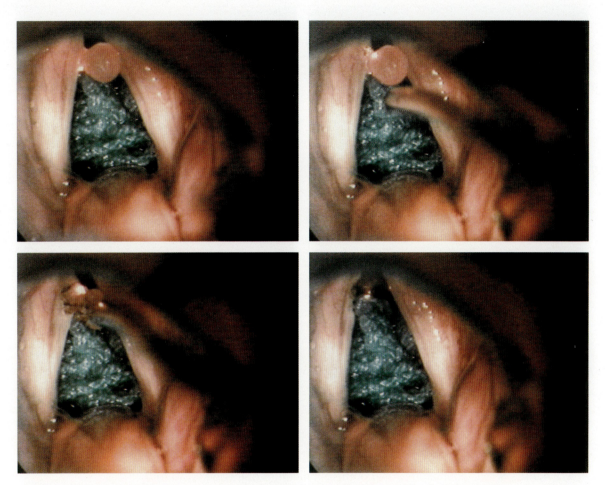

PLATE 4.22: Pedunculated edematous polyp of the anterior third of the left vocal fold.

1	2
3	4

1. Exposure of the polyp: edematous pedunculated polyp of the anterior third of the left vocal fold.
2. Impact of the anterior base of the peduncle: power 8 watts, fire continuous.
3. The polyp is grasped with an A-forceps.
4. Removal of the lesion for histological examination; the excision bed is smoothly cleansed with an icy cottonoid.

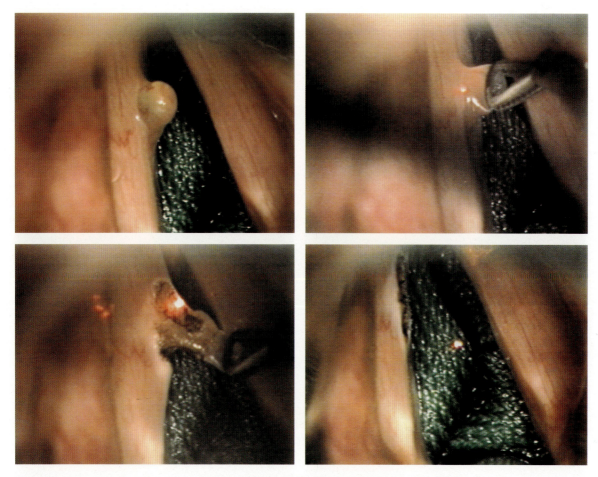

PLATE 4.23: Sessile edematous polyp of the middle third of the left vocal fold.

1	2
3	4

1. Exposure of the polyp: edematous pedunculated, edematous polyp of the middle third of the left vocal fold.
2. Grasping with the A-forceps, the polyp is pulled smoothly into the center of the glottic space, perpendicular to the free edge of the vocal fold.
3. Laser impact from front to back: power 7 watts, continuous fire. The laser beam shoots from the anterior to the posterior base implantation of the peduncle.
4. Removal of the lesion for histological examination. The excision bed is smoothly cleansed with an icy cottonoid.

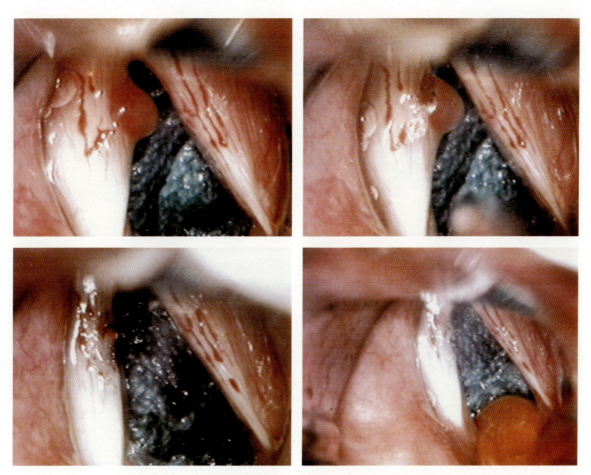

PLATE 4.24: Angiomatous, hemorrhagic sessile polyp of the left vocal fold.

1	2
3	4

1. Exposure of the polyp: angiomatous, hemorrhagic sessile polyp of the left vocal fold.
2. Impact of the anterior border of the implantation base of the polyp: 7 watts (because of vascularization), continuous fire. Laser vaporization is on the superior border of the free edge of the vocal fold, from front to back.
3. After removing the specimen for the histological sample, coagulation of the polyp artery (4 watts, 0.10 second).
4. The excision bed is smoothly cleansed with an icy cottonoid.

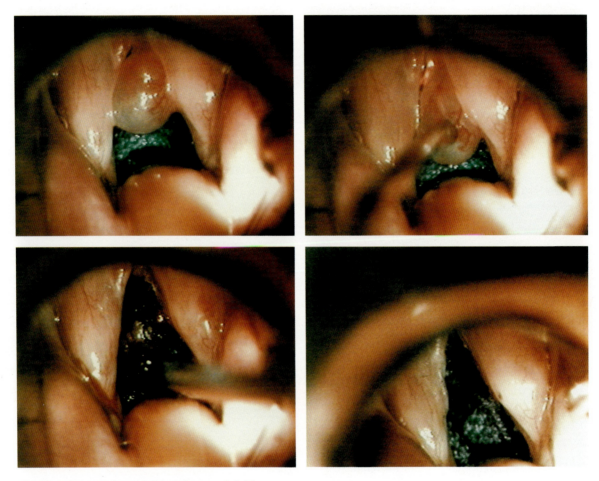

PLATE 4.25: Polyp of the right vocal fold.

1	2
3	4

1. Exposure of the polyp.
2. The A-forceps grasps the polyp smoothly on the posterior glottic space to isolate the anterior implantation of the polyp.
3. Ablation from front to back.
4. The vocal anatomy is restored.

CYSTS

A. Definition

Intracordal cysts appear as small spheres on the margin of the vocal fold. They are mostly caused by an obstruction of a glandular duct where mucus is in retention. These are commonly seen in adults.

B. Location

- The yellow cystic mass is typically observed in the middle third of the vocal fold. The mass may bulge medially, as well as on the superior surface.

- The cyst is often seen in young adult women, particularly in professional voice users.

C. Etiology and Histopathogeny

1. Etiology

Intracordal cysts are caused by the obstruction of a glandular duct. Because there is no other way for the mucus to escape, the cyst may grow larger with time. This mucous retention cyst may be confused with vocal nodules, particularly if the patient develops a lesion on the contralateral vocal fold at the point of contact, giving the appearance of a "kissing nodule."

2. Pathogenesis

- A cyst increases the mass and stiffness of the cover, whereas the transition layers and the body are not affected.

- Increased average airflow is expected because of elevated offset flows and elevated peak flows.

3. Macroscopic Aspect

Cysts present a unique, smooth, surface tumefaction more frequently situated on the free border of the vocal fold.

4. Histology

- Vocal fold cysts are located in the superficial layer of the lamina propria.

- Cysts are classically divided into two types:

    Retention cysts, lined with cuboidal or flattened epithelium resulting from the occlusion of a glandular excretory canal

    Malformation cysts, lined with a ciliated pseudo-stratified or squamous epithelium.

They are sometimes associated with a lymphoid stroma if located in the epiglottis.

Small cysts contain a clear fluid. When they mature, larger cysts contain a thick ropy fluid of milky or yellowish color.

D. Clinical Approach

1. Primary Symptoms

- ☐ Hoarseness
- ☐ Lowered pitch
- ☐ Voice fatigue

2. Tele-Video-Naso-Fiberscope and Telescope

Identification of a cyst can be very difficult. These mucous retention cysts may be confused with vocal nodules, and in the past the diagnosis was sometimes not made until the patient was examined at surgery under the operating microscope. Thanks to stroboscopy, that is no longer true. However, the appearance of fullness of the vocal fold and dilated capillaries raise the suspicion of a cyst. Glottal closure is incomplete. In maximum closure, an "hourglass" shape is observed.

3. Stroboscopy

Stroboscopy is very helpful in the diagnosis of the cyst. It is the main exploration.

The vocal fold distended by the cyst exhibits a loss of vibrations manifested by the absence of mucosal wave on videostroboscopy. It can also demonstrate an adynamic focus at the site of the cyst.

Greater aperiodicity and reduced glottal closure have been well described (Kitzing, 1985). Vibration of the two vocal folds is asymmetrical, especially over the area of the cyst, and depends on its volume.

Mass stiffness of the cover is increased. Cysts often impair glottic closure.

Videostroboscopy is also very important to appreciate the change in vibratory activity after surgery.

4. Electroglottography (EGG)

The closing phase of the vocal folds is slower than normal on EGG.

5. Spectrography

- ☐ Fundamental frequencies are modified in hard cysts with lower pitch.
- ☐ The spectral energy distribution is aperiodic.
- ☐ Harmonics are always decreased on high frequencies and can sometimes disappear.
- ☐ Formants are less individualized.
- ☐ Signal-to-noise ratio is increased.

E. Conclusion

- The result in the immediate postoperative period is generally good. The vocal fold quickly resumes its normal mass, and these patients tend to have excellent anatomical and functional results.

- The aim of laser phonosurgery is to remove the sac and prevent recurrences. There are two laser techniques:

  1. Removing the cyst and the epithelium above it (see Plates 4.32 and 4.33)
  2. Removing the cyst without the epithelium (Plate 4.36B)

- The sac of the cyst must be totally removed to prevent recurrence.

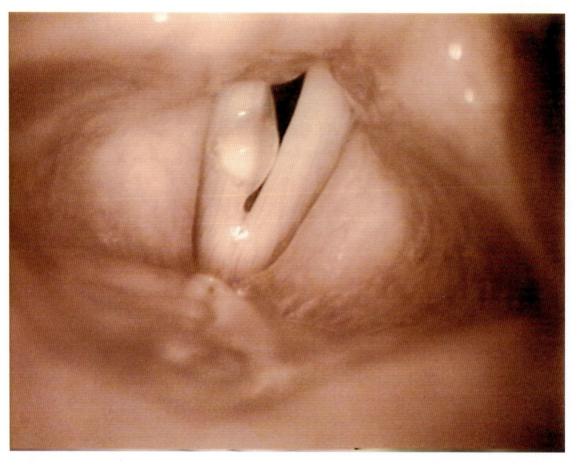

PLATE 4.26: Intracordal cyst of the right vocal fold during phonation. Tele-videoscope. Leakage is important during vibrations.

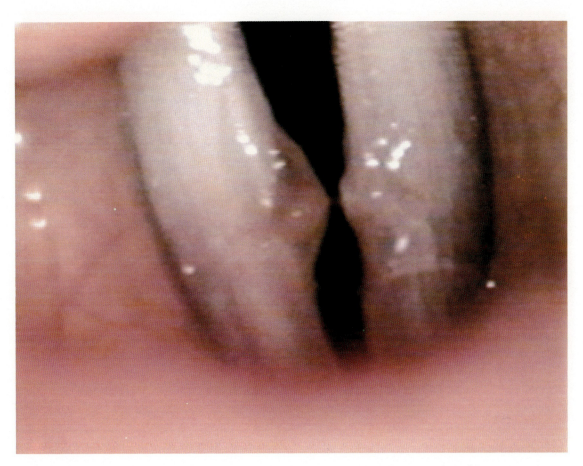

PLATE 4.27: Right vocal fold cyst with a contralateral secondary lesion. Tele-videoscope.

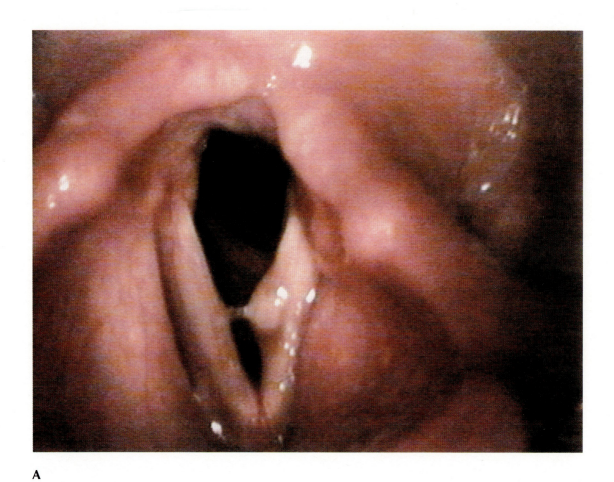

A

PLATE 4.28: **A.** Left vocal fold cyst with asymmetrical vocal process. Tele-videoscopy.

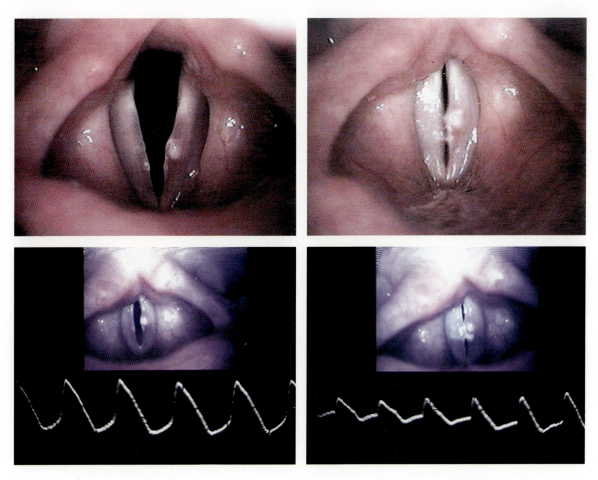

B. Left vocal fold cyst (epidermoid cyst):

1	2
3	4

1. During breathing.
2. During phonation.
3. During stroboscopy with EGG: low pitch, open phase is increased.
4. Stroboscopy with EGG: high pitch, open phase is increased.

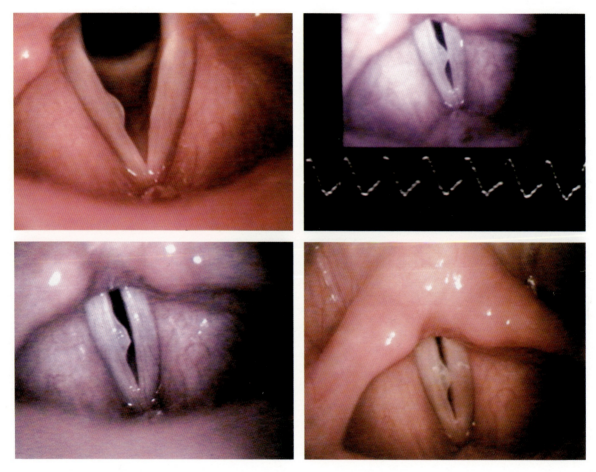

A

PLATE 4.29: A. Cyst of the right fold. Tele-videoscopy.

1	2
3	4

1. During breathing. No secondary lesion is visible.
2. During stroboscopy with EGG: Vibrations are regular, as the EGG display shows.
3–4. Stroboscopy shows the perfect isolated cyst.

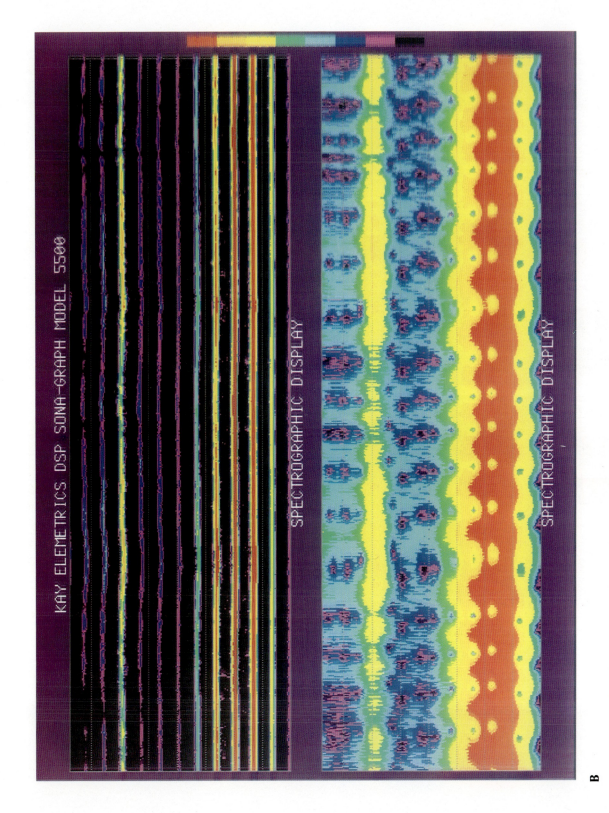

B. Spectrography of an intracordal cyst: Almost normal, as suggested by the EGG.

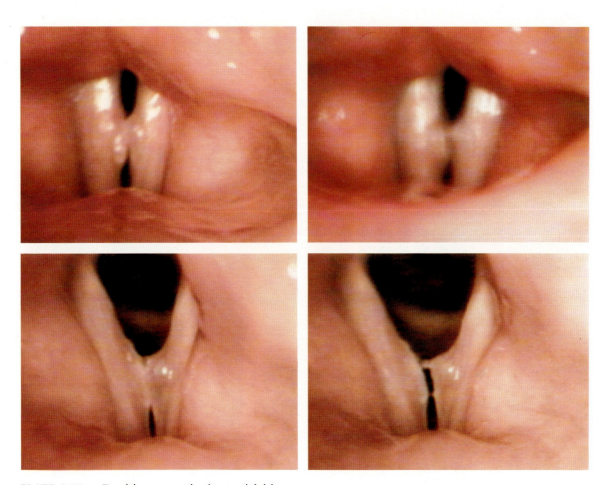

PLATE 4.30: Double cyst on both vocal folds.

Laryngeal Pathologies: CYSTS

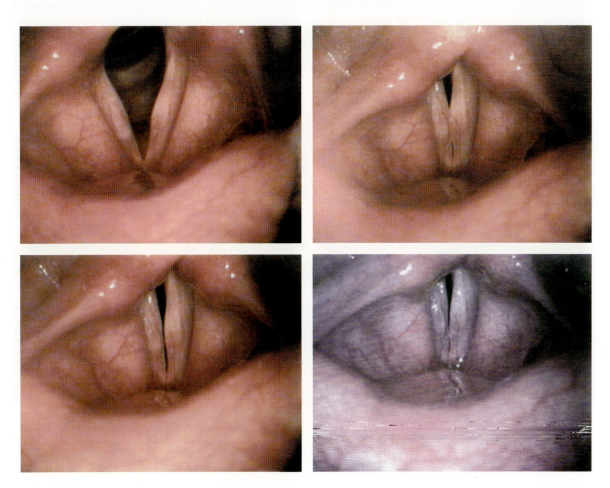

A

PLATE 4.31: A. Bilateral cyst of the vocal folds.

1	2
3	4

1. During breathing,
2, 3, and 4. During stroboscopy: posterior chink.

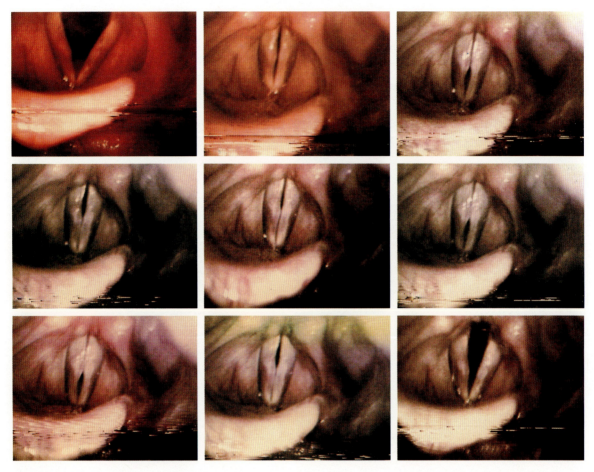

B

B. Bilateral cyst. Same case as Plate 4.31A.

1	2	3
4	5	6
7	8	9

1. Breathing phase.
2. Beginning of stroboscopy: Vibrations are particular: the mechanical properties of the vibratory mass show two different kinds of movements, separated by the cyst: anterior and posterior vibrations.
3. Anterior free edges are open.
   Posterior are closed.
4. Posterior are open.
   Anterior are closed.
5. Vice versa.
6, 7, and 8. Vibratory cycles go again and again, divided in two parts.
9. End of phonation

These signs are specific and characteristic of bilateral intracordal cysts.

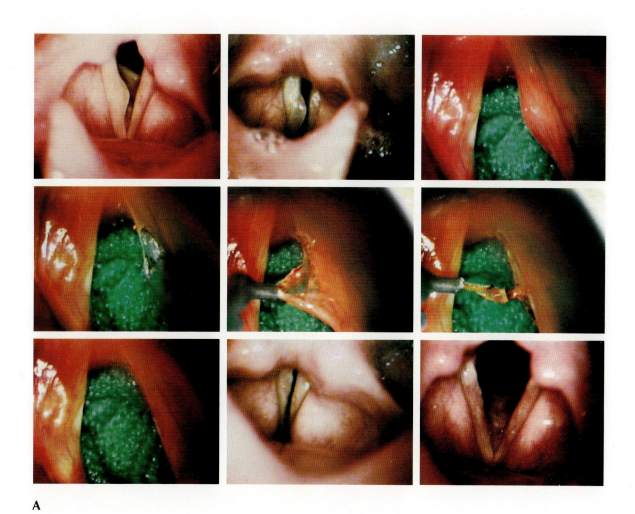

A

PLATE 4.32: **A.** Cyst of the right vocal fold.

1	2	3
4	5	6
7	8	9

1. Cyst as seen in tele-videoscopy during breathing.
2. During phonation.
3. Laser microsurgery. Exposure of the larynx.
4. Aperture of the cyst with the laser microspot.
5. The A-forceps grasps the surface of the cyst and the epithelium and pulls it toward the glottic space.
6. Last laser impact: microspot, 1.5 watts.
7. Perfect glottal anatomy is restored.
8. Tele-videoscopy during phonation, 10 days after surgery.
9. During breathing, 10 days after surgery.

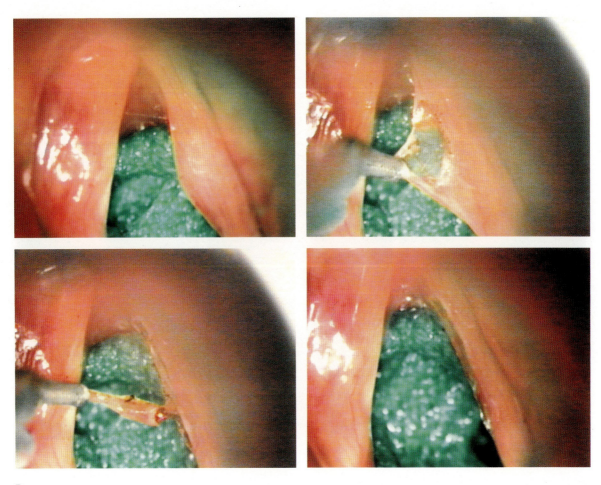

B

B. A closer look at the cyst of the right vocal fold and the technique for removing the epithelium.

1	2
3	4

1. Exposure of the larynx.
2. Laser impact.
3. Removal of the cyst with the epithelium.
4. End of procedure (icy cottonoid cleans the excision bed).

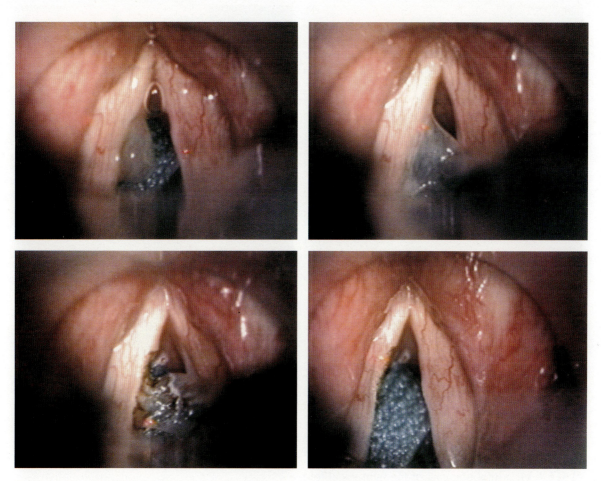

PLATE 4.33: Mucoid cyst: laser microsurgery showing technique for removing the epithelium.

1	2
3	4

1. Larynx exposure: mucoid cyst of the left vocal fold originating from the entire free edge (superior and inferior lips).
2. The triangle-shaped A-forceps grasps the cyst.
3. Impact of a classic laser spot (7 watts, continuous mode).
4. End of procedure.

Atlas of Laser Voice Surgery

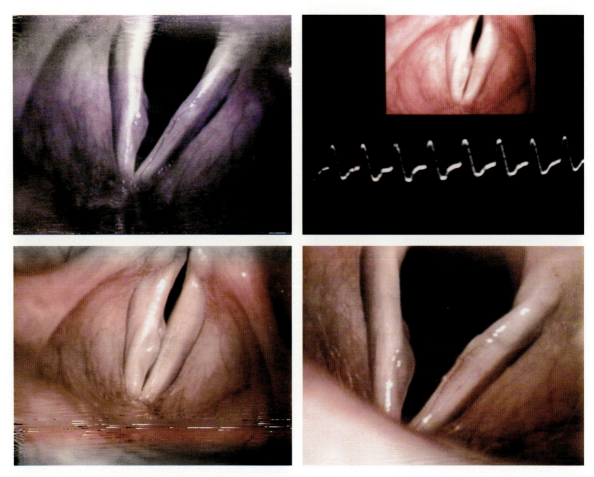

PLATE 4.34: Bilobular cyst of the right vocal fold.

1	2
3	4

1. During breathing, we observe a bilobular cyst of the right side, a micro-varix parallel to the free edge of the left side of the vocal fold.
2. During phonation with EGG: closure phase is increased.
3. During phonation: a posterior chink is seen.
4. Closure during breathing shows a small edema on the left side.

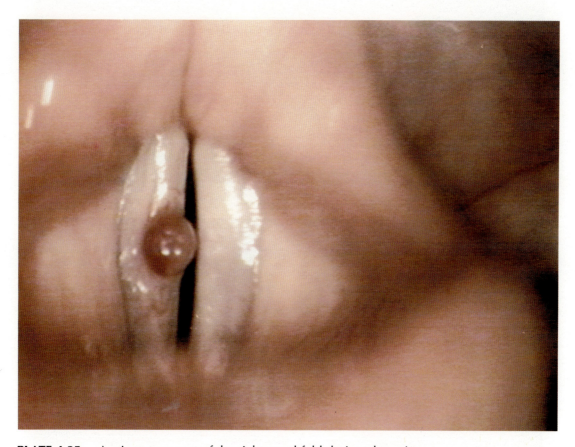

PLATE 4.35: Angiomatous cyst of the right vocal fold during phonation.

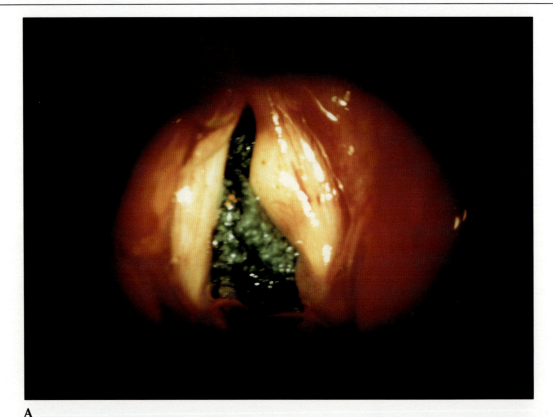

A

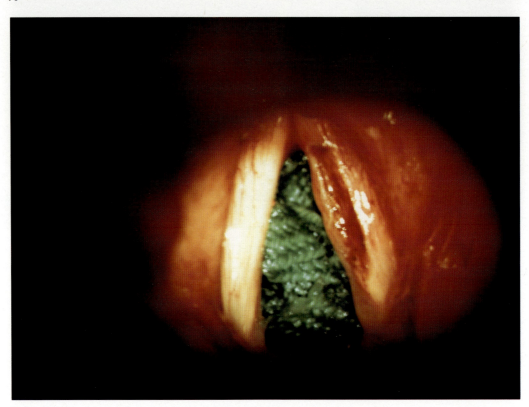

B

PLATE 4.36: **A.** Exposure of the cyst. **B.** An incision is performed from front to back to open the Reinke's space and to remove the cyst without removing the epithelium. The sac is removed during procedure.

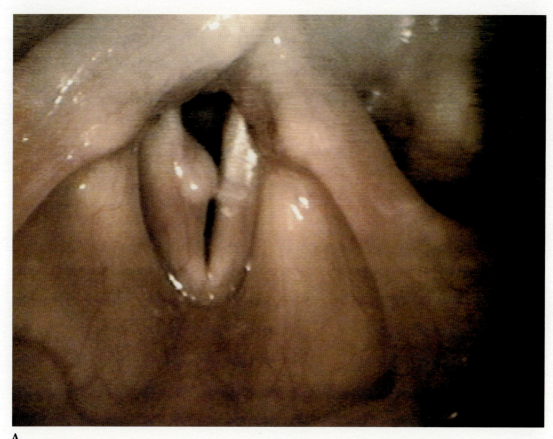

A
PLATE 4.37: **A.** Cyst of the right vocal fold located deep under the epithelium.

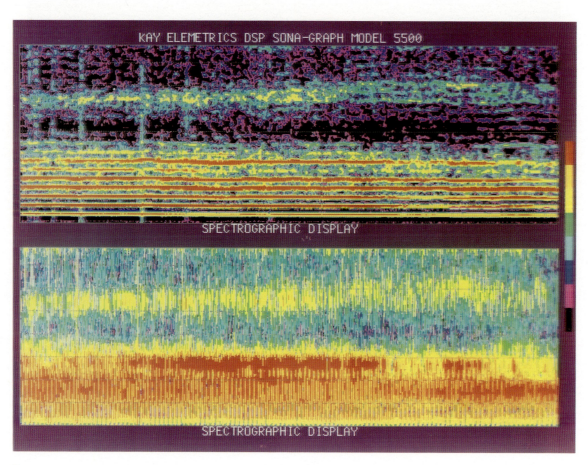

B

B. Spectrography: noise is very increased. Harmonics are just visible for the 7 first levels.

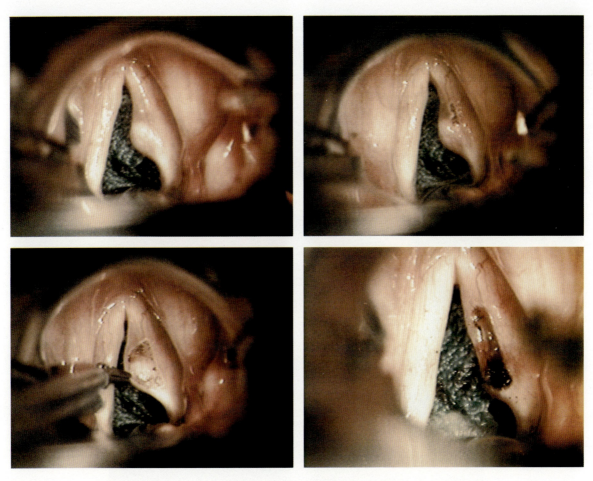

C

C. Cyst removal without removing the epithelium.

1	2
3	4

1. Before surgery: intracordal cyst on the right side.
2. Impact with the CO_2 Laser, using the microspot: Power 1.5 watts, spot size 120 microns opening the superior face of the epithelium near the cyst.
3. An A-forceps grasps the superior face of the epithelium. The flap is maintained to remove the cyst without removing the epithelium.
4. After laser surgery, the bed of the cyst is cured, and the cyst is removed with the sac. The flap is intact.

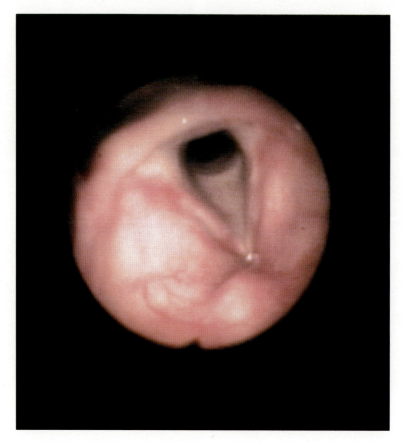

D

D. Results shown by tele-video-endoscopy 6 weeks after laser surgery.

Laryngeal Pathologies: CYSTS

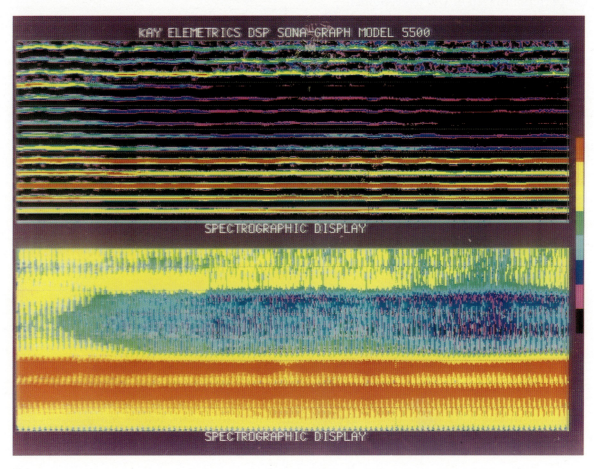

E

E. Spectrography 6 weeks after surgery. Noise has disappeared, and signal-to-noise ratio is normal. Harmonics are almost normal.

GRANULOMAS

A. Definition

Granulomas are benign lesions induced by healing granulomatous tissue secondarily epithelialized. They develop after microtrauma of the microperichondrium of the arytenoids.

We can distinguish two different types of granuloma:

1. Direct trauma: intubation
2. Indirect trauma: reflux, vocal attack with voice abuse, coughing or sneezing.

B. Location

Granulomas are almost always found on the posterior third of the vocal process. Unilateral or bilateral, they often are asymmetric.

C. Etiology and Histopathogeny

1. Etiology

Most of the time, granulomas are a complication of surgery under general anesthesia with intubation. They generally occur after trauma to the vocal process during intubation or extubation.

They may also occur after prolonged intubation. The contact of the vocal process and the endotracheal tube may provoke a bilateral granuloma. Contact ulcers are asymmetrical, bilateral, found more commonly in males, and may be due to vocal abuse.

They are routinely associated with reflux.

2. Pathogenesis

The mucoperichondrium of the arytenoid is first traumatized, causing significant reaction of the epithelium. The denuded vocal process will heal improperly by creating a granulomatous tissue with its own epithelium.

Duration and intubation technique, reflux, and coughing during and after intubation may induce or increase the frequency of granulomas.

Tracheotomy can be proposed if a long period of endotracheal intubation is needed to avoid vocal process pathology such as granulomas, ankylosis, and tracheomalacia.

3. Macroscopic Aspect

Granulomas consist of mono- or multilobulated, opalescent masses, with a yellow color in long-standing granulomas and a reddish aspect if recent. The surface can be ulcerated. In the early stage, the granuloma is located on the superior surface of the vocal process. In advanced stages, it reaches the superior and inferior surfaces of the vocal process, and during phonation, it grasps the edges of the opposite sides.

4. Histology

Granulomas are composed primarily of well-vascularized bud granulation tissue, which includes fibroblasts, collagenous fibers, leukocysts, lymphocytes, and capillaries. Usually, the cover is eroded by a specific squamous epithelium, with a fibrino-hemorrhagic exsudate. This cover may be keratinized.

D. Clinical Approach

1. Primary Symptoms

- ☐ Patients complain of sore throat, a feeling of foreign body in the throat, swallowing irritations, and—rarely—dysphonia.
- ☐ Small granulomas may remain unknown by the patient and be diagnosed for other purposes.
- ☐ They are usually related to reflux laryngitis.
- ☐ Voluminous granulomas can induce breathiness, hoarseness, or pharyngeal and cervical pains.

2. Tele-Video-Naso-Fiberscope and Telescope

The vocal exploration with videoscopy shows:

a. During breathing:

- A precise location of the granuloma, almost exclusively on the arytenoid
- Fixed or mobile with respiratory movements

b. During phonation:

- The granuloma is rarely seen hidden in the posterior commissure.
- Rarely, when it is voluminous, it may disturb the glottic closure which is incomplete.

c. However, granulomas may occur elsewhere on the vocal folds.
In this case, it is always after vocal fold surgery.

3. Stroboscopy

The mechanical properties of the vocal vibratory mass remain intact.

Vocal fold vibrations are normal except on the posterior third with a voluminous mass.

4. Electroglottography (EGG)

EGG waves are normal because vibrations of the contact area of the vocal folds are intact.

5. Spectrography

No characteristic signs can be described except with large or bilateral granulomas in which the range is narrow with a low intensity and an increased noise parameter.

E. Conclusion

Resection of granulomas is indicated if:

- They are large.
- They disturb breathing.
- They look suspicious.
- After 6 months of therapy (antacids, voice therapy) it still disturbs voice and/or it is painful.
- After surgical resection, recurrence is not rare. However, spontaneous resolution has been observed.

Laryngeal Pathologies: GRANULOMAS

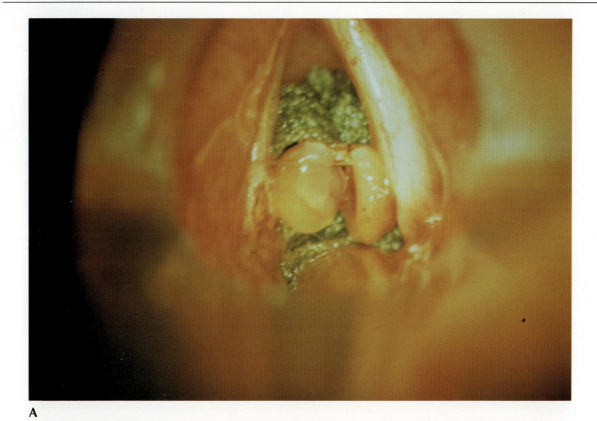

A

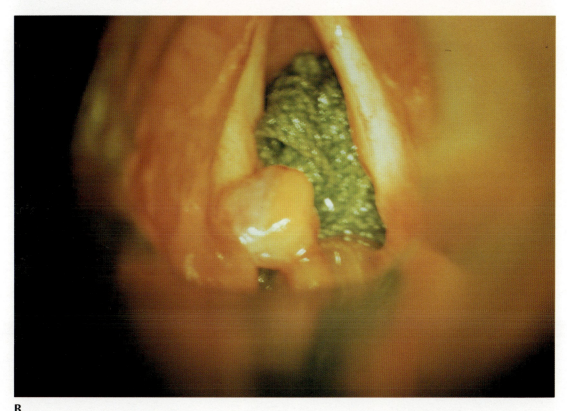

B

PLATE 4.38: **A.** Bilateral granulomas: voluminous and mobile. Ablation from back to front: 7 watts. **B.** During surgery, the right side of the granuloma is removed. Ablation of the left side granuloma. 7 watts. Continuous fire for both.

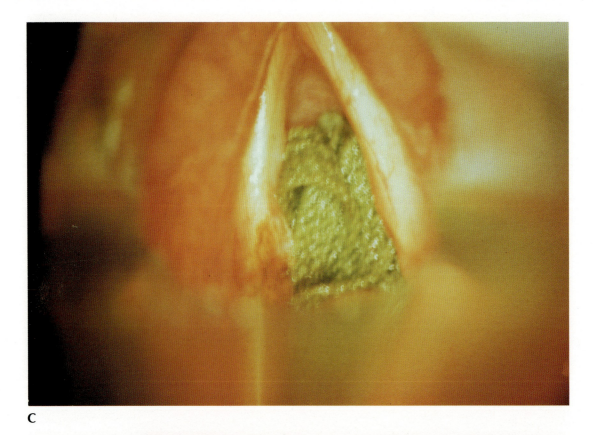

C

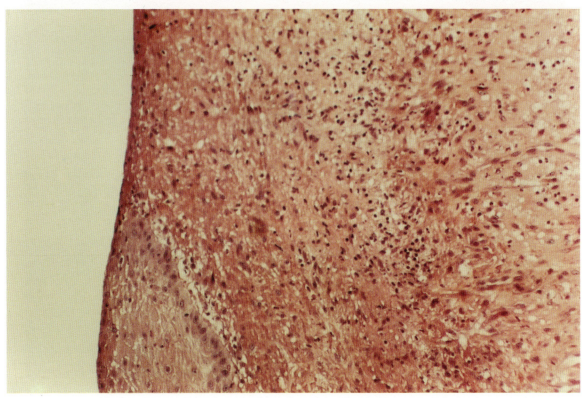

D

C. Immediate postoperative result. **D.** Histology of the granuloma.

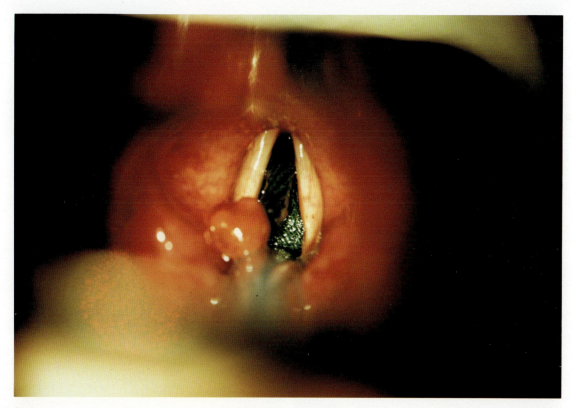

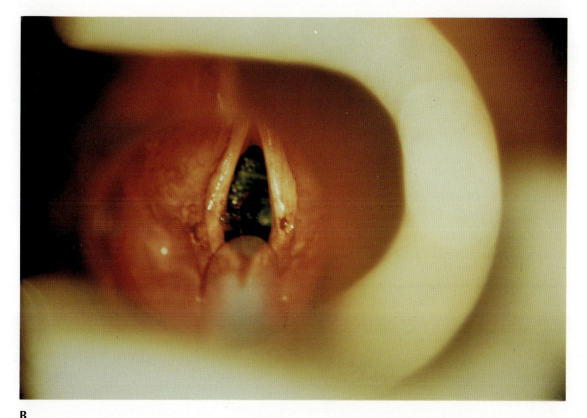

PLATE 4.39: **A.** Post-intubation granuloma. Early stage (reddish). **B.** 7 watts. Continuous fire. Immediate postoperative result.

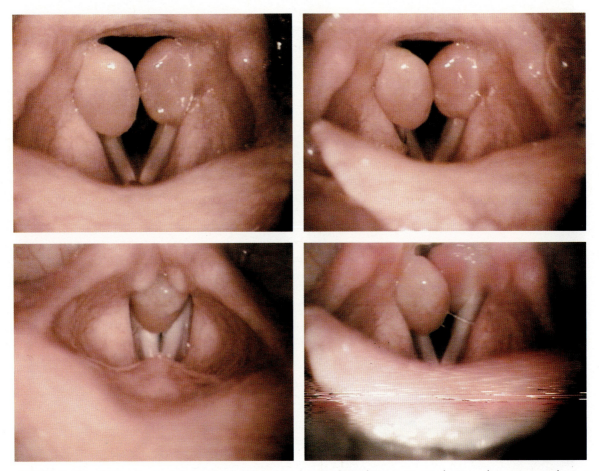

PLATE 4.40: Voluminous bilateral granuloma inducing breathiness (top); during phonation inducing hoarseness (bottom). Tele-videoscopy.

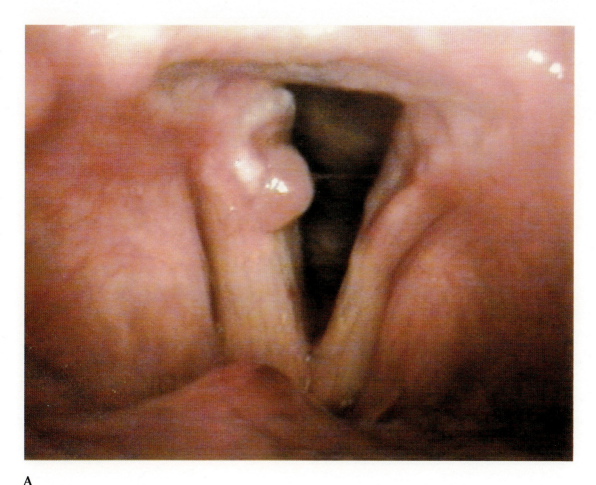

PLATE 4.41: **A.** Unilateral granuloma: right side. Tele-videoscopy.

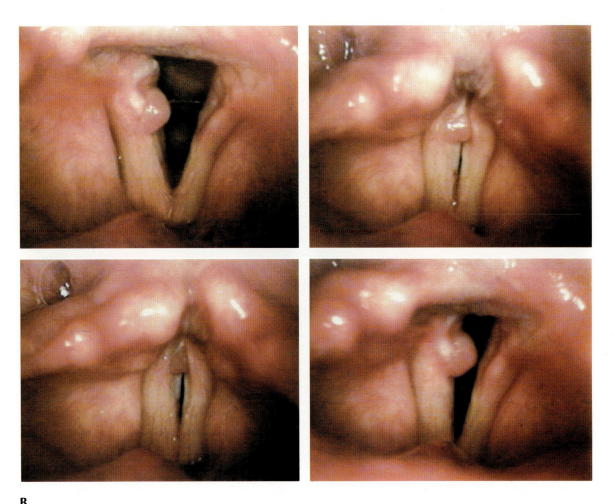

B. During phonation, note the imprint of the granuloma on the opposite side. Tele-videoscopy.

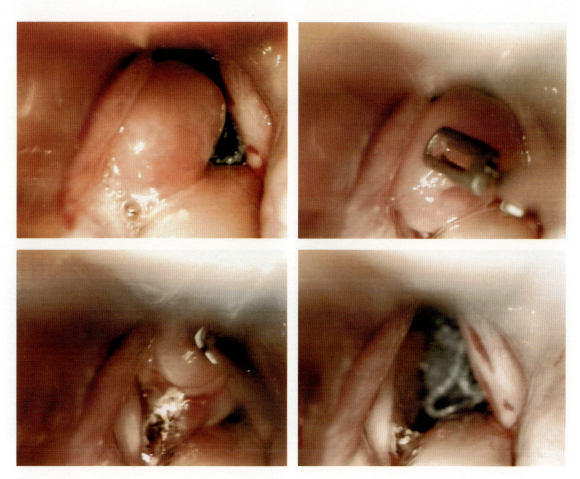

PLATE 4.42: Enormous granuloma of the left vocal fold, showing four steps of laser surgery.

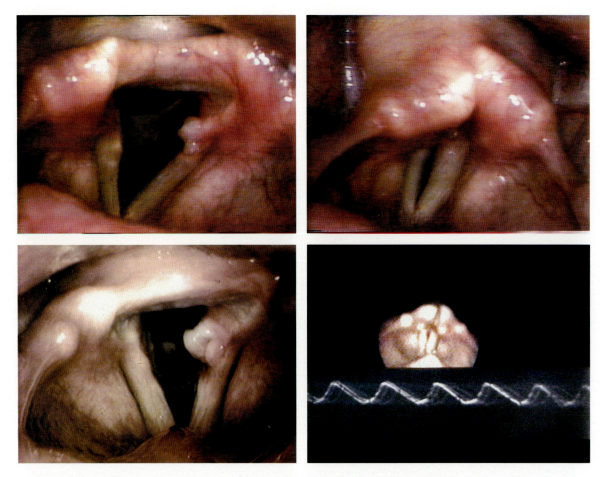

PLATE 4.43: Flat granuloma with an ulcer on the left vocal fold. Tele-videoscopy.

1. During breathing.
2. During phonation, the granuloma is hidden.
3. During breathing.
4. During phonation with EGG.

PAPILLOMAS

A. Definition

- Papillomas are benign lesions that originate from the epithelium, usually involving the lamina propria with a mulberry- or cauliflower-like surface. They may look broad-based, sessile, polypoid, or flat. They appear in both children and adults. They are characterized by an exophitic proliferation of collagenous fibers and squamous cells.

- The difference between juvenile-onset multiple papilloma and adult-onset solitary papilloma depends on their clinical behavior.

- Juvenile papillomas appear in male and female children.

- Papillomas of the adult type usually begin at the age of 20 years. Men are more often affected than women.

B. Location

The glottis is the primary site for papillomatosis. The lesion may occur unilaterally or bilaterally and may spread to the ventricles, subglottic area, and susglottic area.

C. Etiology and Histopathogeny

1. Etiology

Causes are not well understood. Human papilloma viruses (HPVs) 11 and 6 seem to have a role in their development (Abitbol, Mathae, & Battista, 1988).

2. Pathogenesis

The pathogenesis and etiology of laryngeal papillomatosis is beginning to be understood. It looks like co-factors act to prepare the flore of papillomas. Mechanical, infectious, hormonal, genetic, and nutritional factors are involved.

Many studies in the research of co-factors involve carcinomas and papillomas (refer to the section on Carcinoma). Specific elements for papillomas are keratinocyte metabolism in which deficiencies of vitamins A and C, beta carotene, and vitamin E are involved.

Some authors consider immunodeficiency and fungus infection to be the bed of HPV infection. An antigenic relationship to human papilloma viruses can be demonstrated in more than 80% of cases.

3. Macroscopic Aspect

Papillomas appear villous to verrucous.

Papillomas consist of multifocal and confluent lesions in grape-like clusters. They look pink or reddish, rarely white or translucent. Each lobule has a dilated capillary in its center which explains why to "touch it is to make it bleed."

Laser is the best surgical tool for removal of this lesion.

4. Histology

Typically, papillomas are made of folds and crypts.

Papillomas originate from the squamous epithelium. They invade the lamina propria but usually spare the muscles. It is a proliferation of epithelial cells growing in papillary shape. The stroma, rich in fibers, is often inflamed.

Extension is diffuse or multifocal. In adults, papillomas usually are hyperkeratotic.

Papillomas are covered by a multilayered cuboidal epithelium, with large round dark nuclei. An experienced pathologist is needed to analyze samples of papillomas in which mitoses can look like carcinomas.

The basement membrane zone remains intact. Capillary ectasias are often visible at the tips of the papillae.

Malignant transformation occasionally occurs.

D. Clinical Approach

1. Primary Symptoms

Hoarseness is the main symptom in adults, and airway obstruction in children.

2. Tele-Video-Naso-Fiberscope and Telescope

This exploration helps the surgeon determine where the papillomas are located. Most often, it is on the vocal fold, but we must look carefully during breathing and phonation, on low and high pitch, the anterior commissure, the ventricles, and the posterior commissure, mainly the arytenoid epithelium, for evidence of papillomatosis.

This information will help the anesthetist prepare his intubation. A print from the videotape of the vocal fold process is necessary to avoid traumatic intubation and/or laryngoscopy.

3. Stroboscopy

Multilobulated lesions, like papillomas, give a still vibratory mass. The mechanical properties are affected. Vibratory waves and amplitude are disturbed on both sides even if the papilloma is only on one side.

During phonation, closure is incomplete, vibrations are asymmetrical, and the stiffness and the cover are increased.

4. Electroglottography (EGG)

Irregular waveform with no characteristic signs is observed.

5. Spectrography

Harmonics and formants are disturbed with a narrow register, few harmonics, and high levels of noise.

E. Conclusion

Papillomas appear and disappear, in our current stage of knowledge, without significant scientific reasons.

Several therapies have been provided: surgical removal by Harmer in 1903, electrocoagulation in 1968 by Kleinsasser, and podophyllin in 1950 by Hollingsworth. Cryotherapy was used by Andrews, Moss, and Holigerin in 1974. CO_2 laser surgery seems to be the most appropriate tool today.

Laser phonosurgery by microlaryngoscopy must be performed each time it is necessary but:

☐ No bleeding must occur. Icy cottonoid (as many as necessary) must be used to cool the papilloma's bed during the procedure.

☐ Very gentle removal must be done in the glottic space

☐ Only *decortication* is the correct technique to avoid carbonization of the vocal ligament. As a matter of fact, the thermic effect is necessary to avoid bleeding, but needs to be used carefully to avoid burns.

The goal is to remove papillomas without touching the vocal ligament.

It is in the compromise between cutting effect and thermic effect where the experience of the surgeon is important. It is not an easy surgery.

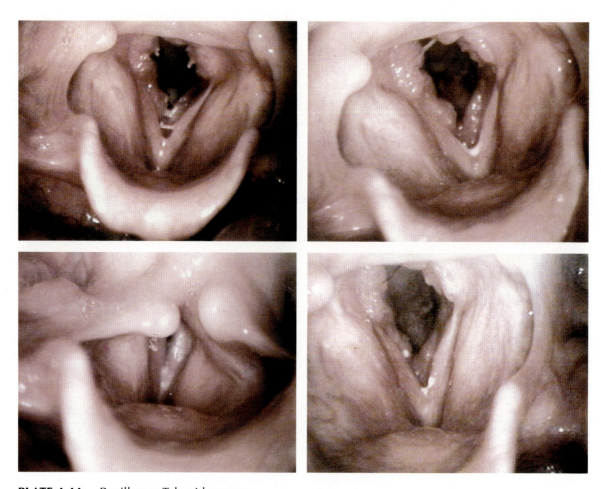

PLATE 4.44: Papilloma: Tele-videoscopy

1	2
3	4

1, 2, and 4. During breathing: papilloma of the inferior lip of the free edge of both vocal folds, of the subglottic anterior commissure, and of the posterior commissure.

3. During phonation: papillomas are not seen.

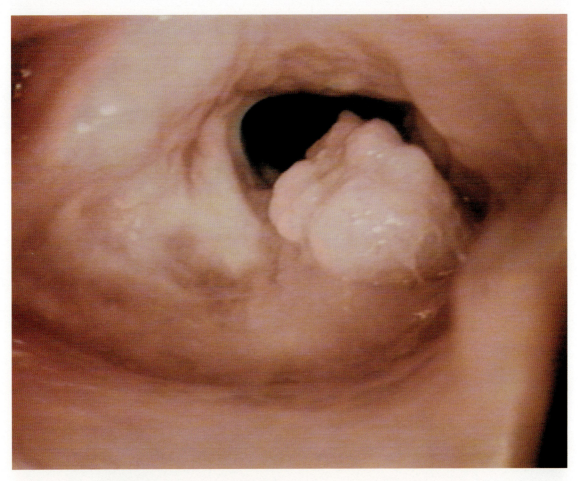

PLATE 4.45: Papilloma of the laryngeal border of the epiglottis. Tele-videoscopy: Papillomas are located on the epiglottis. We also observe a partial laryngeal stenosis.

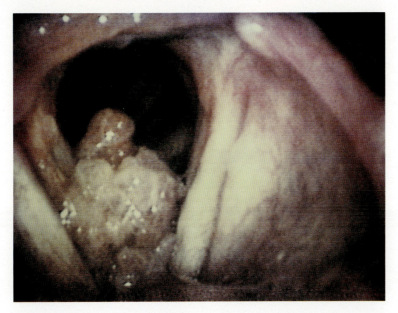

PLATE 4.46: Exophitic papilloma of both vocal folds and anterior commissure. Tele-videoscopy.

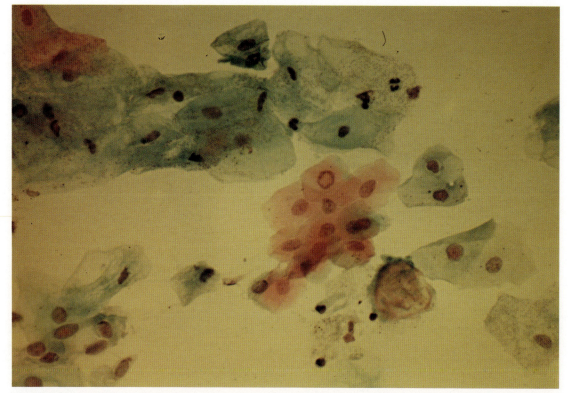

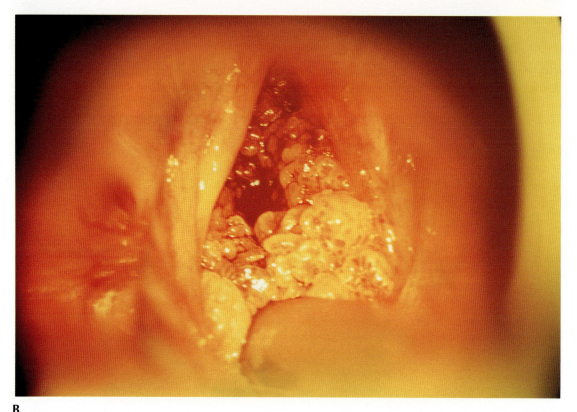

PLATE 4.47: **A.** Papilloma: smear test. Koilocytes can be seen. **B.** Papilloma: laser microsurgical procedure. Larynx exposure. Voluminous papilloma.

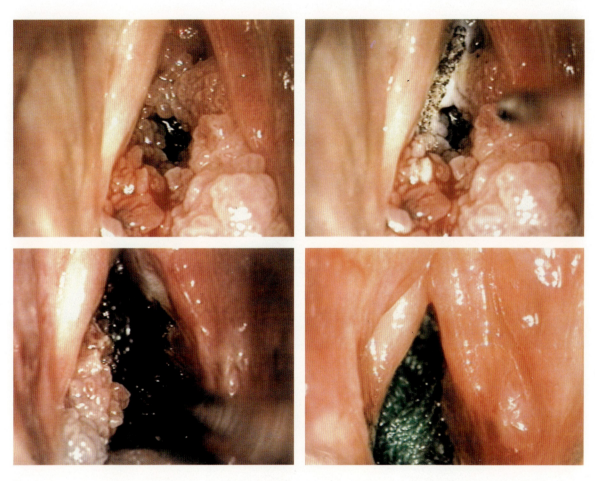

C

C. Laser microsurgery for an obstructing papilloma.

1	2
3	4

1. Larynx exposure.
2. Laser impact from front to back (10 watts, spot size of 300 microns, continuous fire).
3. Removal of the papilloma on the posterior commissure.
4. The integrity of the glottis is restored with no bleeding.

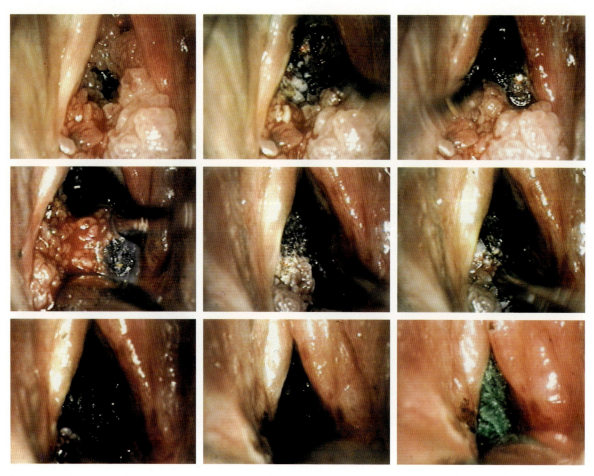

D. Closer look at the same patient in Plates A–C showing nine steps of the laser surgery.

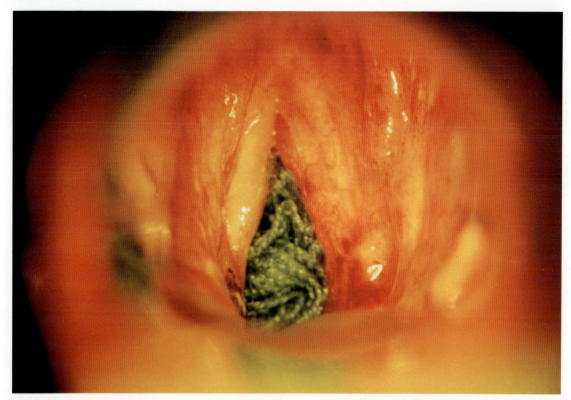

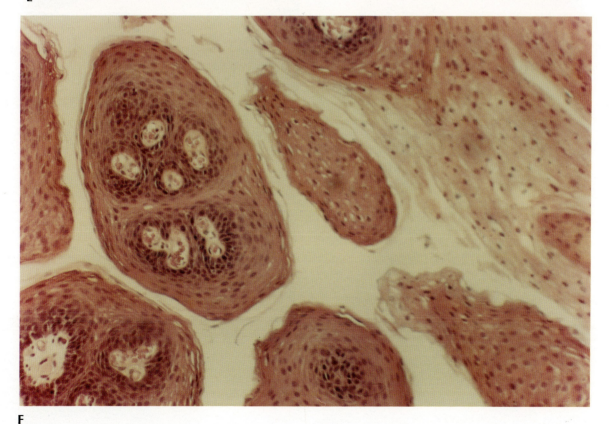

E. Same case after surgery: 7 watts, continuous fire. The glottal anatomy is restored, the vocal ligament remains intact. **F.** Histology of papillomas.

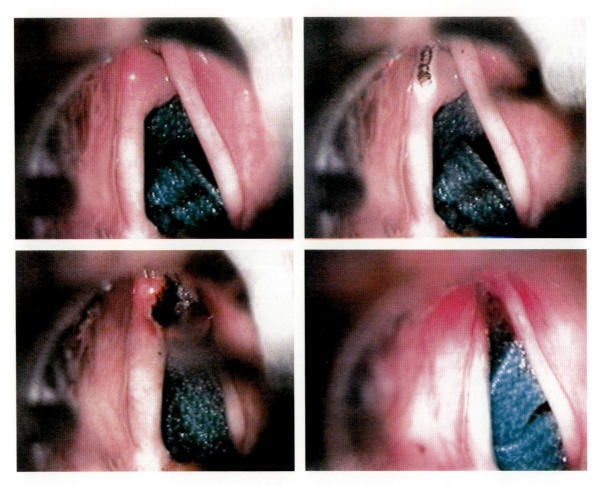

PLATE 4.48: Papilloma of the left vocal fold. Laser microsurgical procedure.

1	2
3	4

1. Exposure of the larynx: Papilloma of the anterior part of the left vocal fold.
2-3. Laser impact of 10 watts, continuous fire. It is a decortication, not a vaporization in situ.
4. End of the procedure. The glottal anatomy is restored.

Laryngeal Pathologies: PAPILLOMAS

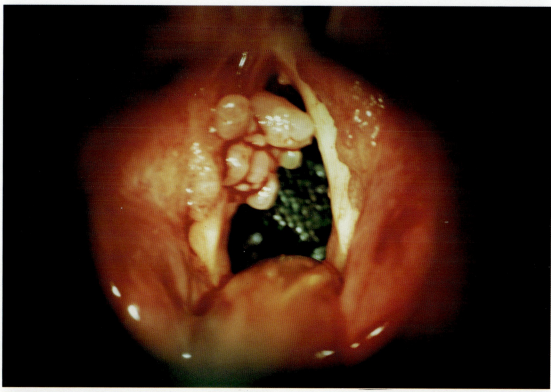

PLATE 4.49: Exophitic papilloma of the left vocal fold and flat papilloma of both ventricles. Laser microsurgery (power: 8 watts, normal spot size).

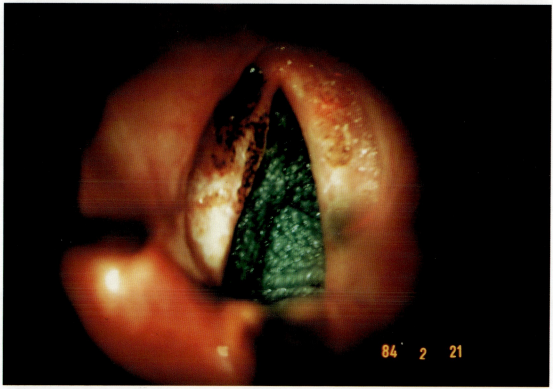

PLATE 4.50: End of surgical procedure shown in Plate 4.49. Papilloma was removed, the vocal ligament remains intact.

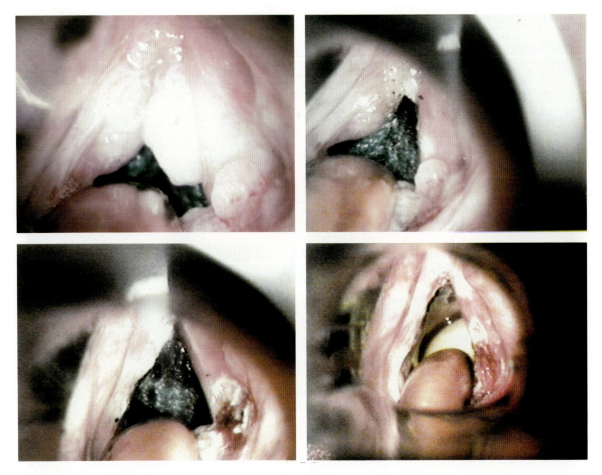

PLATE 4.51: Papilloma of both vocal folds and posterior commissure. Laser microsurgery.

1	2
3	4

1. Larynx exposure: it must be done very carefully to avoid bleeding.
2. Right vocal fold is performed by our "decortication technique" (power: 8 watts, continuous mode, normal spot size).
3. Papilloma of the left vocal fold is removed, then of the posterior commissure.
4. End of procedure.

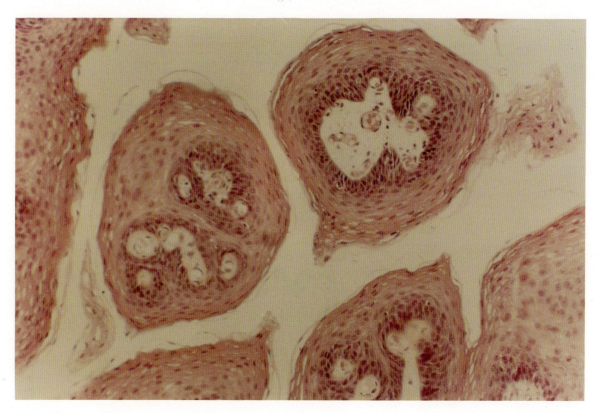

PLATE 4.52: Histology of papilloma shown in Plate 4.49.

Atlas of Laser Voice Surgery

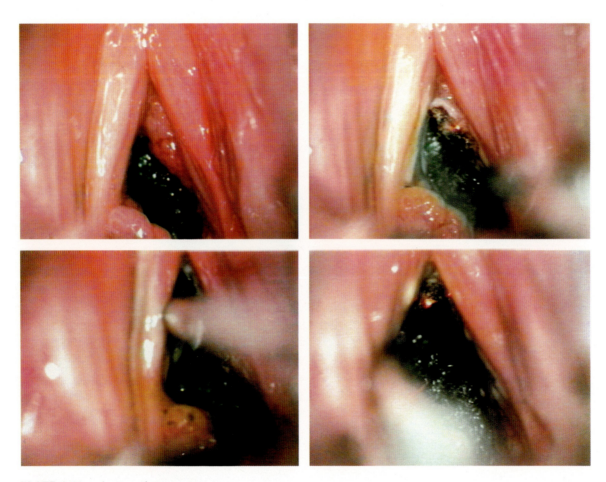

PLATE 4.53: Laser microsurgery:

1	2
3	4

1. Larynx exposure: papilloma of the left lower lip of the posterior commissure and the right lower lip of the vocal fold.
2. Removal of the papilloma: 10 watts, 300 micron spot size, continuous fire, bloodless technique.
3. Removal of the posterior papilloma.
4. End of surgical procedure.

VASCULAR PATHOLOGY

A. Definition

- Capillary ectasia is a varicose dilation of the capillaries of the vocal fold. It is manifested by small dilated vessels. It is a relatively common finding in women.

- Hemangiomas are the most frequent benign tumors of the larynx. Lymphangiomas are rare. They have the same pathogenesis as capillary ectasia. Uni-or bilateral, they are easy to diagnose.

- Hemorrhage of the vocal fold is mostly due to a submucous hemorrhage, involving the entire length of the vocal fold, and due to the rupture of a submucous varix, rarely a muscle hematoma.

B. Location

Vascular lesions are most often located on the superior surface of the vocal folds and close to the free edge. Fifty percent affect one vocal fold only; the other half affect both folds. Small dilated vessels run parallel to the free margin and often end with an angiomatous cluster of variable size.

C. Etiology and Histopathogeny

1. Etiology

Most of our patients with capillary ectasia are female professional singers, and were subjected to considerable vocal strain and hormonal problems.

Hemangiomas are more frequently found in adults than in children.

2. Pathogenesis

The state of filling of the dilated capillaries varies with the demands on the voice, because vocal disorders often appear only after a long period of singing.

Before or during menstruation, if a patient suddenly becomes aphonic, due to a submucous hemorrhage arising from the rupture of a varix, singing is impossible.

3. Macroscopic Aspect

Five different types of vascular lesions of the vocal fold can be observed:

a. Vascular dilatation arising from a thickened capillary situated on the free edge or the superior face of the vocal fold.

b. Several unusual tortuous and irregular ectatic vessels.

c. A combination of hemorrhagic nodules and varices of the vocal fold.

d. Hemangioma presents as a purplish red, telangiectasic, firm, multilobular mass with a sessile or pediculate implantation. In infants, it is subglottic and infiltrating, smooth, compressive, and associated in 50% of cases with skin or visceral lesions.

e. Large submucous hemorrhage.

Capillary ectasia may be associated with other intracordal lesions. It is very important to distinguish an isolated vascular lesion from an ectasia associated with underlying cysts and sulcus vocalis. Videostroboscopy is essential in distinguishing the two.

4. Histology

- Hemangioma: there is a normal epithelium. In the submucosa, large, endothelium-lined lacunae containing blood are present.

- Biopsies cannot be obtained adjacent to the hemangiomas because vessels are vaporized during laser surgery.

D. Clinical Approach

1. Primary Symptoms

- Simple capillary ectasia usually does not have an important effect on the voice because of its location on the superior surface of the vocal fold.

- Large capillary ectasia and hemangioma may alter vocal fold vibration and may modify the timbre of the voice.

The problem can arise after a single incident of excessive voice use, and resolve spontaneously, but, in most cases, it begins insidiously. Patients may complain of voice fatigue due to secondary vasomotor phenomena that occur with prolonged voice use. In this case, surgery is indicated, because of the discomfort experienced by the patient, particularly if he or she is a singer, and also to avoid a hemorrhagic accident that could ruin a career.

2. Tele-Video-Naso-Fiberscope and Telescope

These examinations can easily show the lesion on the superior surface of the vocal fold: small dilated vessels, thickened capillaries, unusual tortuous and irregular ectatic vessels, and large submucosal hemorrhage.

On the other hand, it can be a small angioma, a red, telangiectasic, firm multi-lobulated mass whose implantation is sessile or pediculate or has an infiltrating aspect.

The lesion may also have the appearance of a nodule or a hemorrhagic polyp.

3. Stroboscopy

Stroboscopy will enhance the anatomical aspect. After 2 or 3 minutes of voice production, signs are more obvious, vascular lesions will have increased. An intracordal cyst, however, must be searched for.

4. Electroglottography (EGG)

Irregular patterns have been recorded.

5. Spectrography

Loss of harmonics and intensity are recorded.

E. Conclusion

Operations should not be performed during the acute phase of bleeding into the vocal fold but should be delayed until the blood has been resorbed and the capillary ectasia is clearly visible.

Aspirin avoidance should be prescribed for these patients.

- It is important to inspect the vocal fold carefully to determine any zone of induration that may indicate an intracordal lesion visible by stroboscopy.

- The operation consists of a series of superficial laser vaporizations at several sites along the length of the dilated vessel without touching the free edge of the vocal fold. Most of the lesions are on the superior surface or, rarely, on the upper lip of the free edge of the vocal fold.

After a few weeks, the voice improves. Phoniatric rehabilitation with voice therapy is performed in the pre- and post-operative period.

- We have noticed few recurrences in our patients

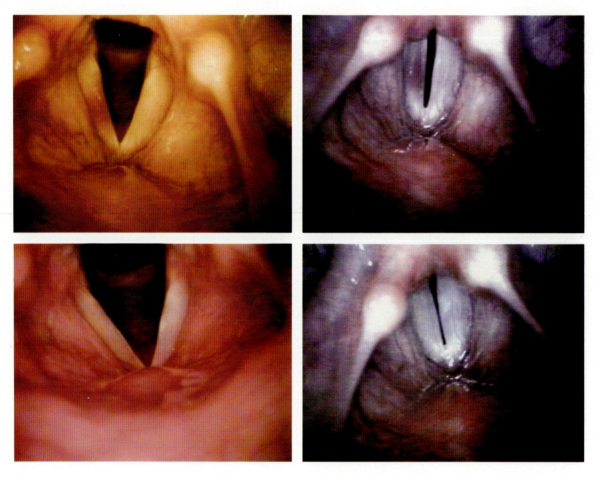

A

PLATE 4.54: **A.** Submucous hemorrhage of the right vocal fold, 1 day before menstruation and follow-up after menstruation (Tele-videoscopy).

1	2
3	4

1. Breathing phase, 1 day before menstruation.
2. Phonation phase, 1 day before menstruation.
3. Breathing phase: 10 days after menstruation.
4. Phonation phase: 10 days after menstruation.

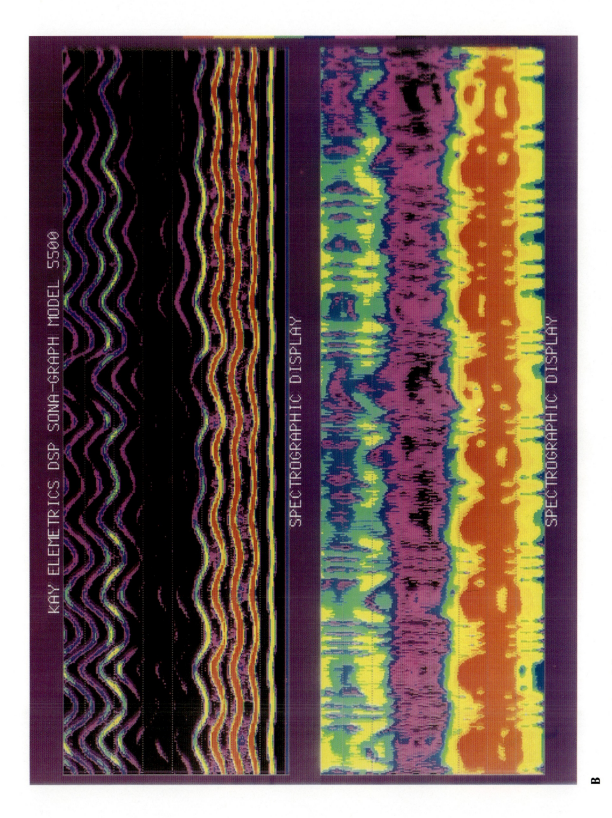

B. Spectrography of the same patient, a 37-year-old mezzo soprano, 10 days after menstruation.

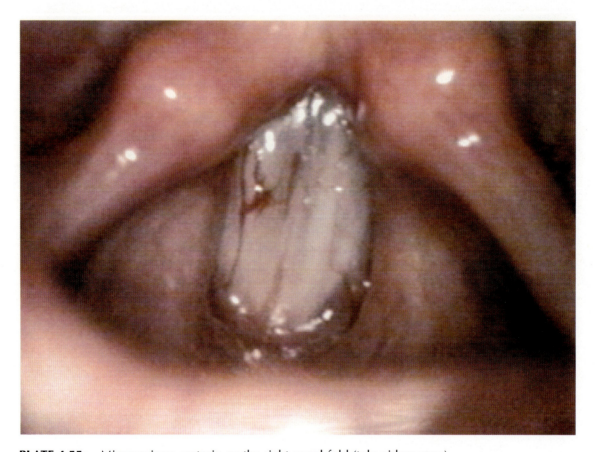

PLATE 4.55: Microvarices: ecstasia on the right vocal fold (tele-videoscopy).

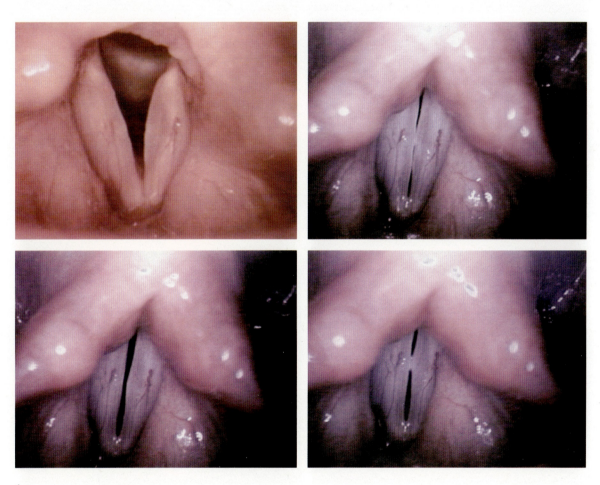

A

PLATE 4.56: Microvarices and edema during menstruation. Tele-videoscopy.

1. Breathing phase.
2–4. Stroboscopy: irregular vibrations and asymmetry.

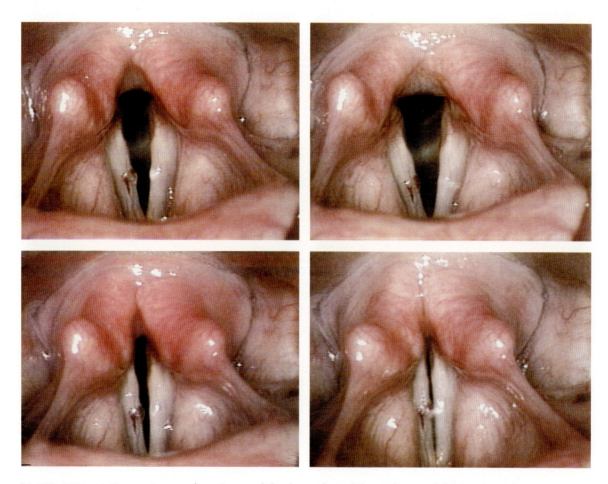

PLATE 4.57: Microvarices and angioma of the free edge of the right vocal fold. Tele-videoscopy.

1	2
3	4

1. During breathing.
2. During breathing after coughing: no more mucus, no secondary lesions.
3–4. Stroboscopy.

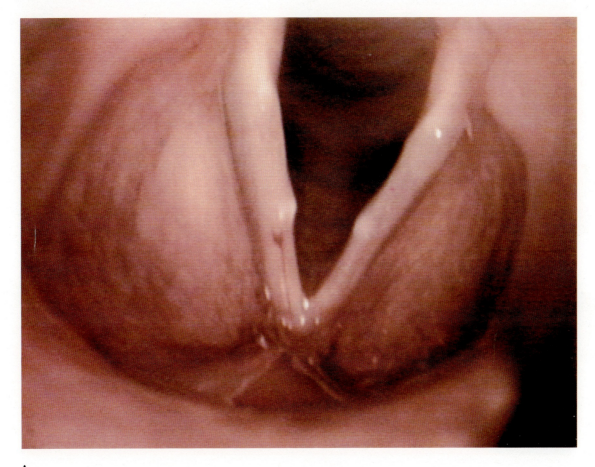

A

PLATE 4.58: **A.** Microvarix and ecstasia on the right vocal fold with soft nodules. Tele-videoscopy during breathing in a popular female singer before menstruation.

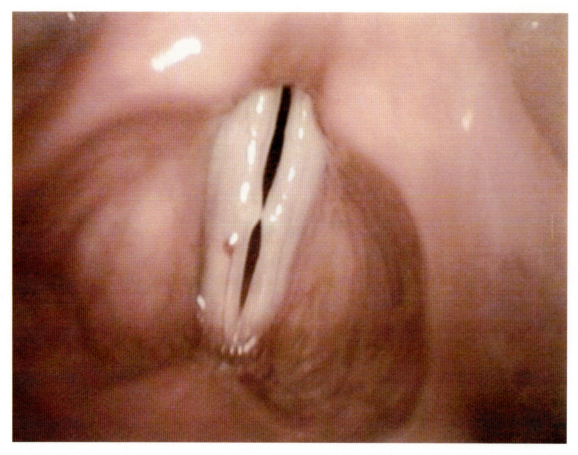

B

B. Case in **A** during phonation. **C.** Spectrography of the same popular female singer: almost normal.

Laryngeal Pathologies: VASCULAR PATHOLOGY

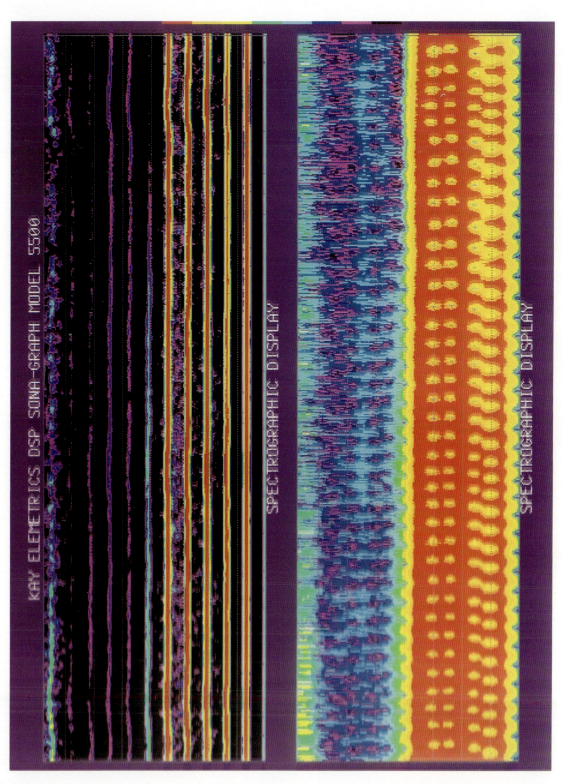

C

231

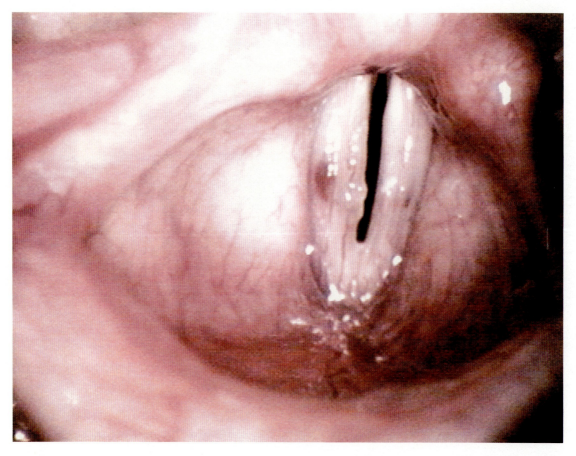

A

PLATE 4.59. **A.** Microvarices and angioma of the right vocal fold, edema of the free edge of the vocal fold: tele-videoscopy during stroboscopy. **B.** Stroboscopy with EGG.

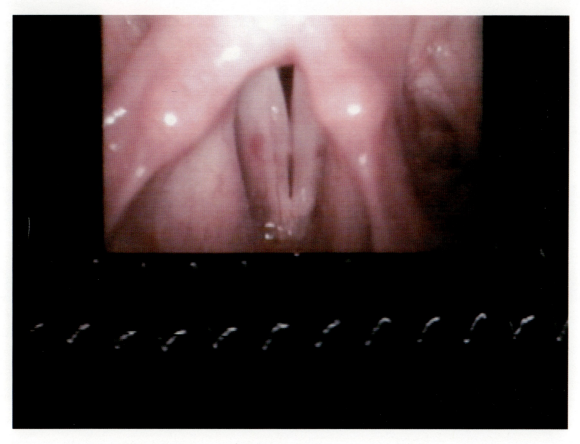
B

Atlas of Laser Voice Surgery

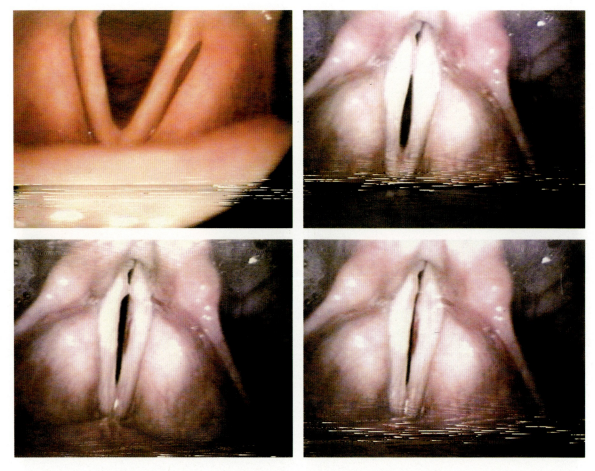

A

PLATE 4.60: **A.** Micro-hemorrhage of the free edge of the left vocal fold. Tele-videoscopy showing the importance of stroboscopy.

1	2
3	4

1. During breathing: no hemorrhage can be seen.
2. During phonation: no hemorrhage can be seen.
3–4. Stroboscopic phases: micro-hemorrhage can be seen of the free edge of the left vocal fold.

Laryngeal Pathologies: VASCULAR PATHOLOGY

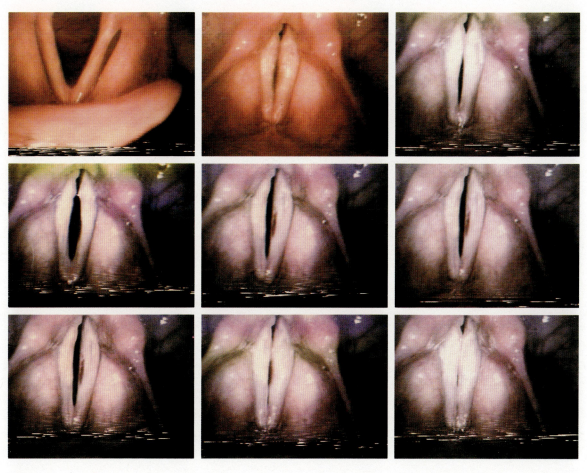

B

1	2	3
4	5	6
7	8	9

B. Micro-hemorrhage of the free edge of the left vocal fold. Nine different steps can be seen: we have to look closely at the free edge to detect such micro-hemorrhages.

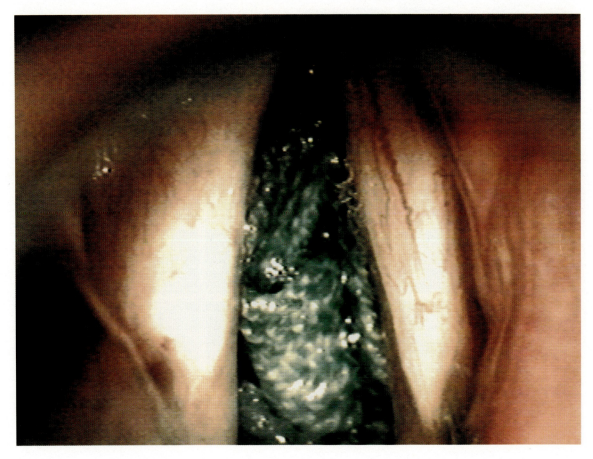

A

PLATE 4.61: **A.** Laser microsurgery: exposure of the larynx. Microvarix and telangiectasia on the right vocal fold. (It was performed 6 months after a hemorrhage.) **B.** Vaporization of the vascular pathology (4 watts, discontinuous fire, 0.1 sec., normal spot size).

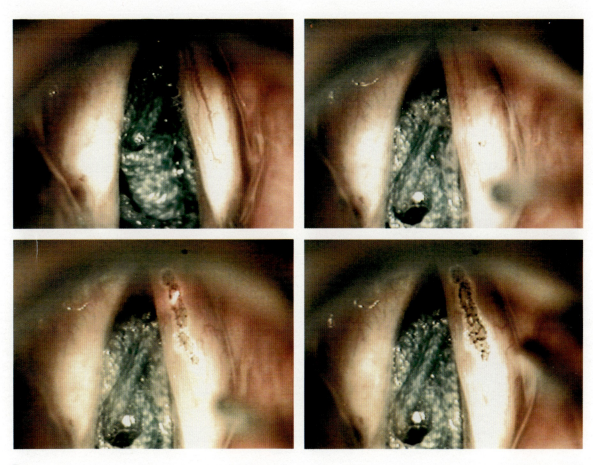

B

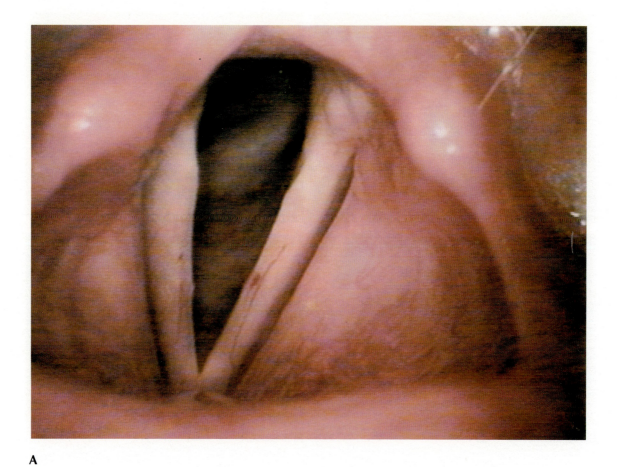

A

PLATE 4.62: **A.** Microvarices and capillary ectasia. Tele-videoscopy during breathing.

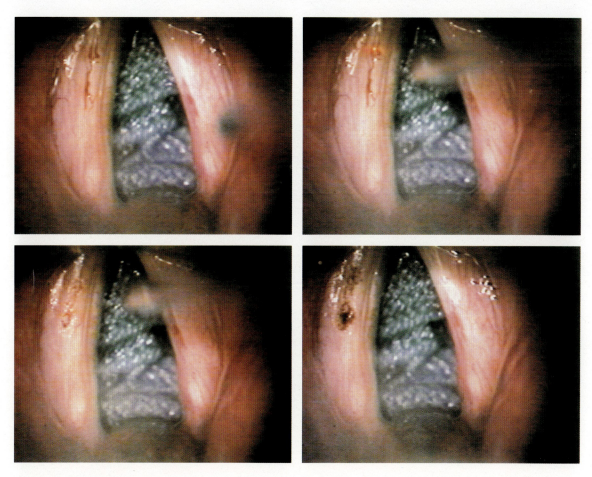

B

B. Laser microsurgery procedure

1	2
3	4

1. Exposure of the larynx
2. Laser vaporization: 4 Watts, 0.1 sec, discontinuous, normal spot size.
3. Fire on the left vocal fold.
4. End of procedure.

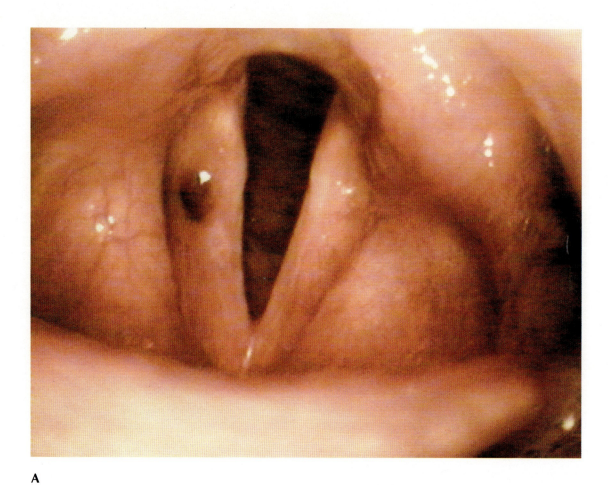

A

PLATE 4.63: **A.** Angioma of the superior surface of the right vocal fold (tele-videoscopy during breathing).

Laryngeal Pathologies: VASCULAR PATHOLOGY

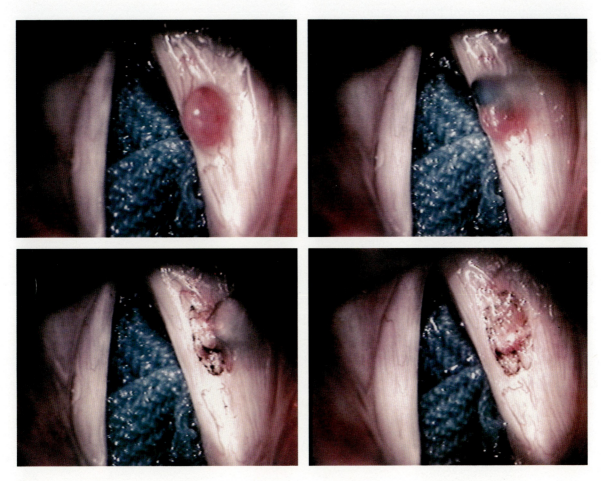

B

B. Laser microsurgery procedure:

1	2
3	4

1. Larynx exposure.
2. Suction nearby the angioma, without touching it.
3. Laser impact, then a microforceps grasps the angioma (7 watts, 300 micron spot size, discontinuous fire).
4. End of procedure. Bloodless.

VOCAL FOLD HEMORRHAGE

A. Definition

It is a submucosal hemorrhage.

B. Location

It is located in the lamina propria, under the epithelium, usually in the middle third of the vocal fold, and it spreads first to the anterior and posterior third of the fold and later to the subglottic area.

C. Etiology and Histopathogeny

1. Etiology

Submucosal vocal fold hemorrhage results from vocal abuse, rarely from intubation.

2. Pathogenesis

Most often it is a rupture of the capillaries (varices). It often appears during premenstrual syndrome.

D. Clinical Approach

1. Primary Symptoms

Hoarseness and voice fatigue are the main symptoms. Generally it is not possible to sing.

2. Tele-Video-Naso-Fiberscope and Telescope

Hemorrhage is observed on the superior surface of the vocal fold located under the epithelium.

3. Stroboscopy

Vibrations are decreased and asymmetrical on the side of the hemorrhage, or vibrations may be absent.

4. Electroglottography (EGG)

Waves are flat and aperiodic, amplitude is decreased.

5. *Spectrography*

- Decreased range with few harmonics and a very narrow register; formants are poor.
- Intensity is low

E. Conclusion

Most patients, after medical treatment, recover totally. Voice rest for 10 days is necessary. Three weeks are needed to restore normal vibration. (See Plate 4.65).

Some patients have sequelae varicose vessels which may be vaporized by laser.

Rarely, hemorrhage persists with enlarged, varicose vessels. These cases, however, need evacuation of the hematoma for satisfactory recovery. Patients are operated on by laser phonosurgery. An incision is made on the upper surface of the vocal fold. A power of 7 watts is used with continuous mode, or a 1.5 watt power with the microspot. The vocal fold is humidified before laser with an iced gauze. The suction will evacuate the hematoma. The mucosal flap is not removed even if it looks bigger than it should be. A total voice rest of 8 days is prescribed after the surgery. Voice recovery takes 4 weeks.

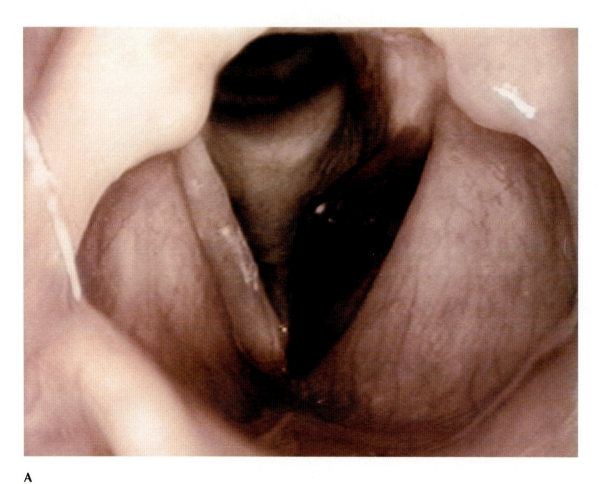

A

PLATE 4.64: **A.** Hematoma of the left vocal fold after hemorrhage (5 weeks of follow-up).

Laryngeal Pathologies: VOCAL FOLD HEMORRHAGE

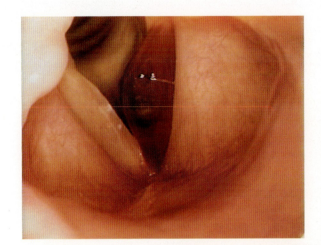
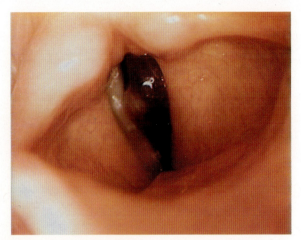
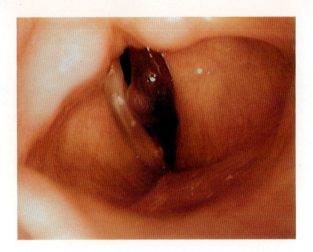

B. A closer look at case in **A** (Tele-videoscopy).

1	2
	3

1. During breathing.
2–3. During stroboscopy.

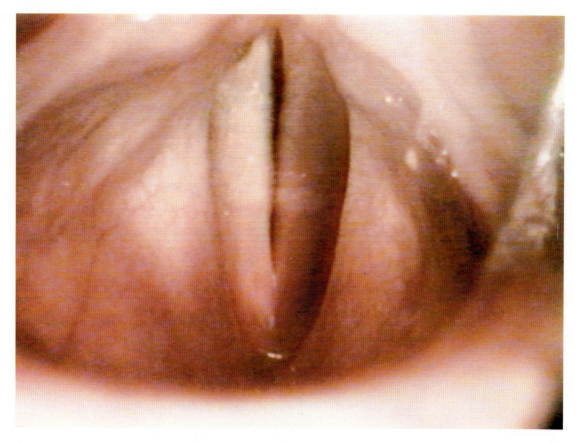

A

PLATE 4.65: **A.** Hemorrhage of the left vocal fold during phonation. Tele-videoscopy. **B.** Same case after medical treatment.

Laryngeal Pathologies: VOCAL FOLD HEMORRHAGE

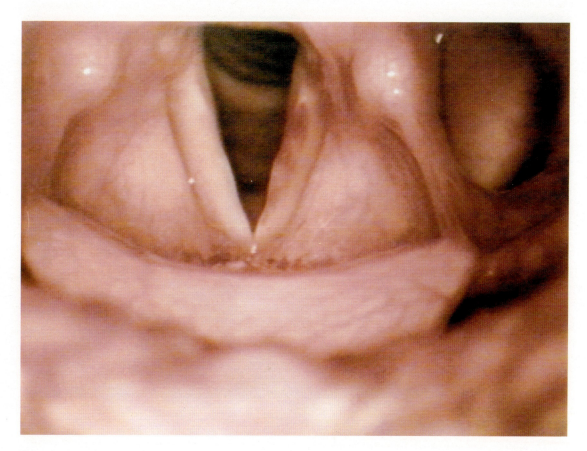

B

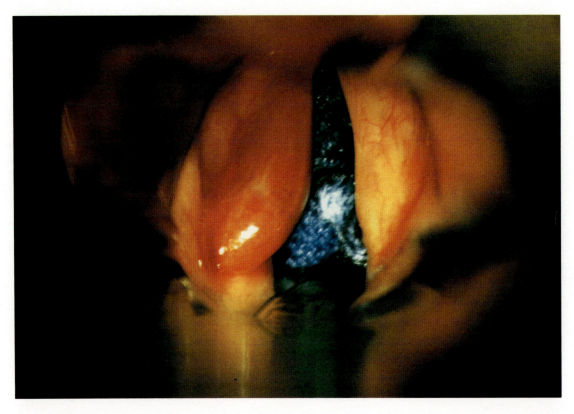

A

PLATE 4.66: **A.** Laser microsurgery procedure: Larynx exposure. **B.** After laser surgery: 7 watts, continuous mode. It is a difficult surgery: the vocal ligament must be avoided.

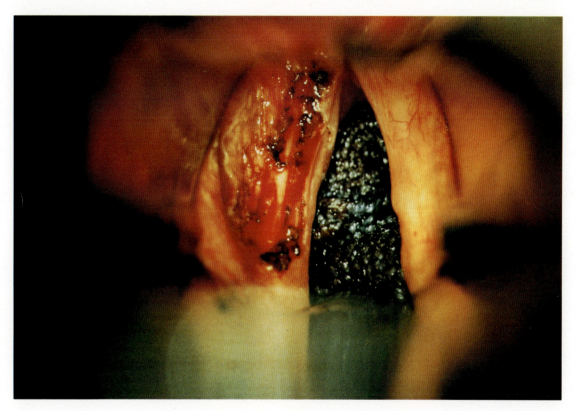
B

REINKE'S EDEMA

A. Definition

Reinke's edema, a particular and very frequent form of chronic laryngitis, which is better known as "laryngité d'aspect myxoedemateux ou pseudomyxome" in the French literature, and as corditis or polypoid degeneration in English. It refers to the build-up of fluid in the first layer of lamina propria of the vocal fold.

B. Location

The edema that characterizes Reinke's edema occurs in the submucosal lining of Reinke's space, which is between the epithelium and the vocal muscle. Most often bilateral and asymmetrical, it is mostly observed on the superior surface of the vocal fold and in the ventricle.

C. Etiology and Histopathogeny

1. Etiology

Edema is a natural reaction of tissue to trauma, pollution, and misuse of the voice. The etiology is unknown, but in addition to vocal abuse, Reinke's edema is most often associated with tobacco use (98%). Chronic diseases of the nose and sinus appear to play a role. It occurs much more frequently in females, especially if they are smokers.

2. Pathogenesis

Reinke's edema may disturb the elasticity of the cover layer, resulting in decreased stiffness and increased vocal mass. Such a reduction in stiffness would allow for greater amplitudes of vibration.

3. Macroscopic Aspect

Even though the endoscopic appearance of Reinke's edema may appear as an edematous polyp extending along the whole length of the vocal fold, in fact, it is not! It separates the vocal ligament and the superficial layer of the epithelium which is thickened. The surface is smooth and the mucosa will appear translucent with a clearly visible capillary network or, on the contrary, the mucosa may be red and angiomatous. The edema is soft and, when laser incised, yields a characteristic yellowish or gelatinous fluid.

The micro-laryngoscopic appearance is very characteristic: both vocal folds are almost always affected, but often to different degrees. The early stage consists of a spindle-shaped swelling of the vocal fold extending from the anterior commissure to the apex of the vocal process. Later, capillaries and thick swelling appear.

4. Histology

Histologic examination reveals a gelatinous fluid in a fine honeycombed network beneath a normal vocal fold's squamous epithelium. In the early stages, the secretion is clear and relatively thin, but in more long-standing cases, the secretion is viscous, yellowish, macroscopically very close to that of a glue ear.

Edema affects the superficial layer of the lamina propria. The mass of the cover is increased, whereas its stiffness is decreased. The transition layers and body are not affected in Reinke's edema. The increase in bulk and reduction of stiffness would contribute to a lowered fundamental frequency of vibration. We have defined three stages: the first stage, reduced vibration compared to normal; the second stage, fewer vibrations; and the third stage, dyspnea with almost no vibrations.

D. Clinical Approach

1. Primary Symptoms

Reinke's edema produces a lower than normal pitch level with or without hoarseness, with or without shortness of breath. These symptoms depend on the significance and extent of the edema.

2. Tele-Video-Naso-Fiberscope and Telescope

A spindle-shaped swelling edema to a total edema of both vocal folds can be observed.

3. Stroboscopy

Stroboscopy shows abnormal vibrations of the two vocal folds. Vocal mass will modify the symmetrical movement.

4. Electroglottography (EGG)

EGG can be normal or abnormal, depending on the stage of Reinke's edema.

5. Spectrography

Fundamental frequencies are lower than expected for the sex and age of the patient. The mean fundamental frequency can reach 108 Hz for females and 90 Hz for males, (Bennett et al., 1987). Harmonics, formants, and signal-to-noise ratios will depend on the stage of the Reinke's edema.

Acoustic signs show an increased frequency and amplitude perturbation as well as the presence of spectral noise. Closure of vocal folds is incomplete from one-third to two-thirds of the vocal fold. In some cases, the vocal fold is totally closed, and the patient is dyspneic.

E. Clinical Classification of Reinke's Edema

Reinke's edema occurs at the very beginning on the upper surface of the vocal folds, in the ventricle, and will be developed on the upper lip, and later on the lower lip of the free edge of the vocal fold. It is nearly always the result of alcohol, tobacco, and voice abuse in subjects with strong personalities.

In our experience, we have noticed a wide variability in symptoms. Dynamic Vocal Exploration and macro-optical inspection of Reinke's space edema defines a better approach of the appropriate therapy. We distinguish three stages of evolution to designate subsequent levels of pathology by the appearance of specific patterns that develop:

1. Stage I

- Voice is hoarse in the morning and has to be warmed up. Voice fatigue appears after an hour of speech. Register is lower than normal.
- Respiratory signs: None.
- No movement of the mucosa can be seen during breathing.
- Vocal folds have proper closure during phonation, and a possible posterior chink.
- Stroboscopic exploration shows a symmetrical vibration with the spindle-shaped swelling edema.
- Spectrography: Fundamental frequencies are lower than normal. Harmonics and formants are almost normal. Signal-to-noise ratio is higher than normal.
- **Therapy:** No surgery. Voice therapy and vocal hygiene are instituted.

2. Stage II

- Hoarseness and voice fatigue are present in the morning. Voice remains hoarse throughout the day.
- Respiration signs: None.
- Vocal folds: Movement of mucosa of the free edge can be seen as butterfly wings during breathing.
- Vocal folds have irregular closure with a prominent posterior chink.

- Stroboscopic exploration shows an asymmetric vibration, sometimes absent vibrations on one vocal fold.

- Spectrography: Fundamental frequencies are very low. Fewer harmonics and formants are seen. The signal-to-noise ratio is fairly high.

- **Therapy:** Voice therapy first for 1 year. If no improvement occurs, laser surgery (lifting of the vocal fold) is performed.

3. Stage III

- Hoarseness, low pitch, low intensity, breathiness, and voice fatigue are observed.

- Respiratory signs are observed: Dyspnea occurs during voice production secondary to effort and blockage of the airway.

- Movements of the mucosa during breathing. Glottic space is obstructed.

- Vocal fold closure is inappropriate.

- Stroboscopic examination does not show any normal vibration.

- Spectrography: Fundamental frequency is about 90 Hz. Harmonics and formant show "ghost patterns." Signal-to-noise ratio is uninterpretable.

- **Therapy:** Laser surgery: First step: Lifting of the vocal fold plus removal of the mucosa. Second step: voice therapy.

F. Conclusion

Reinke's edema does not undergo surgery systematically. It is not at all a question of "plastic surgery of the vocal fold shape," but rather which therapy leads to a satisfactory voice for the patient!

1. We have defined three clinical stages:

In Stage I, no surgery must be performed. Speech therapy and lifestyle changes for 1 or 2 years are the procedures to follow.

In Stages II and III, surgery is necessary. Techniques for the removal of Reinke's edema have changed little since MacKenzie, basically calling for avulsion or stripping of all polypoid tissue from the vocal folds. Conventional techniques involve stripping of a single fold at one sitting with a second procedure performed approximately 5 or 6 months thereafter to avoid denuding approximating surfaces at the anterior commissure and, thereby, reduce the likelihood of web formation. With such techniques, mucosa is almost entirely removed from the free edge of the vocal fold, and the waves of the epithelium take a long time to recover.

2. Surgical Procedure

Lifting of the vocal folds by laser surgery, to our knowledge, was first described by us in 1981. CO_2 laser is employed to bloodlessly incise the superior surface of the vocal folds, beginning 1 mm from the edge of the false vocal fold, and stopping 1 mm before the anterior and posterior commissure. Suctioning removes a characteristic yellowish and gelatinous fluid. (With a normal spot size, a power of 10 watts is used, discontinuous fire time of .10 of a second; with a microspot we use a power of 1.5 watts and the same discontinuous fire.) When the glue is removed, a small icy cotton pad saturated with naphtazoline-xylocaine is used to cleanse the excision bed. Once evacuation is complete, an empty epithelial sac remains. Tension is gently applied to the redundant epithelium. This flap is lifted as in face lift. The excess epithelium from the sac is trimmed with the laser by the microspot beam as necessary. The reconstructed layer of epithelium is noted to completely cover the superior surface of the vocal fold and the bed of the ventricle. There is no trauma on the free edge of the vocal fold. It is a "no-touch" surgery that avoids damage to free edge of the vocal fold and the anterior-posterior commissure.

Both sides also may be performed during the same procedure. This technique allows the lateral polypoid surgery without fear of web formation because the region of anterior commissure is not violated. Postoperative healing reveals epthelializations in 10 to 21 days. Voice rest is necessary for 10 days. Video-fiberstrobolaryngoscopy shows perfect objective results of the lifting of the vocal folds—pitch is higher and, on the telephone, ladies are no longer called "Sir."

Recurrence of Reinke's edema is very rare after surgery.

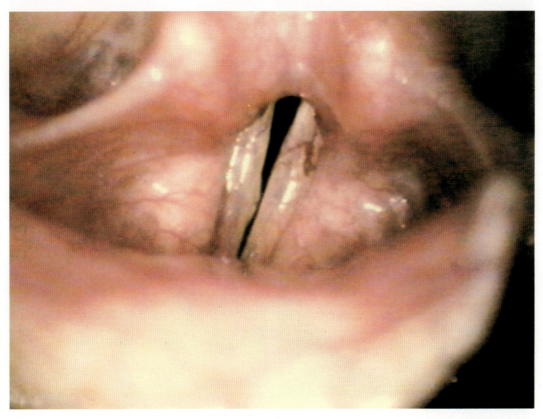

PLATE 4.67: Reinke's edema, stage 1, during phonation. Closure of the vocal folds shows a posterior chink. Tele-videoscopy.

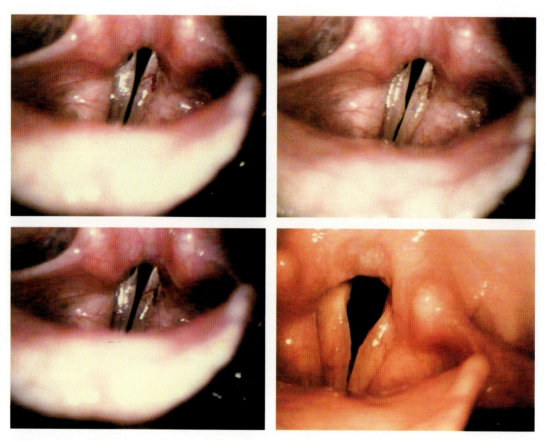

PLATE 4.68: Reinke's edema, stage 1. Tele-videoscopy during stroboscopy.

1	2
3	4

1, 2, and 3. Vibratory mass is slightly stiff, has left amplitude, and vibrations are asymmetrical.

4. During breathing.

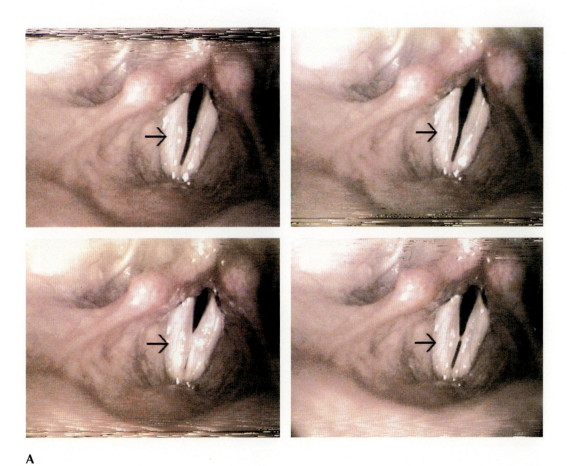

A

PLATE 4.69: **A.** Reinke's edema, stage 1. Tele-videoscopy during stroboscopy: The right vocal fold has fewer vocal waves mucosa than the left. Vibrations are irregular in high pitch. Pianissimo is impossible.

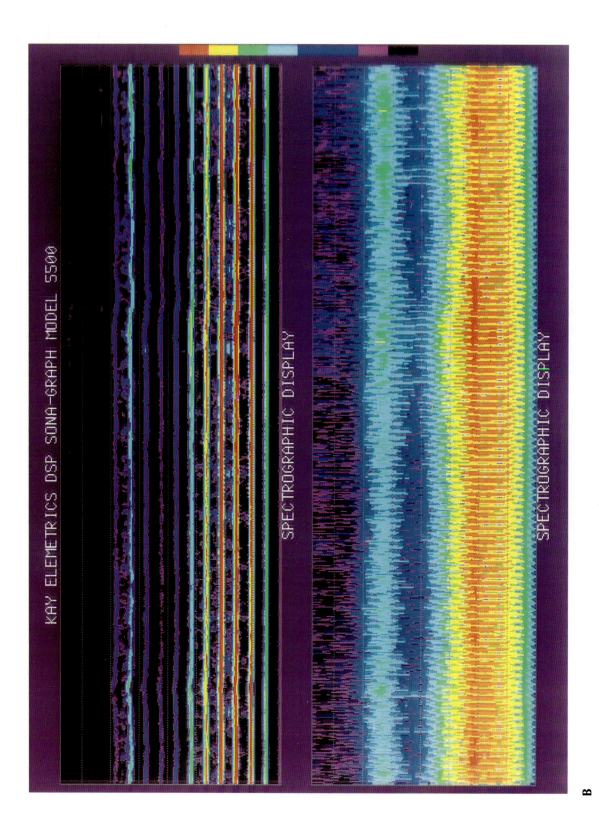

B. Spectrography shows reduced harmonics and formants. Noise level is increased.

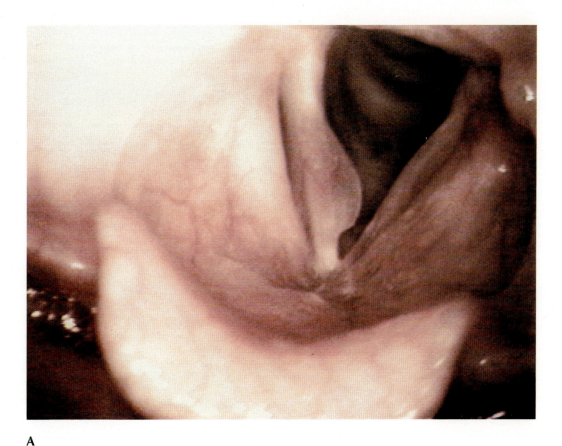

PLATE 4.70: **A.** Fusiform edema: breathing in a case between stages 1 and 2.

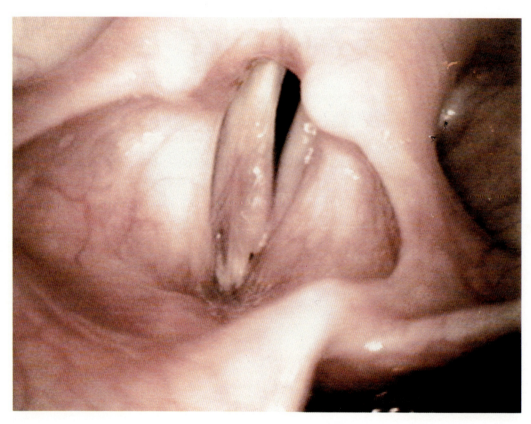

B

B. Phonation in the same case. **C.** Spectrography of case shown in **A** and **B** shows reduced range and few harmonics. Formants remain correct.

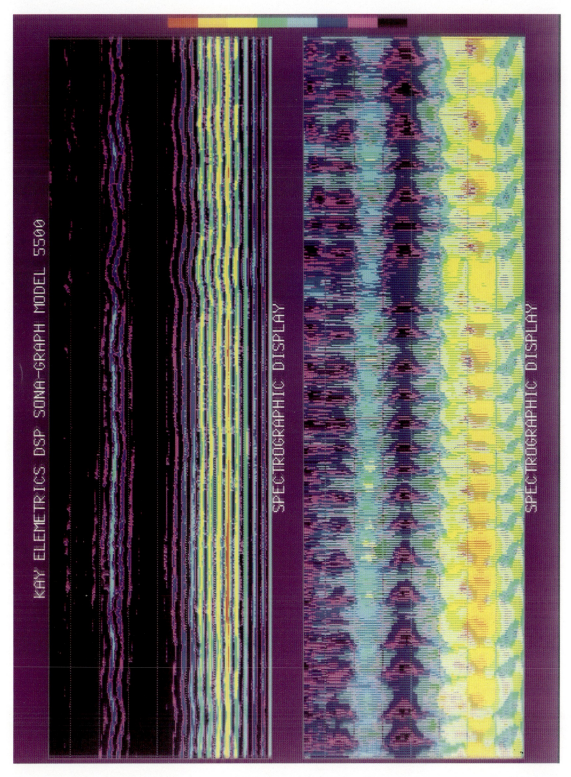

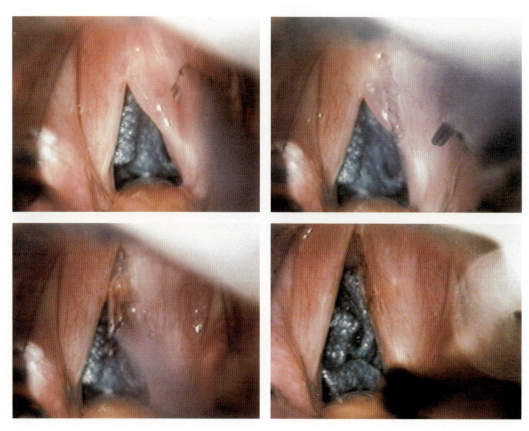

D

D. Laser microsurgery for fusiform edema.

1	2
3	4

1. Exposure of the larynx, visualization of a fusiform edema of the right vocal fold, mobile with the A-forceps.
2. Laser incision from front to back to remove the edema and the mucosa, with the laser, power 7 watts, continuous mode.
3. Removal of the sample: it is totally different from the lifting technique.
4. End of the procedure: the glottal anatomy is restored.

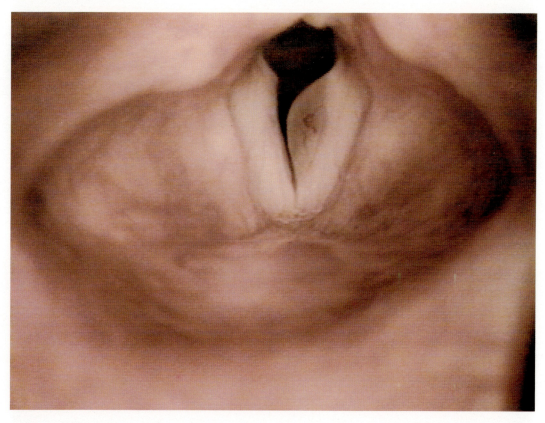

PLATE 4.71: Reinke's edema, stage 2. Tele-videoscopy shows edema of the left vocal fold with a capillary ectasia during breathing.

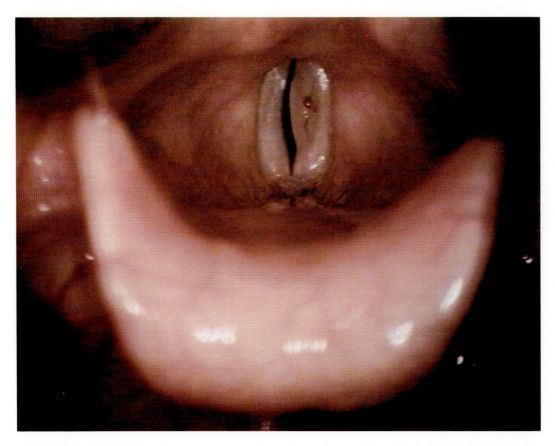

PLATE 4.72: During phonation (same case shown in Plate 4.71), the edema gives an imprint on the opposite vocal fold.

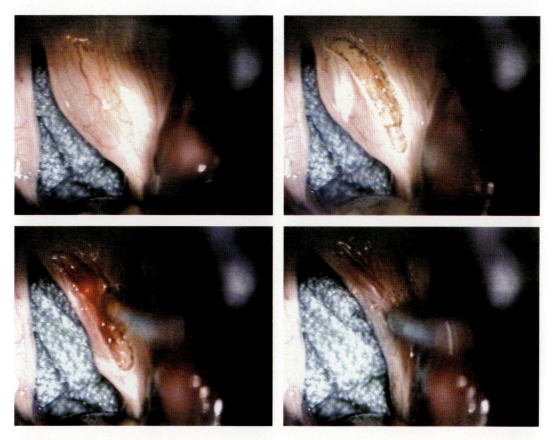

PLATE 4.73: A. Reinke's edema, stage 2, during laser phonosurgery:

1	2
3	4

1. Exposure of the larynx.
2. Incision with the laser (7 watts, continuous mode) of the superior surface of the vocal fold, 2 mm inside the false vocal fold.
3. Micro-suction of the glue.
4. End of the procedure.

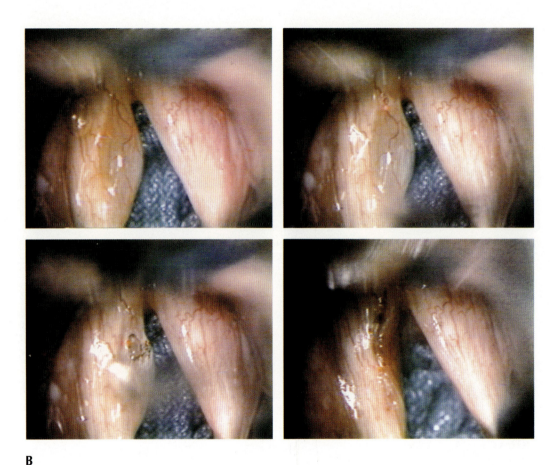

B. Reinke's edema, stage 2, during laser surgery of the left vocal fold: The same procedure is performed.

Laryngeal Pathologies: REINKE'S EDEMA

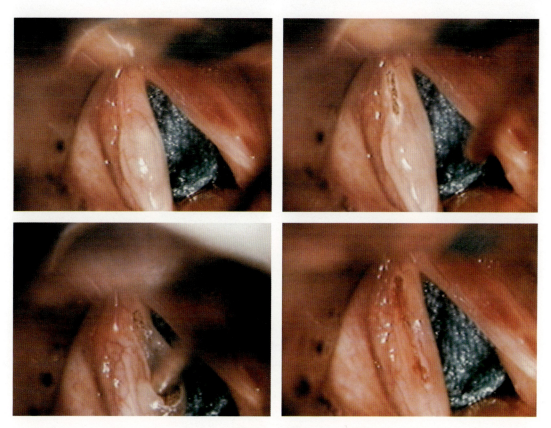

PLATE 4.74: Reinke's edema, stage 2, during laser microsurgery.

1	2
3	4

1. After exposure of the larynx, the right vocal fold has already been operated, during the same procedure, by the laser microsurgery lifting technique. The left vocal fold is now operated.
2. Incision of the mucosa of the superior surface of the vocal fold (7 watts, continuous mode). The incision is stopped in the middle third of the vocal fold.
3. Microsuction is performed.
4. End of the procedure.

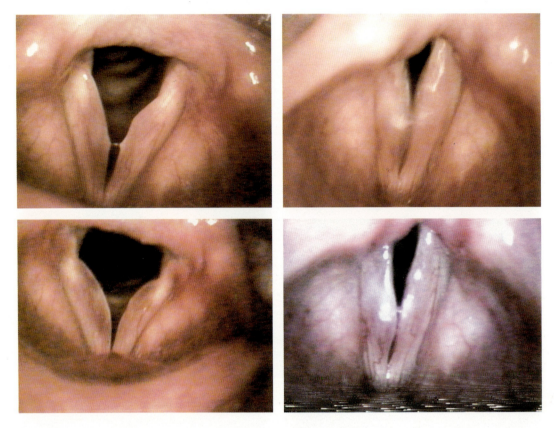

A

PLATE 4.75:   **A.** Reinke's edema, stage 2. Tele-videoscopy.

1	2
3	4

1. During breathing: both vocal folds touch each other in inspiration.
2. During phonation: posterior chink.
3. During expiration, the edema is well seen.
4. During stroboscopy: the posterior chink is emphasized.

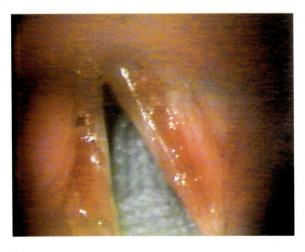

B

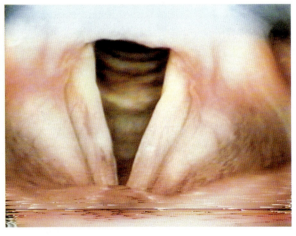

C

B. During laser microsurgery, lifting of both vocal folds, 10 watts, continuous mode. **C.** Results of surgery shown by tele-videoscopy 4 weeks after the surgical procedure.

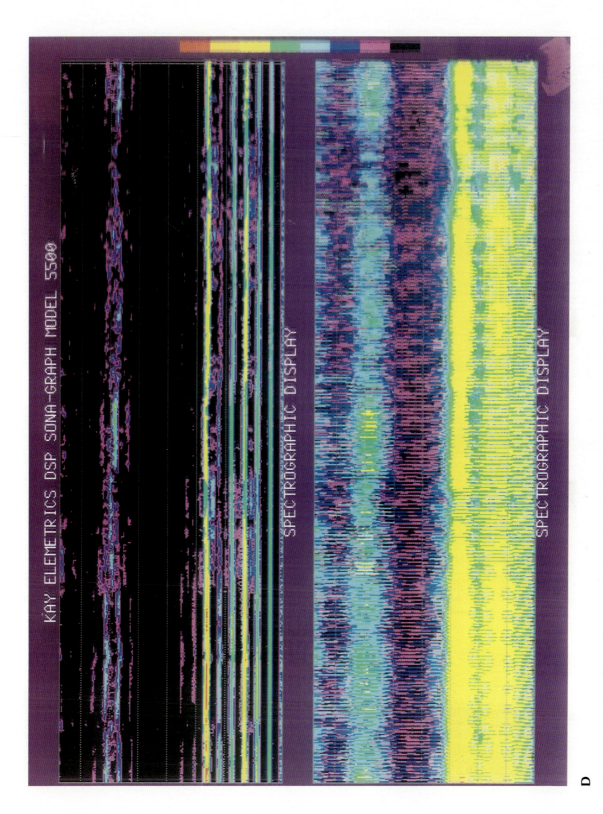

D. Spectrography of case shown in **A–C** before laser microsurgery: reduced range, harmonics are few, no high frequencies; formants are reduced.

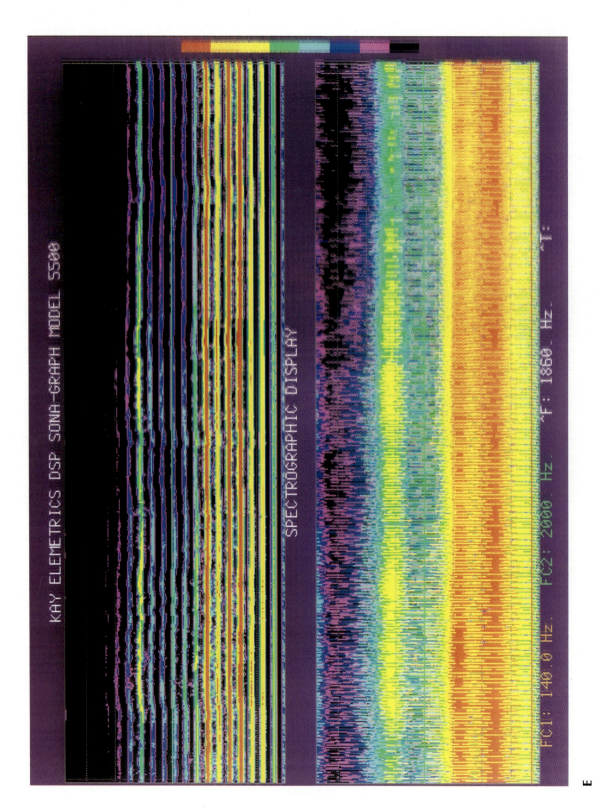

E. Spectrography of case shown in **A–D** after laser microsurgery: almost all harmonics have been recovered.

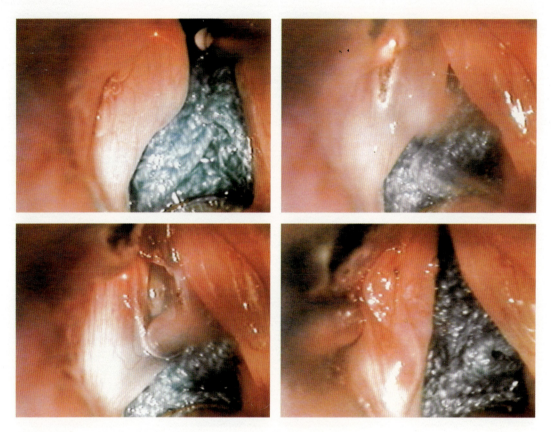

PLATE 4.76: Reinke's edema, stage 2. Laser microsurgery.

1	2
3	4

1. Larynx exposure.
2. Laser impact of 7 watts, continuous mode, on the upper surface of the vocal fold.
3. Microsuction.
4. The microflap is sealed with a laser low power impact.

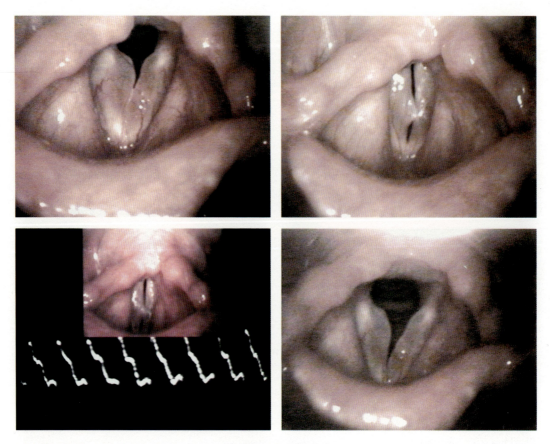

PLATE 4.77: Reinke's edema, stage 3. Tele-videoscopy.

1. During inspiration: the edema is important; the free edges touch each other.
2. During phonation: edema is compressed.
3. Vibratory mass has almost a regular wave (as we can see on EGG).
4. During expiration.

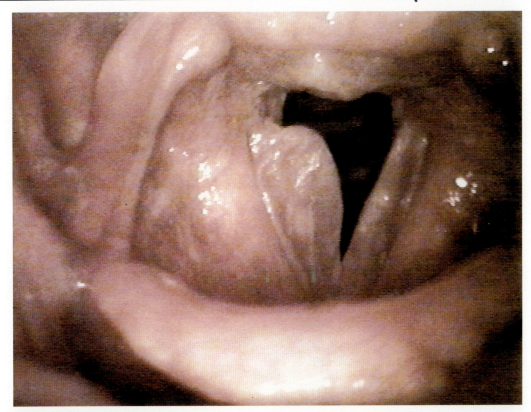

PLATE 4.78: Reinke's edema, stage 3. Tele-videoscopy during breathing.

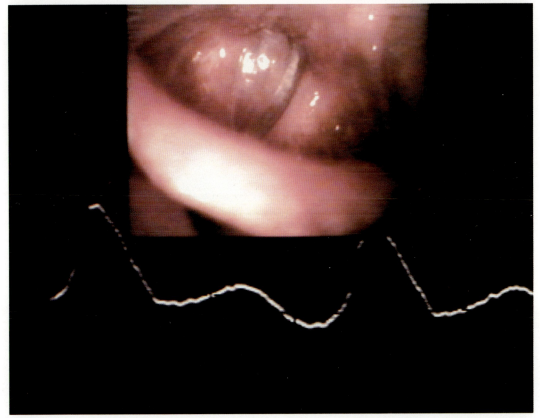

PLATE 4.79: During phonation (same case shown in Plate 4.78), with EGG which has regular waves, with a long open phase.

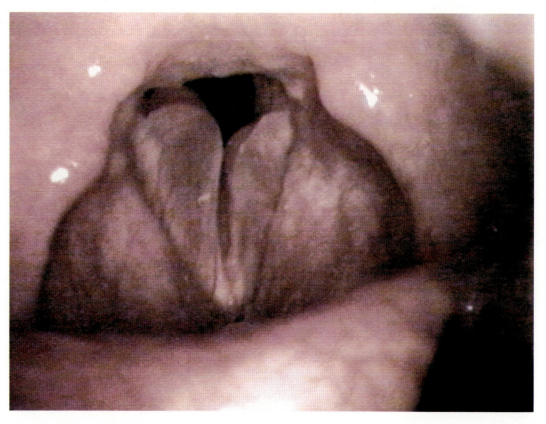

A

PLATE 4.80: **A.** Reinke's edema, stage 3. Tele-videoscopy. The free edges touch each other during breathing. It is a double edema involving the entire free edge of the vocal fold. **B.** Spectrography. Harmonics have almost disappeared. There is a high level of noise.

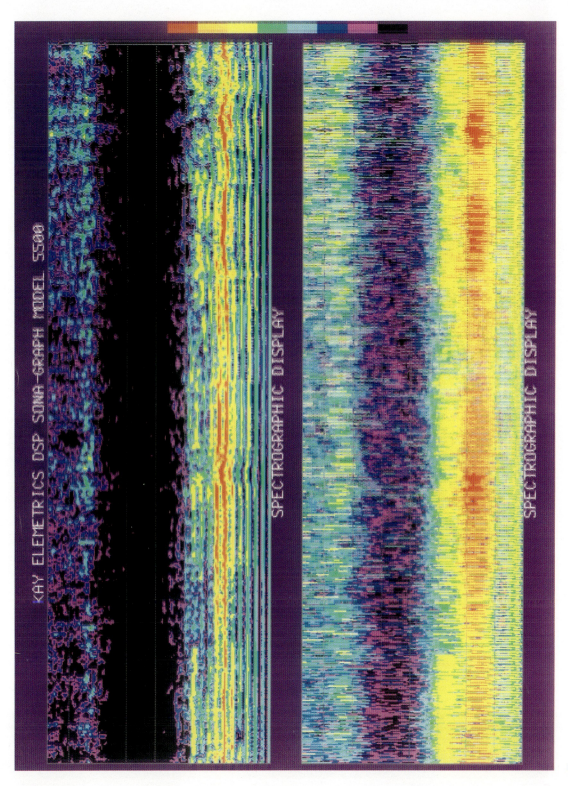

Atlas of Laser Voice Surgery

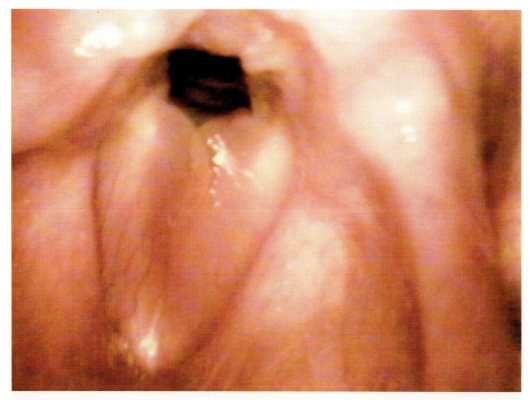

A

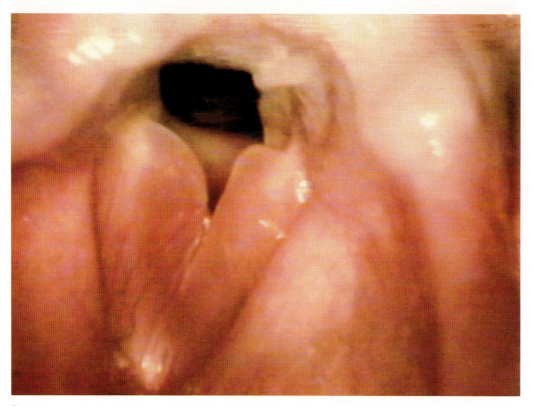

B

PLATE 4.81: **A.** Reinke's edema, stage 3. Tele-videoscopy during inspiration. **B.** During expiration, it looks like butterfly wings.

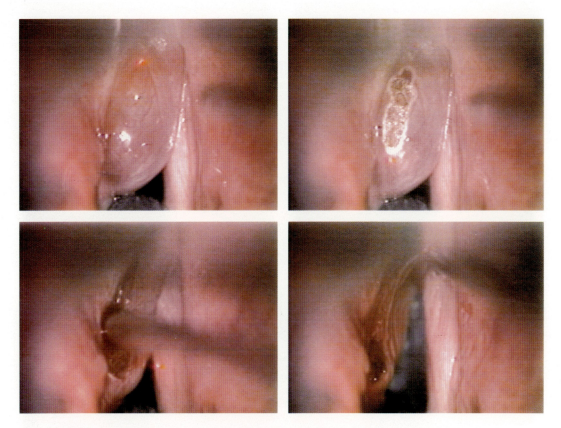

PLATE 4.82: Reinke's edema. Laser microsurgery: lifting of the left vocal fold.

1	2
3	4

1. Exposure of the larynx with visualization of the laser spot.
2. Incision parallel to the free border: the laser impact is on the superior surface of the vocal fold. It starts 3 mm behind the anterior commissure and 3 mm in front of the posterior commissure.
3. Microsuction, removing excess of mucosa.
4. End of procedure.

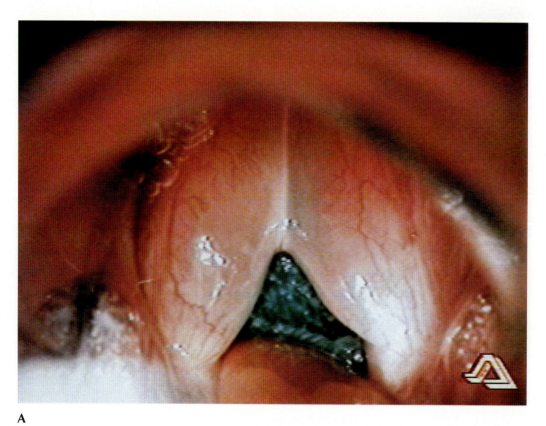

A

PLATE 4.83: **A.** Reinke's edema, stage 3. Laser microsurgery. Larynx exposure: a green gauze is put under the vocal folds, protecting the tube and the cuff; the gauze is wet and icy.

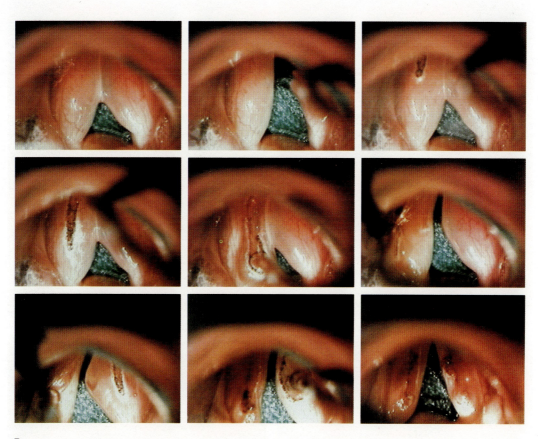

B. Same patient as **A**.

1	2	3
4	5	6
7	8	9

1. Exposure of the larynx.
2. Palpation of the edema with the A-forceps.
3. Laser impact starts from the anterior part of the superior surface of the vocal fold, nearby the ventricle (7 watts, continuous mode).
4. End of laser incision.
5. Suction.
6. End of the procedure for left vocal fold.
7. Beginning of the right vocal fold operation with the same technique.
8. Microsuction.
9. End of the entire procedure.

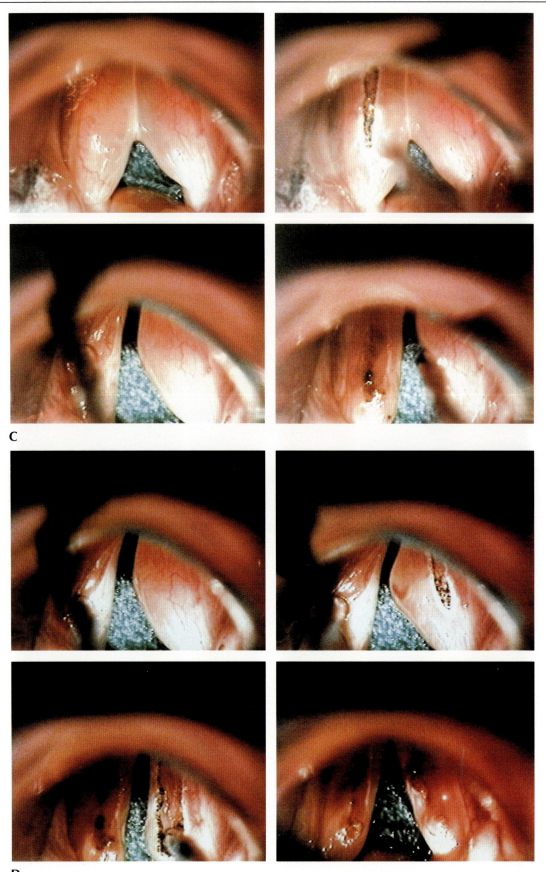

C. A closer look at the procedure in **B**. **D.** Another look at the procedure in **B**.

CHRONIC LARYNGITIS

A. Definition

Chronic laryngitis is a common pathology in adults. Laryngitis is an acute or chronic inflammation of the vocal folds and larynx, causing dysphonia.

B. Location

Chronic laryngitis is found on the laryngeal epithelium. Most often it appears on the vocal folds (on the squamous epithelium). Any type of infection or pollution may cause laryngitis. We will describe only chronic laryngitis in this chapter. Acute laryngitis may be cured by medical treatment and rarely results in chronic laryngitis.

C. Etiology and Histopathogeny

1. Etiology

Many factors are involved in the outcome of chronic laryngitis: tobacco, alcohol or drug intoxication, environmental agents (inhalation of toxic dusts or vapors), upper respiratory tract infections and vocal abuse are often associated. In rare instances, tuberculosis should be considered.

2. Pathogenesis

Laryngitis affects the cover of the vocal folds by increasing its stiffness, with little effect on the mass of the vocal folds.

Acute laryngitis resulting from bacterial infection is not directly related to vocal abuse. However, it does affect voice production and indirectly may be aggravated by vocal abuse. Chronic abuse will lead to persistent inflammation and perhaps result in a thickening of the vocal folds. It may also lead to permanent changes, such as nodules, polyps, or hypertrophy of the laryngeal epithelium.

Airflow and air pressure are elevated in laryngitis, especially if there is incomplete glottic closure.

3. Macroscopic Aspect

Chronic laryngitis leads to mucosal changes, particularly on the vocal folds. The great diversity of endoscopic findings has led to numerous clinical classifications which are very complex because they do not refer to a specific etiologic, histologic, therapeutic, or prognostic element. The polymorphism of the endoscopic finding is the expression of the transformation of the superficial epithelium and the submucosal layer.

Keratotic epithelium initially presents as slightly raised, poorly defined greyish areas. As the thickness of the horny layer increases, the lesion takes on a characteristic pearly white color. The keratosis may be flat or exophytic, as in the case of hyperkeratotic papilloma.

Keratotic areas are principally observed on the free border and superior surface of the anterior half of one or both vocal folds. The foci of keratosis contrast with the inflammatory redness of the adjacent mucosa covered by normal epithelium. The combination of the different stromal and epithelial changes varies constantly from place to place and in time. This explains the pictures, more often composite, seen in micro-laryngoscopy, which do not correspond to traditional red and white laryngeal pachydermis.

From an endoscopic point of view, erythroplasia may mean a simple inflammation or carcinoma. For some, leukoplakia means keratosis, for others, a combination of keratosis and dysplasia. Only histological examination of the mucosa, particularly of the epithelial cells in the deep layers, permits accurate diagnosis between benign and malignant lesions, because keratin is like a mask covering the underlying epithelial lesion.

4. Histology

The most important changes that occur in the submucosa are in the stroma. Localized or diffuse edema is always an important component of inflammation and gives the lesion its hypertrophic appearance. Edema may be associated with more or less marked inflammatory infiltration consisting of lymphocytes and plasmocytes and, in the case of acute exacerbation, also of polynuclear neutrophils.

Vascular changes are often found, consisting of dilatations or proliferation which give an erythematous appearance to the mucosa. If inflammation persists, fibrosis appears progessively. Submucosal glands may be involved in the inflammation, but their morphological changes are very discrete.

The superficial epithelium is thickened due to hyperplasia of the basal layer. The epithelial cristae thicken and lengthen, giving the epithelial base a wavy appearance (acanthosis). Nonkeratinized pavement epithelium may develop focal or diffuse keratosis or horny metaplasia. This keratinization may be ortho- or para-keratotic, with preservation of the horny layer nuclei. In contrast to normal epithelium, which is translucent, keratotic epithelium thickens and becomes opaque.

D. Clinical Approach

1. Primary Symptoms of Laryngitis

Primary symptoms include marked roughness or hoarseness in the voice with accompanying discomfort and dryness in the throat. When secondary to infection, the hoarseness may persist for some time after the infection has been controlled. Continued heavy use of the voice during this time may contribute to the laryngitis and continued hoarseness. The pitch levels of the voice may appear to be higher than normal, and it will be difficult to speak in a loud voice. It is a breathy voice with voice fatigue.

2. Tele-Video-Naso-Fiberscope and Telescope

Laryngitis shows a marked redness and small, dilated blood vessels may be visible on the inflamed vocal fold.

3. Stroboscopy

The vocal folds may show greater asymmetry and aperiodicity, with reduced mucosal waves and incomplete vibratory closure if there is a posterior chink. The propagation of the mucosal wave is diminished. A jerk-like movement of the mucosal wave has been noted, in which the wave appears to travel along part of the surface at one speed, then changes its speed for the remainder of its travel. The movement may also be called biphasic.

Acoustic signs show a greater or smaller than normal frequency and amplitude perturbation. Phonation range is reduced. Maximum sustainable intensities may be much lower than normal. Spectral noise in the voice is increased. Intensity is reduced.

4. Electroglottography (EGG)

The EGG signal may show marked variability from one cycle to the next, although closure times may be normal. Electroglottographic levels would be expected to be normal or slightly elevated.

5. Spectrography

Fundamental frequencies may be either elevated or reduced. This may be related to the severity of the cordal involvement. Harmonics and formants are few. The range is reduced.

E. Conclusion

Chronic laryngitis, if untreated, may result in serious complications, including dry laryngitis, characterized by marked atrophy of the mucosa of the larynx. There is a lack of vocal fold lubrication due to the reduction or absence of glandular secretions. The vocal fold becomes dry and sticky, associated with a chronic cough. Sometimes, laryngeal crusting may result, requiring a surgical removal.

Laryngitis may become a premalignant lesion. Beside the laser biopsy with the microspot by microlaryngoscopy, smear testing is a technique of choice to follow up these patients. Nevertheless, the more important question we have to answer to is:

"Is it a premalignant lesion?"

This is why CO_2 laser technique is suited for the treatment of this disease.

Laser phonosurgery by microlaryngoscopy requires an experienced pathologist to study the frozen sections during the operation.

- **Simple dysplasia** (hyperplastic, acanthotic, keratinized epithelium) usually will need a "decortication," but sometimes a type 1 cordectomy is needed (refer to Cancer section).

- **Moderate to severe dysplasia** may occur in laryngitis and need a type 1 cordectomy.

In our experience, before any laser phonosurgery, a trial of medical therapy must be performed. Antibiotics, antifungal agents, and antacids are prescribed for 4 weeks. During this month of treatment, vitamin A therapy also is prescribed. Also, the patient is advised not to smoke and not to drink alcohol.

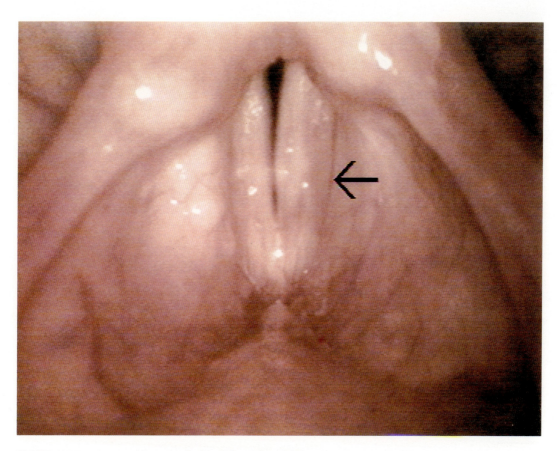

PLATE 4.84: Laryngitis catarrhalis. Tele-videoscopy.

Atlas of Laser Voice Surgery

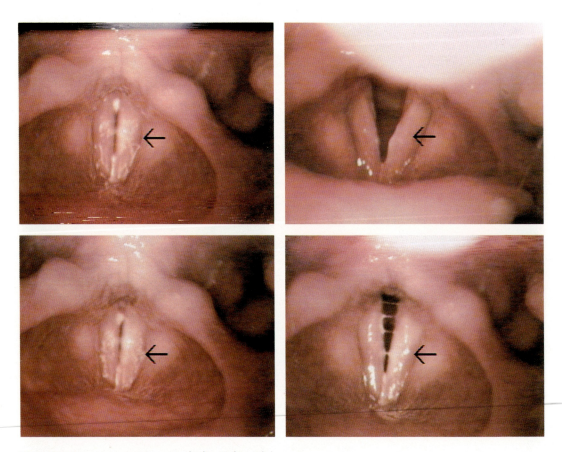

PLATE 4.85: Laryngitis catarrhalis. Tele-videoscopy.

1	2
3	4

1. During phonation: The left vocal fold does not vibrate.
2. During breathing: Swelling of the epithelium.
3. During phonation: Mucus is sticking to the free edge of the vocal fold.
4. During breathing: Dyspnea due to the infection.

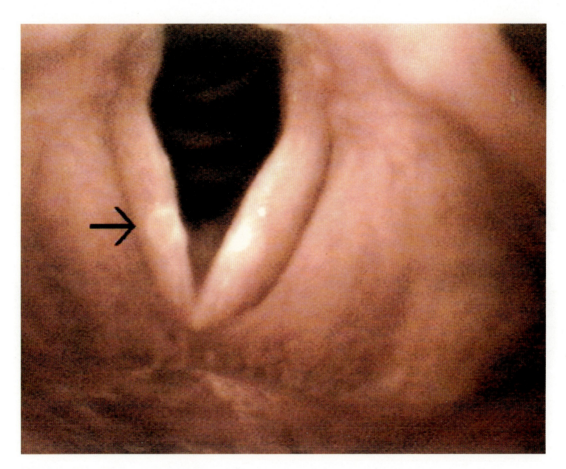

PLATE 4.86: Herpetic laryngitis.

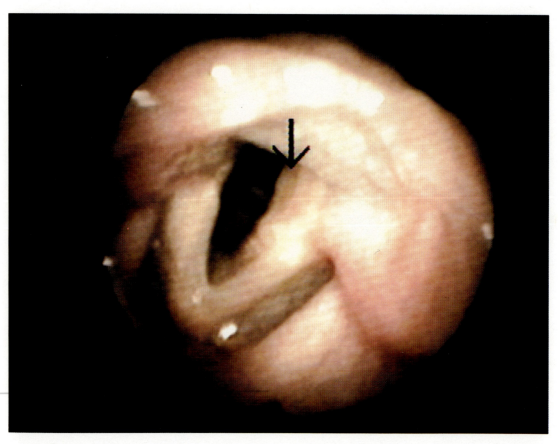

PLATE 4.87: Tuberculosis before medical treatment. Tele-videoscopy.

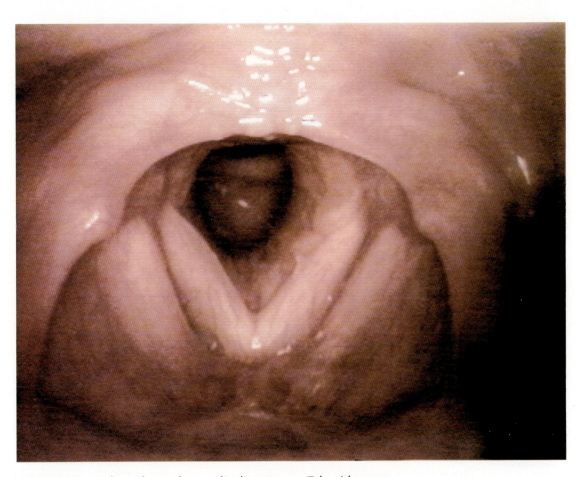

PLATE 4.88: Tuberculosis after medical treatment. Tele-videoscopy.

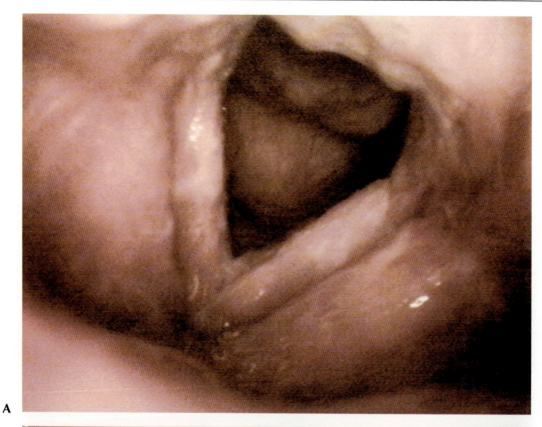

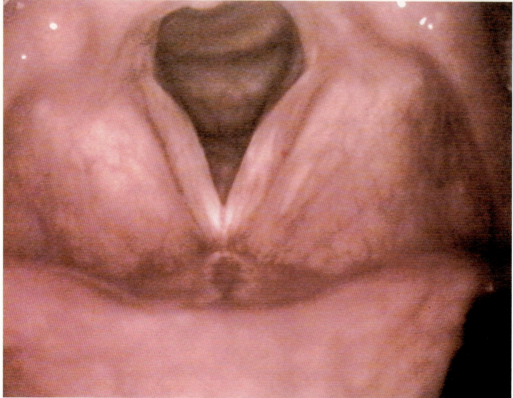

PLATE 4.89: **A.** Chronic laryngitis due to tobacco. Tele-videoscopy before medical and laser microsurgery. **B.** Same case 3 months after decortication of both vocal folds and a complementary medical treatment (vitamin A). Tele-videoscopy.

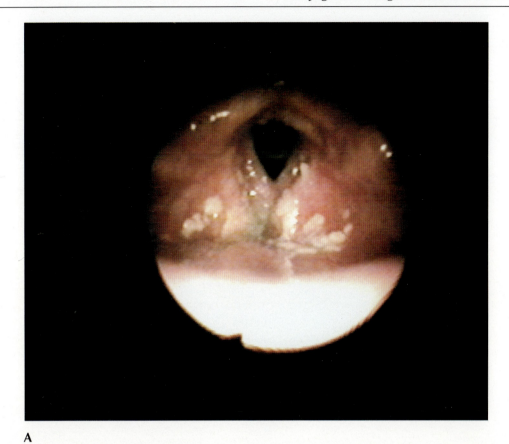

PLATE 4.90: **A.** Fungus infection. Laryngitis of both vocal folds plus susglottic area. Reflux. Tele-videoscopy. **B.** Smear test of the vocal fold: fungus can be seen (filamentous structures).

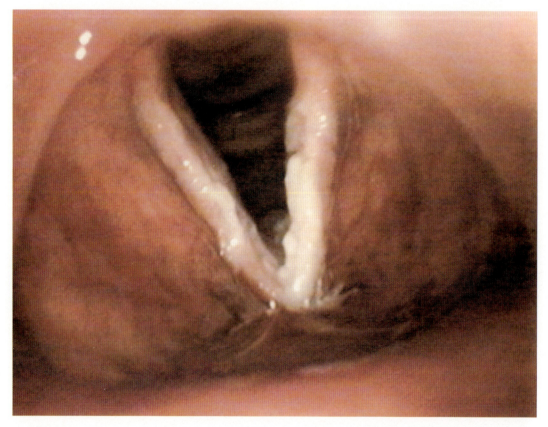

PLATE 4.91: Fungus laryngitis with pachydermia of both vocal folds. Tele-videoscopy before medical treatment.

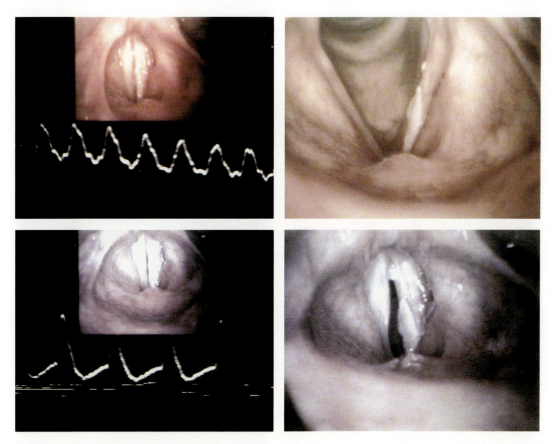

PLATE 4.92: Fungus laryngitis shown in Plate 4.91 after medical treatment.

1	2
3	4

1. During phonation with EGG: regular waves. Increasing of the closing phase.
2. During breathing: only pachydermy of the left vocal fold can be seen, which needs laser microsurgery.
3–4. During stroboscopy: asymmetrical waves can be seen with a partial rigidity of the left vocal fold.

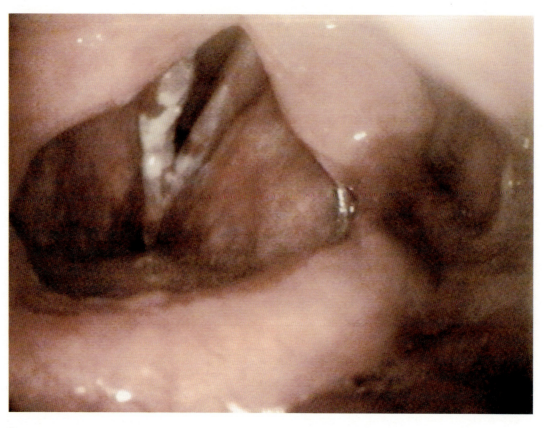

A

PLATE 4.93: **A.** Pachydermic laryngitis of both vocal folds. Bilateral decortication must be performed. **B.** Spectrography: reduced range, few harmonics, and few formants can be seen on the display.

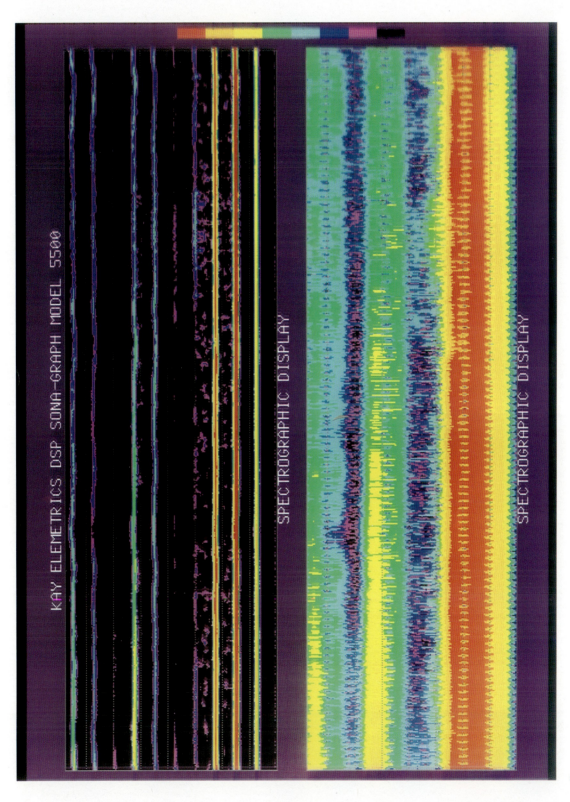

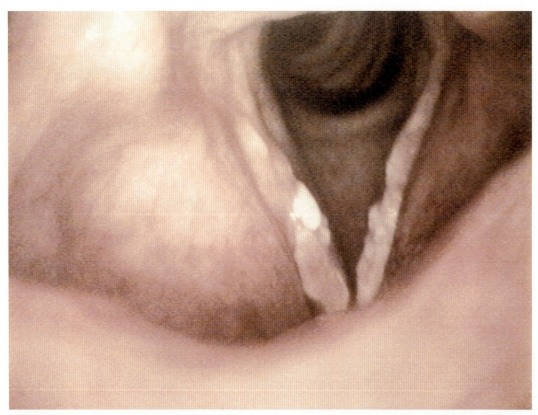

PLATE 4.94: Hyperkeratotic laryngitis during breathing. Tele-videoscopy.

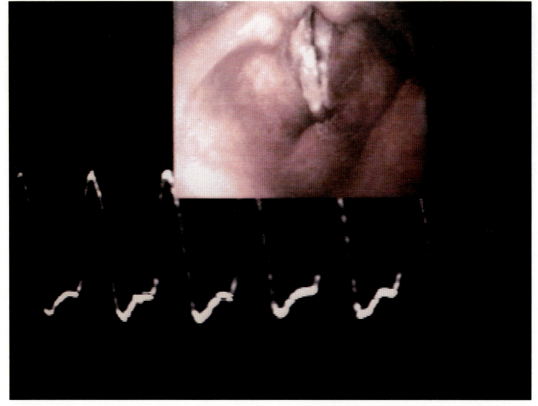

PLATE 4.95: During phonation: EGG is regular, the vibrations are regular but asymmetrical.

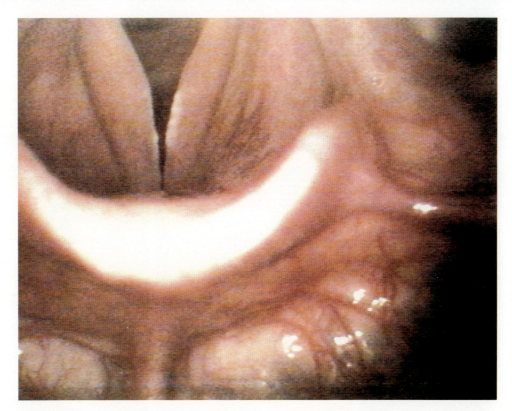

PLATE 4.96: Leukokeratotic laryngitis after medical treatment. Tele-videoscopy during breathing.

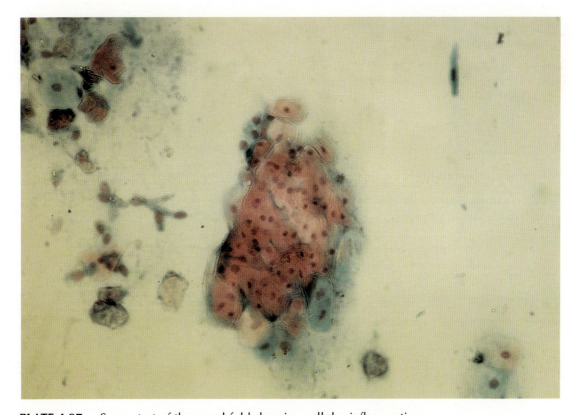

PLATE 4.97: Smear test of the vocal fold showing cellular inflammation.

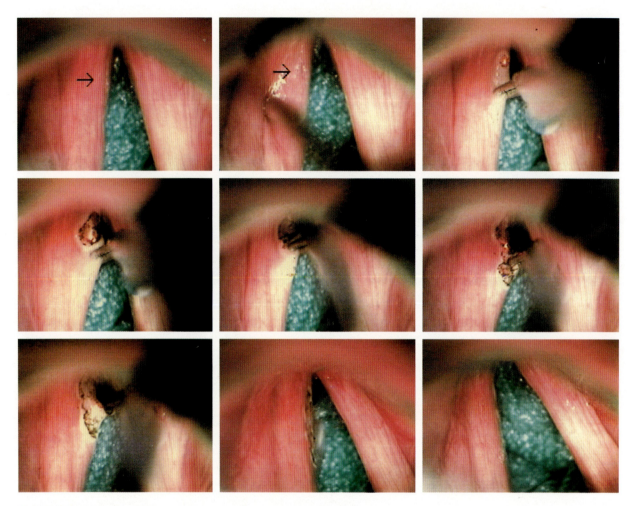

PLATE 4.98: Laser microsurgery procedure:

1	2	3
4	5	6
7	8	9

1. Exposure of the larynx: leukokeratotic lesion is on the free edge.
2. The A-forceps pushes the superior surface of the vocal fold to gain a better view on the free edge.
3–7. Laser impact 7 watts, continuous modes. The A-forceps grasps the lesion smoothly and pulls it toward the glottis.
8–9. End of the procedure. Icy cottonoid to remove the char tissue.

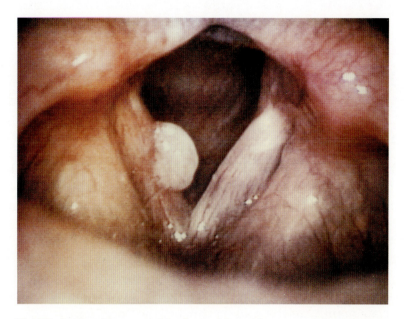

PLATE 4.99: Hypertrophic laryngitis with a suspicious lesion. Tele-videoscopy.

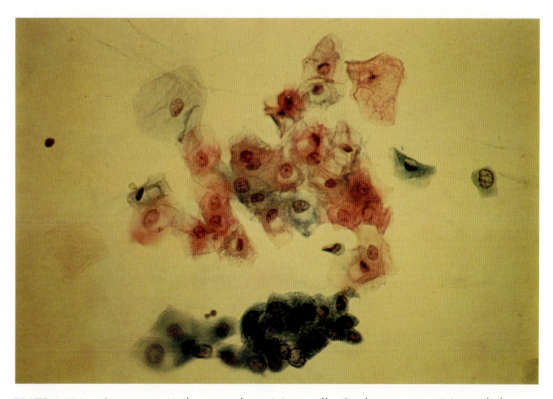

PLATE 4.100: Smear test: Koilocyst and suspicious cells. Cordectomy type 1 is needed.

MALIGNANT TUMORS OF THE VOCAL FOLDS
CARCINOMA IN SITU, T1N0, AND T2N0

A. Definition

Malignant tumors, carcinoma of the vocal fold, are specifically epidermoid carcinomas. They are specific because of the few lymphatic vessels found in the vocal folds. They are sparse and lie mostly at the beginning in the submucosal space.

B. Location

Malignant tumors rarely involve both vocal folds. They usually are unilateral and occur mainly on the middle third of the vocal fold.

C. Etiology and Histopathogeny

1. Etiology

- More than 97.5% of patients are smokers and users of alcohol. Irritants such as formaldehyde or other chemicals and contaminants can be involved as co-carcinogens, as can factors such as human papilloma virus (HPV), AIDS, or immunologic disturbances.

- Synergy of the use of alcohol and smoking increases the risk of endolaryngeal cancer by more than 50%.

- Eighty percent of these tumors are found in males of 40–65 years of age.

2. Pathogenesis: Co-factors

Nutritional deficiency, which results in abnormal metabolism of keratinocytes, favors persistent colonization by HPV. Vitamin A and vitamin C deficiencies have been often associated with laryngeal dysplasia, and also with cervical dysplasia.

Studies in the United States and Japan have shown the important effect of beta-carotene as an epithelial protector to prevent severe dysplasia. Vitamin A deficiency leads to epithelial metaplasia and can be associated with the development of a carcinoma. Low magnesium concentration in erythrocytes and serum is found in patients with laryngeal carcinoma. Carcinomatous tissue contains higher concentrations of magnesium than normal tissue. It has been speculated that magnesium deficiency might contribute as a co-carcinogen.

Tobacco has a direct effect on the laryngeal epithelium. More than 95% of laryngeal cancers are linked to smoking. Nicotine from tobacco may not possess any carcinogenic effect. However, burning the tobacco releases tar from which, so far, about a dozen polycyclic aromatic hydrocarbons have been isolated. These are known to have a carcinogenic effect through their derivatives, methylcholanthrene or benzopyrene.

These substances reach the cellular surface of the epithelum via the smoke and are dissolved in saliva. Breakdown of these carcinogens by arylhydrocarbon hydroxylase produces the actual carcinogenic epoxides that bind to the DNA and RNA molecules. The process of the cancer development is subject to all possible influences: type of tobacco, temperature and speed of burning, length and intensity of exposure to the carcinogen. The period and quantity of tobacco consumption are directly related to the risk of laryngeal carcinoma. The earlier a person begins to smoke and the more he smokes, the higher the risk of developing a carcinoma in the exposed area.

Alcohol has an indirect effect. It is suspected that alcohol either potentiates other carcinogens, damages the epithelium, causes a deficiency of riboflavin, or disturbs the synthesis of immunoglobulin. Statistically, there is a synergy between alcohol and tobacco. It increases the risk of laryngeal cancer; with exposure to both factors, the risk increases about 50% more than the increase predicted if the effects were simply additive.

3. *Macroscopic Aspect*

- Carcinoma often hides under a fungus infection or a chronic hyperplastic laryngitis (20% of cases).

- With glottic keratosis, ulceration covered with fibrin, the surface may be irregular, mammilated and polypoid, or scattered with keratotic plaques and hemorrhage.

- Glottic carcinomas spread along the epithelium and rarely invade deeper structures in the beginning.

4. *Histology*

The epidermoid carcinoma presents four variable aspects:

a. Well-differentiated carcinomatous, squamous, hyperkeratinized cells focally conserving their polarity.

    b. Undifferentiated with only strings of anarchical cells visible.

    c. Rarely, fusiform cells looking like sarcoma.

    d. Occasionally, adenocarcinoma or lymphoma are found.

According to the American Joint Commission on Cancer Staging, the stage of carcinoma is related essentially to the invasion of the basal membrane zone. In the glottis:

    a. Carcinoma in situ (CIS): The basal membrane zone is spared; the lesion, originating from the epithelium, is located in the superficial layer of the lamina propria.

    b. Micro-invasive carcinoma or T1N0: The basal membrane zone is destroyed, the corium is invaded. The lamina propria is involved, as well as the Reinke's space with or without the entire vocal ligament. The muscles are spared.

    c. Invasive carcinoma or T2N0: the basal membrane zone and the superficial layer of the muscles are involved. No cases have presented with impaired vocal fold mobility.

    d. A particular case: verrucous carcinoma: Macroscopically, it looks like an invasive lesion; histologically, there is rarely an invasion of the vocal fold muscles.

D. Clinical Approach

1. Primary Symptoms

The glottic space is mobile. Only CIS, T1N0M0, and T2N0M0, will be described.

T refers to the volume and the histological site

N refers to the involvement of the lymphatic nodules

M refers to metastasis

None of our cases had nodules in the neck, dyspnea, or dysphagia.

- Hoarseness is the main sign for a lesion located on the middle third and the anterior commissure. Often it begins like a laryngitis but it does not improve after treatment.

- Voice fatigue and persistent dysphonia in a patient who smokes is a signal for the laryngologist to proceed with closer inspection of the vocal folds, especially if there is otalgia.

2. Tele-Video-Naso-Fiberscope and Telescope

- By fibervideoscopy, mobility of the larynx and limits of the tumor from front to back and top to bottom are well observed. The superior limit with the lateral recess of the ventricle, the inferior limit with the conus elasticus, the 2 mm of the anterior commissure, and posterior vocal process are particularly studied because lymphatic vessels are located there.

- By telescopy, the aspect of the tumor is more precisely analyzed; the volume of the roots and the limits of the lesion are evaluated. The macroscopic findings indicate the stage of the carcinoma. Then, the type of cordectomy can be decided. If the tumor spreads to the ventricle, to the anterior or posterior commissures, or to the subglottic area, a microlaryngoscopy for diagnosis is carried out. Laser cordectomy is contraindicated.

3. Stroboscopy

- **Stroboscopy is essential in diagnosis. A small lesion is always suspicious if the aspect of the vibration looks like a surfboard on a wave.** A flat lesion that does not vibrate, and is white or reddish in color. If it resists medical treatment after 3 weeks of follow-up, a smear test or a biopsy must be done. A type I cordectomy is carried out.

- The tumor interferes with the vibratory mass. A gap can be observed with irregular closure during vibration.

In large lesions, the entire vocal fold does not vibrate.

4. Electroglottography (EGG)

It is very irregular.

5. Spectrography

Patterns are irregular. Harmonics and formants show a narrow register, few harmonics, and high levels of noise. Signal-to-noise ratio is usually low.

C. Conclusion

1. For Early Stage Cancer, Stroboscopy Is Essential

Any patient with a malignant lesion must have a smear test if there is doubt about a fungus infection; and after 3 weeks of medical treatment, a laser microlaryngoscopy surgery with frozen section must be carried out. The type of treatment will be suggested during videotelescopy and decided during laser surgical procedures with the help of the pathologist.

Laser cordectomy by microlaryngoscopy was popularized by the CO_2 laser technique, early recognition of premalignant stage by telestroboscopic exploration, and the improved health education of the general exploration. But, in any case, fundamental rules must be followed for laser microlaryngoscopy cordectomy.

2. Three Types of Cordectomy

We have developed a personal protocol of laser surgery with three types of cordectomy.

1. **Type 1:** Mucosa and corium are removed.

2. **Type 2:** Mucosa, corium, and superficial muscle layers are removed, and the false vocal fold is usually removed to have an unobstructed view of the floor of the ventricle.

3. **Type 3:** Mucosa, corium, and thyroarytenoid muscles are removed up to the perichondrium, and the false vocal fold is also removed. Coagulation of posterior arteries is often necessary (See Plates 4.101 and 4.102).

The false vocal fold may hide lesions sheltered in the ventricle. That is why it must be removed.

Techniques are the same for any type of cordectomy:

- The lens angle from the microscope to the vocal fold is 90°.

- The shooting starts: the attack angle is 90°, perpendicular to the free edge, on the horizontal plane, from the free border to the ventricle to start and finish the cordectomy.

- A straight fire, parallel to the free border, is performed with the laser from the anterior angle to the posterior angle of the vocal incision. It starts 2 mm behind the anterior commissure. It ends 2 mm before the posterior commissure. A rectangular sample is removed.

A second-look laser microsurgery may be necessary 2 months later if any healing looks suspicious. An acute follow-up is needed. Acoustic signs are not significant because the voice is hoarse anyway. Tele-videoscopy and fiber-videoscopy are the main explorations.

Is it a premalignant lesion or a carcinoma?

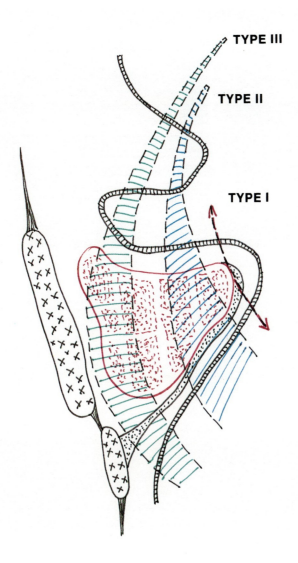

PLATE 4.101: Diagram of three types of cordectomy.

The importance of the pathologic study by frozen section is critical:

1. **Simple dysplasia** means a hyperplastic, acanthotic epithelium. It is keratinized, but regular, with differentiation of cells in all layers and no nuclear atypia. Here a "decortication" is performed because the dysplasia is a reflection of a chronic hyperplastic disease of the laryngeal epithelium, with keratin in some cases. We cannot guarantee that it will remain benign. These lesions must be regarded as possible premalignant tumors.

2. **Moderate to severe dysplasia** adds nuclear atypia to what we just described. Here, more than ever, an experienced pathologist is needed, and these lesions must be very carefully analyzed. A Type 1 cordectomy or a "decortication" is performed.

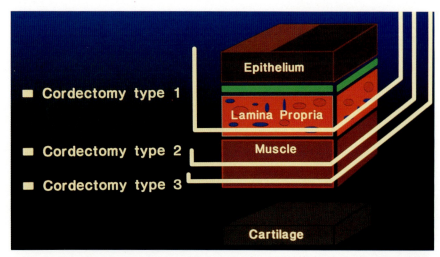

A

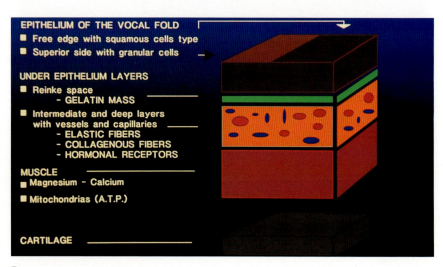

B

PLATE 4.102: **A.** Diagram showing impact of laser in three types of cordectomy. **B.** Differentiation of tissue layers in three types of cordectomy.

3. **In carcinoma in situ**, a Type 1 cordectomy is performed. We must have a frozen section. If necessary, a Type 2 cordectomy may be completed during the same laser surgery.

4. **T1N0** usually needs a Type 2 cordectomy. Sometimes after the results of the frozen section are analyzed, a Type 3 cordectomy is carried out.

5. **T2N0** usually needs a Type 3 cordectomy; and if the lesion spreads to the anterior or posterior commissure, additional treatment should be provided.

These techniques may be completed by a second laser surgery and/or radiotherapy if recurrences appear.

Laser microlaryngoscopic surgery of carcinoma of the vocal fold requires early detection. Most are revealed by stroboscopic exploration and smear tests. As a matter of fact, if early detection to diagnose a premalignant lesion is necessary to prevent most of the invasive carcinomas, a few of them, principally those appearing on a hyperplastic laryngitis, may grow directly from the basal membrane zone as an invasive carcinoma.

In our experience with laser microlaryngoscopy, if lesions from the anterior or posterior commissure need a complementary treatment and are contraindications for laser surgery, carcinoma in situ, T1N0, and T1N0 of the middle third have very satisfactory results.

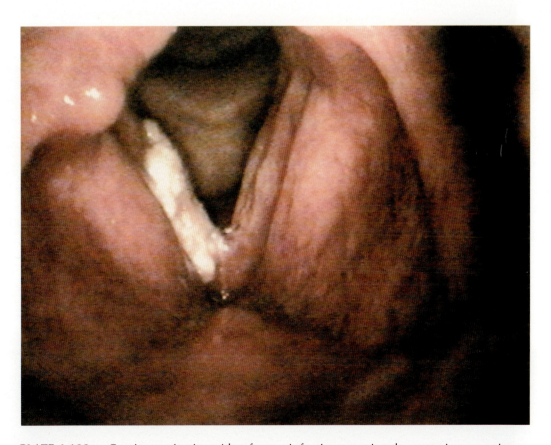

PLATE 4.103: Carcinoma in situ with a fungus infection spearing the posterior commissure (Telescope).

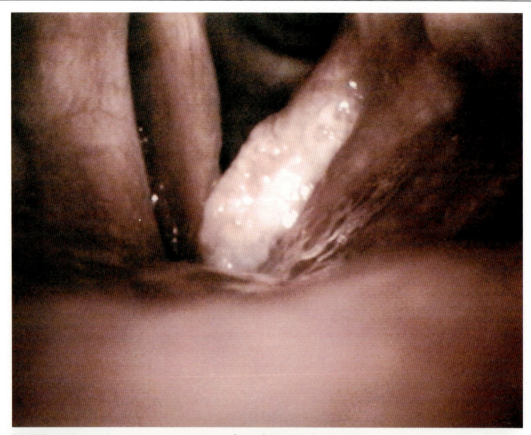

PLATE 4.104: Verrucous carcinoma Tele-videoscope.

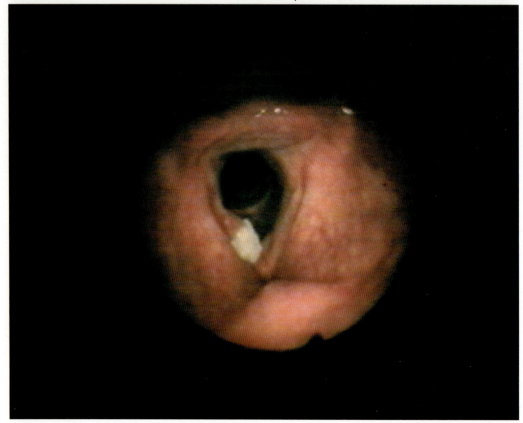

PLATE 4.105: Verrucous carcinoma Tele-videoscope.

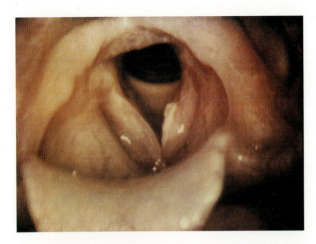

PLATE 4.106: T1N0 carcinoma Telescope.

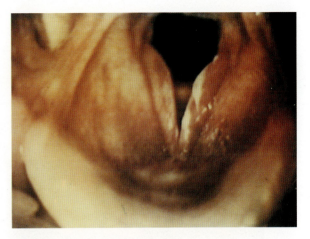

PLATE 4.107: T1N0 carcinoma.

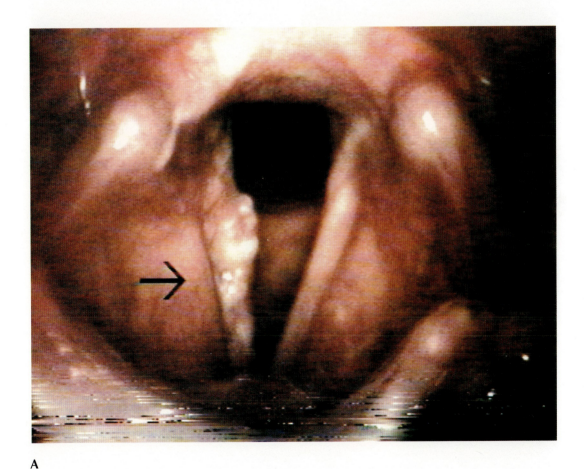

A

PLATE 4.108: **A.** T2N0 carcinoma on right vocal fold.

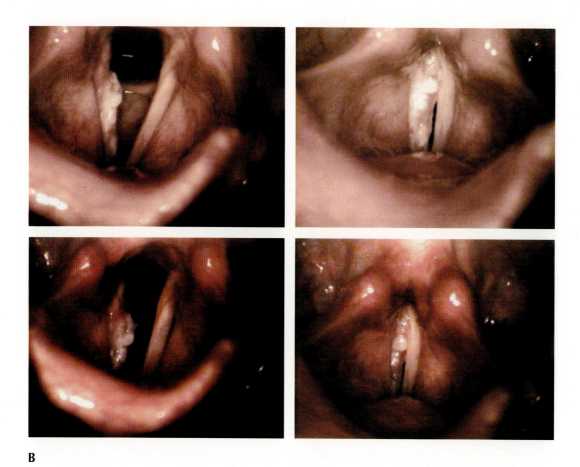

B. Hyperkeratotic carcinoma T2N0, Tele-videoscope. **C.** Spectrography of hyperkeratotic carcinoma. Narrow register, few harmonics in the upper part, F_0 + 3–4 harmonics. Loss of register + sounds.

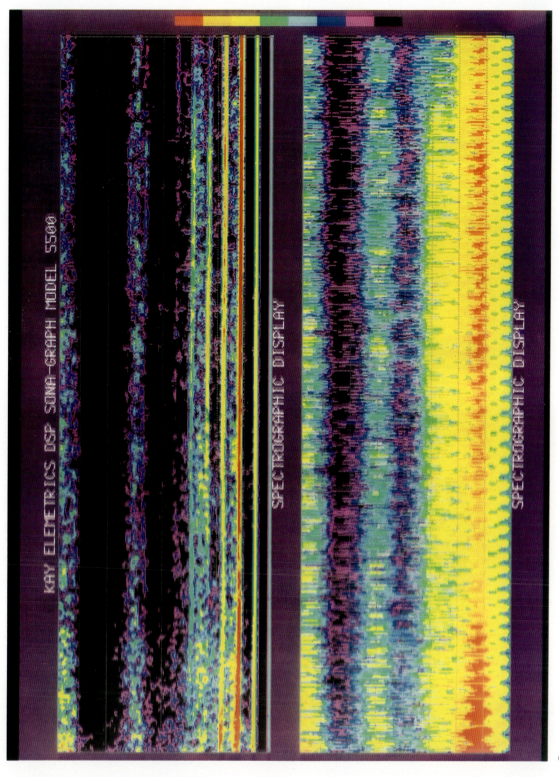

Atlas of Laser Voice Surgery

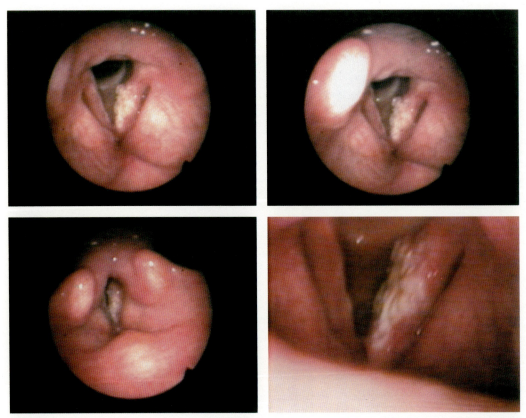

PLATE 4.109: T2N0 carcinoma on the left vocal fold.

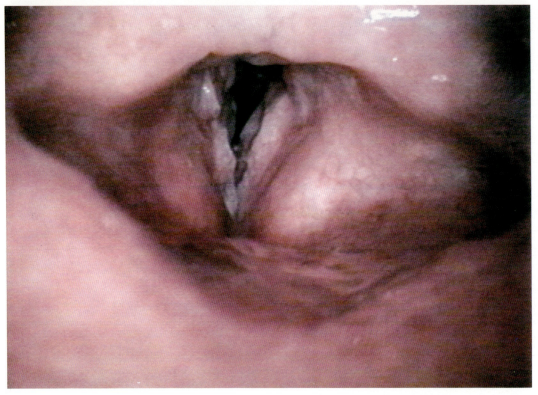

PLATE 4.110: T2N0 bilateral carcinoma with anterior commissure (a contraindication for laser surgery).

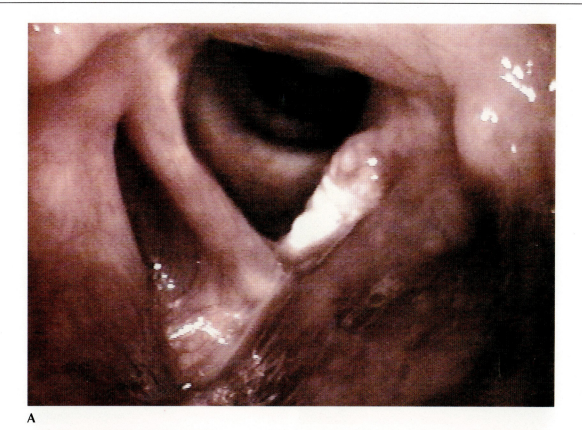

A

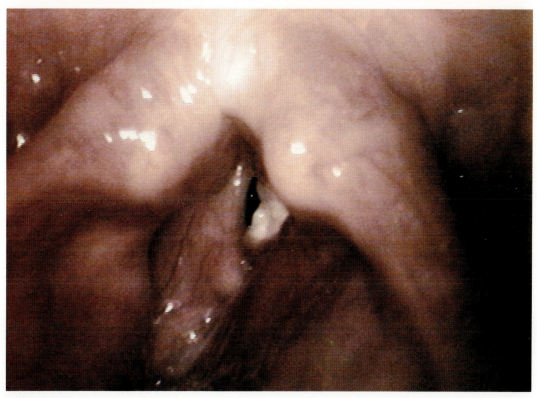

B
PLATE 4.111: Recurrence of carcinoma 3 months after left cordectomy **A.** Telescope during breathing. **B.** Telescope during phonation.

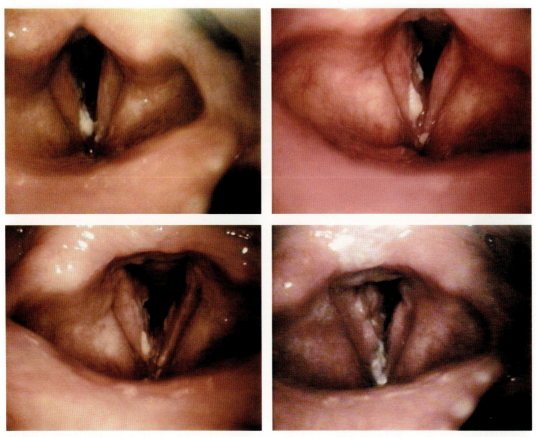

PLATE 4.112: T2N0 unilateral carcinoma of the right vocal fold with anterior commissure (a contraindication for laser surgery).

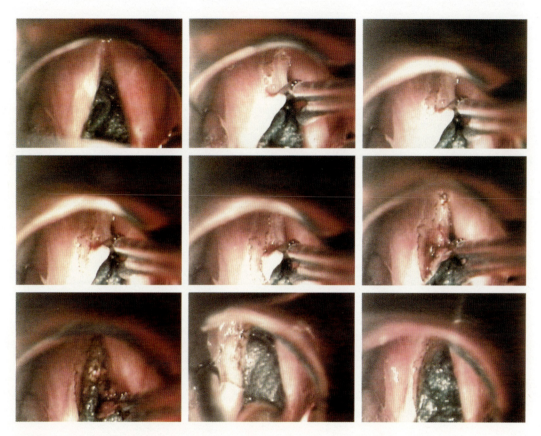

PLATE 4.113: Cordectomy type I: left side.

1	2	3
4	5	6
7	8	9

1. Before surgery.
2. Grasping of the vocal fold inside the glottic space and impact of microspot at 90° on the anterior commissure.
3. Parallel laser cut to the border line.
4. Parallel laser cut to the border line with a slight bleeding due to microspot.
5. Spot size is changed to normal spot because of bleeding: laser cut.
6. Up to the anterior commissure.
7. Pulling the vocal fold into the glottic space with the A-forceps.
8. Check of the bed of the cordectomy.
9. End of surgery.

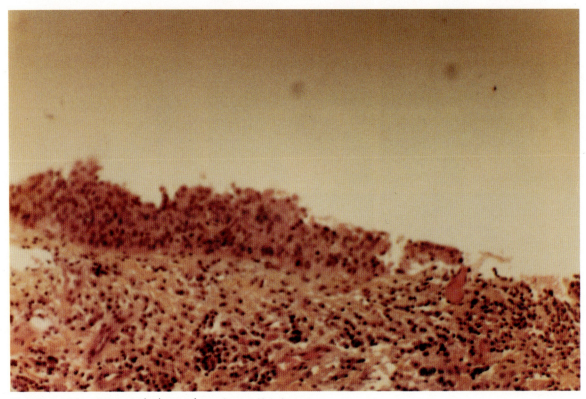

PLATE 4.114: Histopathology of carcinoma in situ.

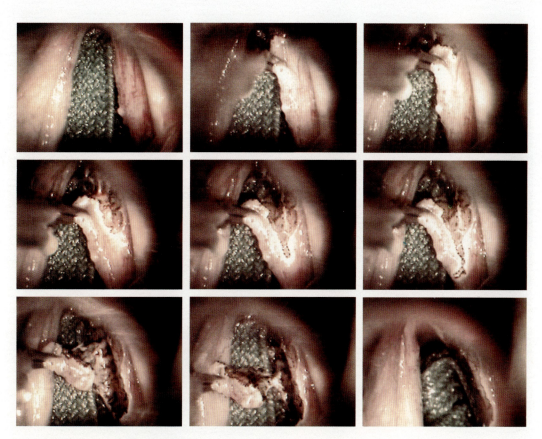

PLATE 4.115: Cordectomy type I: right side.

1. Before surgery.
2. First impact of a microspot at 90°.
3. Angle of 90°.
4. Parallel to the free edge, laser cut: microspot.
5. No char tissue is seen, perfect laser line.
6. Angle of 90° coming back to the free border.
7. The A-forceps grasps the sample and pulls it inside the glottic space.
8. Last impact to remove the fold.
9. End of surgery.

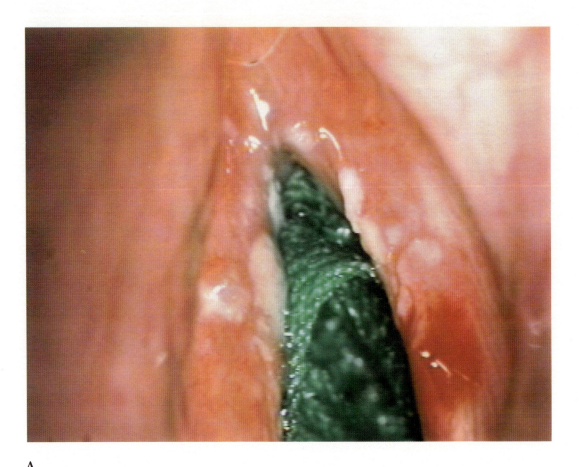

A

PLATE 4.116: **A.** Micro-invasive carcinoma with chronic laryngitis. Double cordectomy type II is performed.

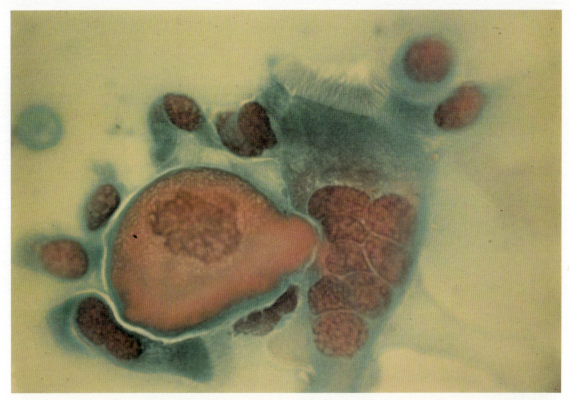

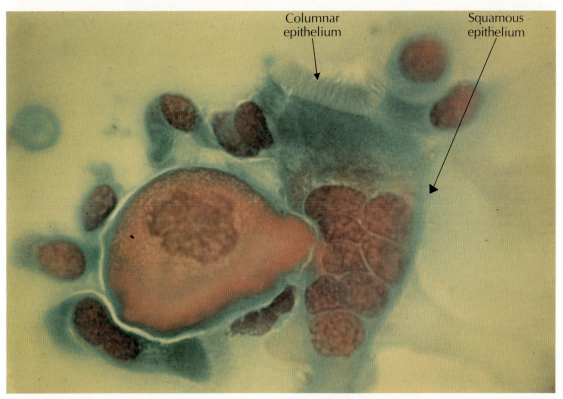

B. Smear test of a micro-invasive carcinoma with the transitional zone between the squamous and the columnar ciliated epithelium. **C.** Columnar ciliated cells and squamous carcinoma cells.

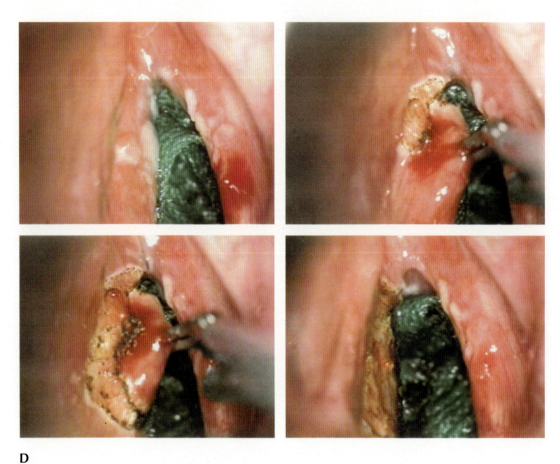

D. Double cordectomy type II (see also **E**).

1	2
3	4

1. Visualization of the vocal folds with the anterior commissure.
2. Incision from front to back after grasping the middle third of the vocal fold with the A-forceps.
3. Incision parallel to the free border is performed. The A-forceps pulls the sample into the glottic space.
4. After surgery of the left vocal fold.

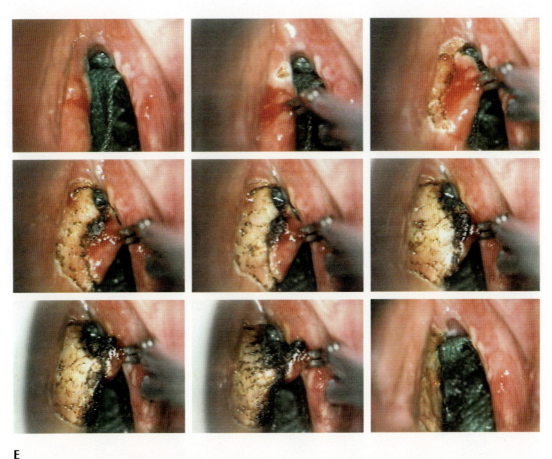

E. Cordectomy type II (same case as **D**).

1	2	3
4	5	6
7	8	9

1. Visualization of the vocal folds with the anterior commissure through the microspot.
2. First impact: 90°.
3. Incision parallel to the free border.
4. Last impact of the epithelium going to the free border: 90°.
5. A-forceps pulls the vocal folds inside and down the glottic space. The vocal ligament starts to be removed.
6. The muscle starts to be fired.
7. Muscle is removed superficially.
8. Last impact: no bleeding is observed. Signal is given for a frozen section
9. After surgery, char is removed with a cotonoid. The excision bed is smoothly cleansed.

Commentary: Laser power is 7 watts, classical spot size, continuous fire. The false vocal fold is not removed because pulling the vocal fold with the A-forceps is enough to detect any lesion of the superior surface of the vocal fold.

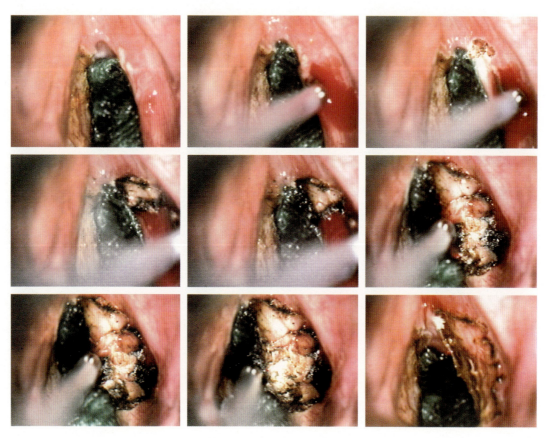

F

F. Double cordectomy type II (see **D**, **E**, and **G**).

1	2	3
4	5	6
7	8	9

1. Exposure of the vocal folds: left side is already done, the right side is undergoing laser surgery: the anterior commissure is spread.
2. On the middle third a small hemorrhage is observed.
3–7. Same technique as described in E.
8. A coagulation is done on the posterior arytenoid artery.
9. After surgery, anterior commissure is intact as is the posterior commissure.

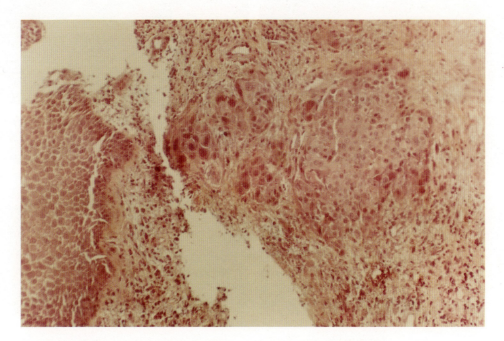

G. Histopathology of the micro-invasive carcinoma shown in **D–F**.

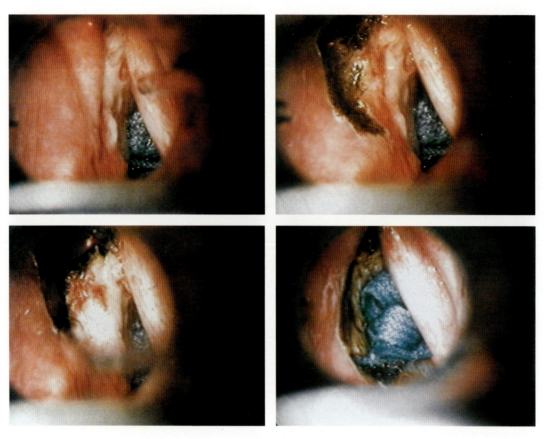

A

PLATE 4.117: A. Cordectomy type II.

1	2
3	4

1. Exposure of the vocal fold and anterior and posterior commissures.
2. False vocal fold ablation.
3. Visualization and impact of the laser on the true vocal fold. The lesion invades the superior surface of the vocal fold.
4. The excision bed is bloodless, no coagulation is needed. The bed of the vocal fold is smoothly cleansed.

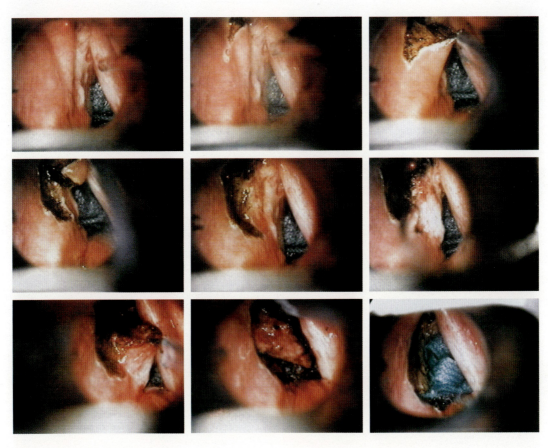

B

B. Cordectomy type II for carcinoma T1N0.

1	2	3
4	5	6
7	8	9

1. Exposure of the glottic area; anterior commissure is spared, as well as posterior commissure.
2. Removal of the false vocal fold.
3. Middle impact.
4. The A-forceps grasps the false vocal fold and pulls it into the glottic space.
5. The false vocal fold is removed. The superior surface of the vocal fold is visualized and leukoplakia is observed. It needs cordectomy type 2.
6. Vocal fold is grasped and pulled into the glottic space.
7. Cordectomy is performed from front to back, sparing the anterior commissure.
8. The sample is removed and the frozen section is carried out.
9. The excision bed is smoothly cleansed.

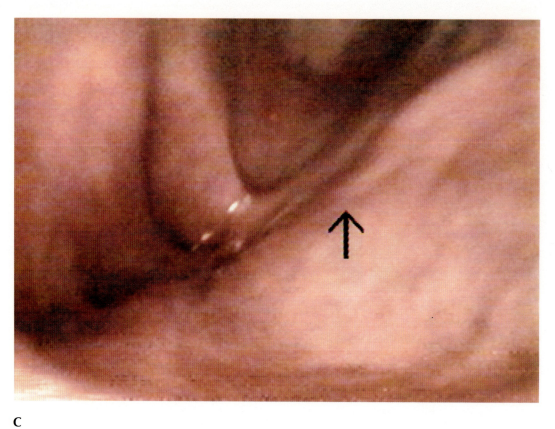

C. Vocal fold aspect 5 years after left cordectomy.

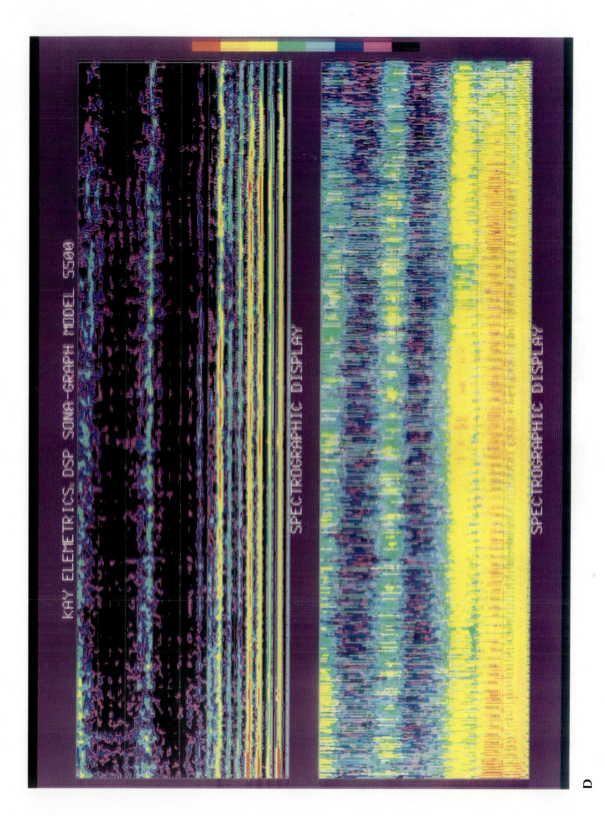

D. Spectrography: F_0 + 9 partial frequencies; voice is improved.

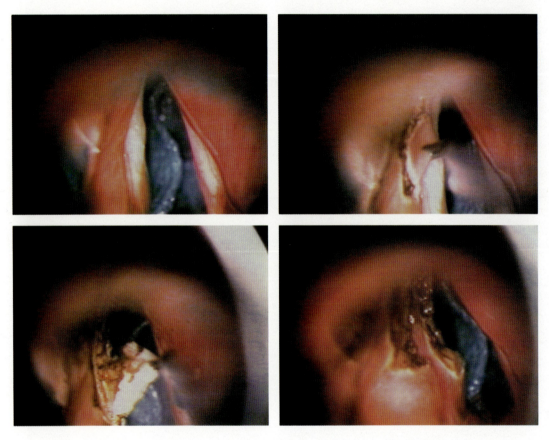

A

PLATE 4.118: **A.** Cordectomy type II for carcinoma T1N0.

1	2
3	4

1. Exposure of the glottic area, carcinoma on the smear test is diagnosed. The vocal fold is not well observed. The false vocal fold must be removed.
2. Removal of the false vocal fold. The A-forceps grasps it and pulls it toward the glottic space.
3. The vocal fold is removed from front to back and a frozen section is carried out.
4. Exposure of the glottic space after surgery.

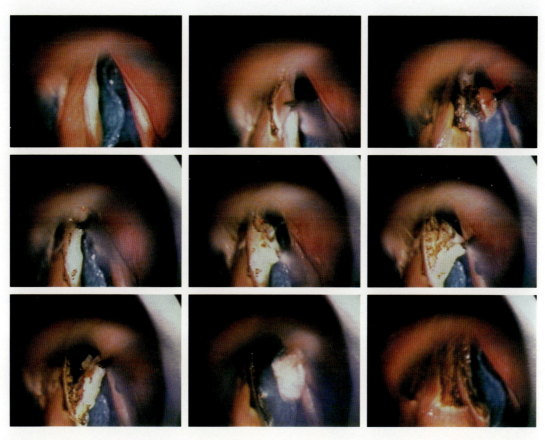

B. Cordectomy type II for carcinoma T1N0.

1	2	3
4	5	6
7	8	9

1. Exposure of the vocal fold: carcinoma.
2. False vocal fold is removed.
3. A-forceps takes it off.
4. Exposure of the two vocal folds. The lesion does not spread in the ventricle. It is limited.
5. The A-forceps grasps the vocal fold and pulls it into the glottic space. A 90° angle of shooting is used to start and the impact goes parallel to the border.
6. Parallel impact to the border.
7. On the posterior incision, 90° angle impact.
8. Removal of the vocal fold, sample, and frozen section.
9. Exposure of the larynx: anterior commissure and posterior commissure are spread. No bleeding is observed. No coagulation was necessary.

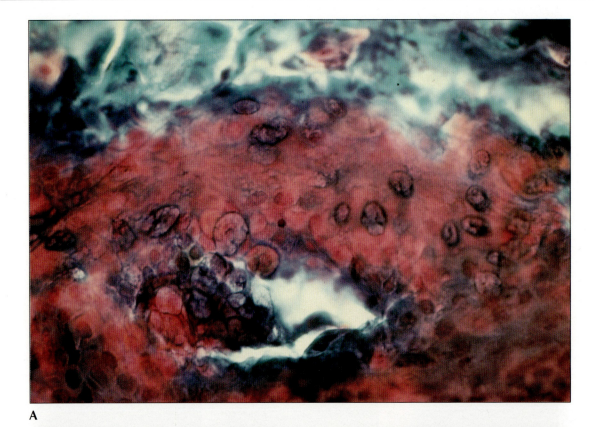

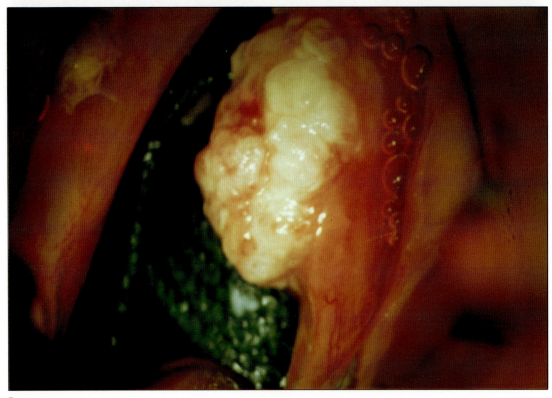

PLATE 4.119: **A.** Smear test of carcinoma. **B.** Invasive carcinoma. View of the larynx showing carcinoma of the right vocal fold. Cordectomy type III is performed.

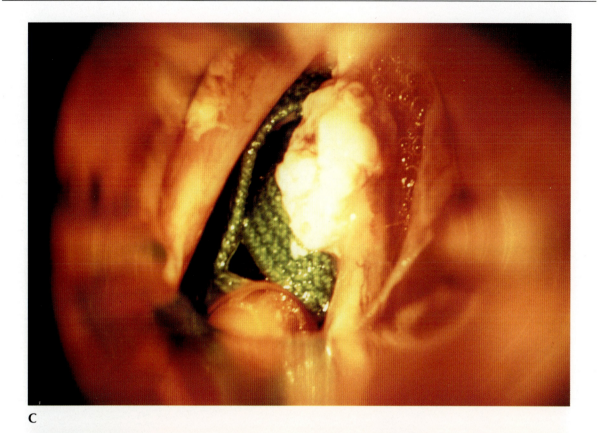

C

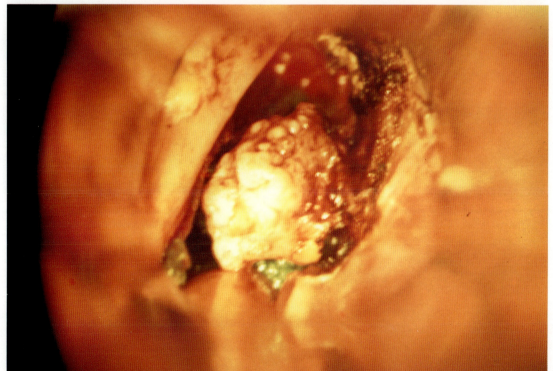

D

C. Laser surgery is performed. A total cordectomy, type III, after removal of the false vocal fold. **D.** Ablation of the vocal fold with the muscles.

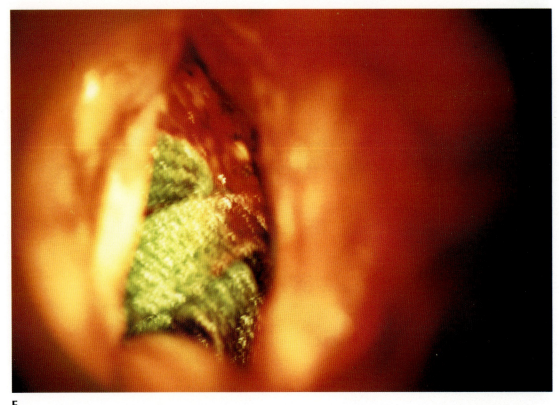

E

E. The excision bed is bloodless and smoothly cleansed. The frozen section has diagnosed an invasive carcinoma.

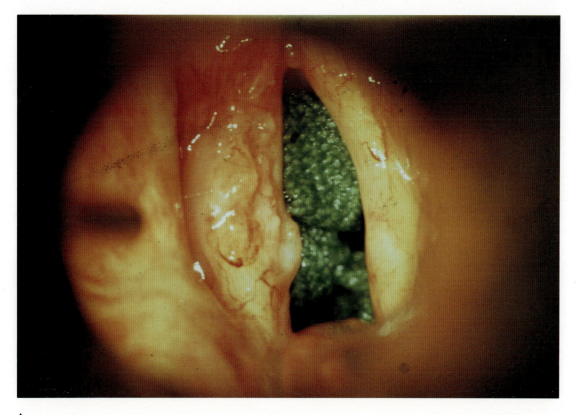

A

PLATE 4.120: **A.** Invasive carcinoma: cordectomy type III. Visualization of a left vocal fold carcinoma. The anterior and posterior commissure are spared.

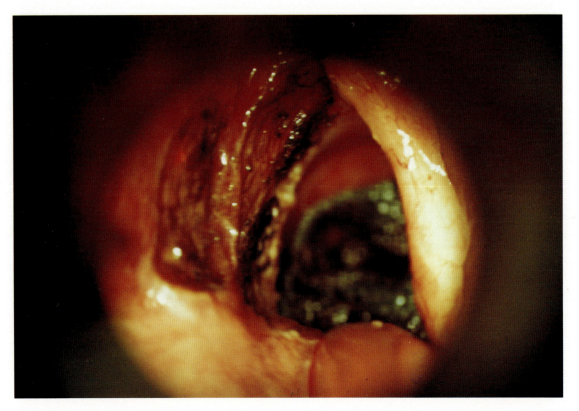

B

B. Total cordectomy (left) is performed. We can see on the bottom of the upper part the false vocal fold muscle.

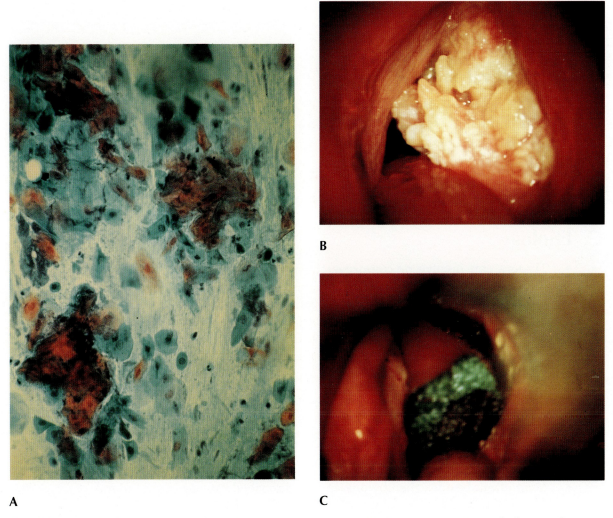

PLATE 4.121: **A.** Smear test: cytology of verrucous carcinoma. **B.** Verrucous carcinoma before cordectomy type III. **C.** Verrucous carcinoma after cordectomy. The false vocal fold is removed, true vocal fold also.

PARALYSIS OF VOCAL FOLDS

A. Definition

Recurrent laryngeal nerve paralysis may be unilateral or bilateral, in adduction or in abduction, depending on the network of muscles affected.

The causes are various, the consequences are always immobility of the vocal folds with amyotrophy.

B. Location

1. Unilateral paralysis

Unilateral paralysis occurs mostly in women and, in our experience, 74% on the left side, in adduction or abduction.

2. Bilateral paralysis

The vocal folds are almost always in adduction, creating dyspnea.

C. Etiology

- Tumors can involve or compress the vocal nerve, for example, nodules, tumors of the base of the skull, and carcinoma of the nasopharynx and esophagus. The left recurrent nerve is more often affected because of its anatomy. A tumor in the left chest may give left vocal fold paralysis. In neck tumors, such as cancer of the thyroid gland, both recurrent laryngeal nerves may be affected. Trauma from mechanical stretching of the nerve during surgery can also occur.

- After thyroidectomy, carotid surgery, or cardiac and left lung surgery, vocal fold paralysis may appear due to section of the recurrent nerve.

- Viruses are involved but have not been proved as a cause of this neuritis (upper respiratory infection, mononucleosis, herpetic virus).

- Most often, besides the obvious causes described, no etiology is found for paralysis of a vocal fold; it often is an idiopathic paralysis.

D. Clinical Approach

1. Primary Symptoms

- Unilateral paralysis produces hoarseness and breathiness, rarely diplophonia.

- Bilateral paralysis causes breathiness and severe dysphonia, sometimes with stridor.

2. Tele-Video-Naso-Fiberscope and Telescope

- Unilateral paralysis is observed in adduction or abduction. Amyotrophy is often obvious after surgical section of the laryngeal recurrent nerve.
- Bilateral paralysis is observed in adduction, mainly after surgical procedures.
- In the glottic level, the affected vocal fold seems to be under the healthy vocal fold.

3. Stroboscopy

- In unilateral paralysis in abduction, there is no sign because the vocal folds do not close.
- In unilateral paralysis in adduction, vibrations with irregular amplitudes, asymmetry, and aperiodic waves and weak vocal fold closure are observed.
- In bilateral paralysis in adduction, the vocal vibratory mass produces irregular waves that are aperiodic but symmetrical during phonation.
- In any kind of paralysis, stroboscopy shows that the energy of the sounds is the airflow when vocal folds touch each other by the Bernoulli effect.

4. Electroglottography (EGG)

EGG patterns reveal a short closure phase and a long open phase. Waves are almost flat.

5. Spectrography

- A reduced register with few or no harmonics is seen. Noise is high.
- Voice intensity is weak.

E. Conclusion

1. **Unilateral paralysis in adduction** will not need a surgical treatment. Voice therapy is necessary, and the results are satisfactory.
2. **Unilateral paralysis in abduction** may require phonosurgery for augmentation if voice therapy fails.

Gelfoam paste, collagen, or fat may be used for augmentation. These materials tend to undergo partial or total resorption. During the procedure, the integrity of the epithelium and the lamina propria, such as the visco-elasticity of the vibratory mass, must be preserved as much as possible. The material is injected in the upper surface of the middle third of the vocal fold. The vocal fold is displaced toward the midline, without changing its level, to ensure the closure of the glottic space during phonation.

Teflon can be injected but may cause complications, such as granuloma. Teflon particles may migrate to the entire vocal fold muscle and also to nodes, lungs, or kidneys. We have reported one case.

Teflon also may induce a foreign body reaction with subsequent development of giant cells and fibrous tissue. In our series, 17% of patients developed granulomas.

Other techniques, described by Isshiki (1974) and modified by Tucker, of external laryngeal surgery also give excellent results in good hands. Reinnervation (Tucker technique) seems to restore the tonus of the vocal fold muscle, even if it does not always restore mobility, and combined with laryngeal framework surgery gives good results.

3. In **bilateral adduction paralysis**, laser arytenoidectomy remains the best technique to reestablish the airway. There must be two surgical goals:

- Retain the voice
- Restore the breath

We speak with the anterior portion of the vocal fold; we breathe with the posterior portion. In fact, it is not as simple as that. In the endoscopic technique, we remove the arytenoid and the posterior vocal fold process without affecting the anterior two thirds of the vocal folds: it is a cordotomy and an arytenoidectomy.

The procedure is performed by laser-laryngoscopy with a classical spot size of 400 microns. The left arytenoid is removed from front to back, external to internal site, after cortisone injection in the cricoarytenoid joint. Coagulation of the posterior arteries is done, for which the laser is used with a power of 10 watts, using continuous mode to ablate the arytenoid.

We do not vaporize the cartilage, but take it off.

Results of this laser surgery are satisfactory.

Paralysis of the Vocal Folds

The goal of laser phonosurgery is to:

- restore an efficient closure of the glottic space
- allow vocal fold vibration
- preserve the airflow

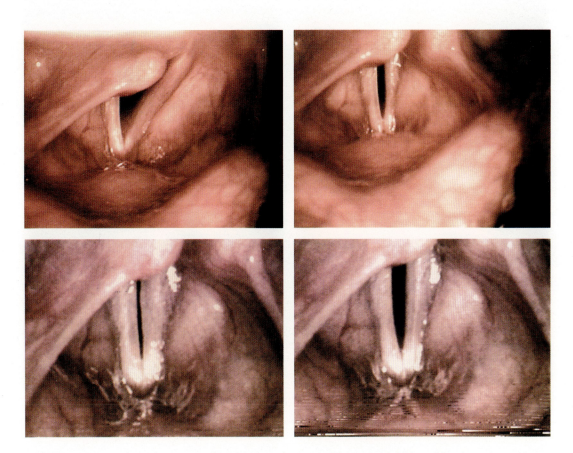

PLATE 4.122: Tele-videoscopy showing paralysis of right vocal fold in adduction: no surgery; voice therapy.

1	2
3	4

1. Breathing phase: right arytenoid falls into the vocal process.
2. Vocal attack.
3. Vibrations of the vocal folds are observed.
4. End of phonation.

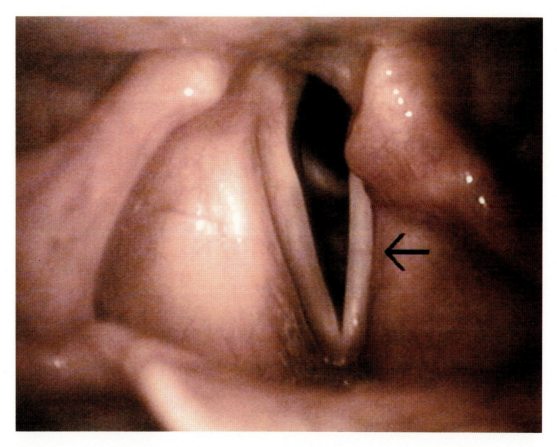

A

PLATE 4.123: **A.** Tele-videoscopy showing paralysis of left vocal fold in abduction after thoracic surgery: Amyotrophy of the left vocal fold (breathing phase).

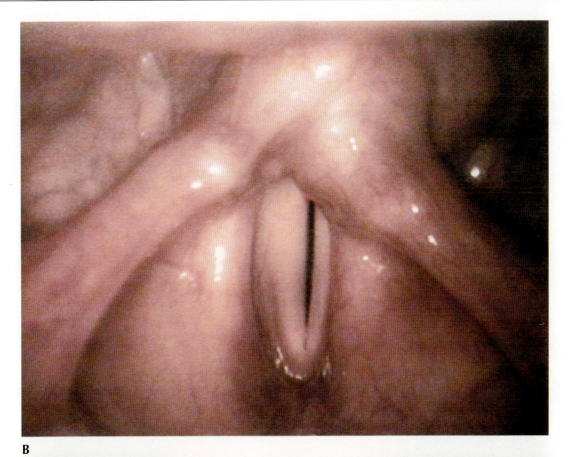

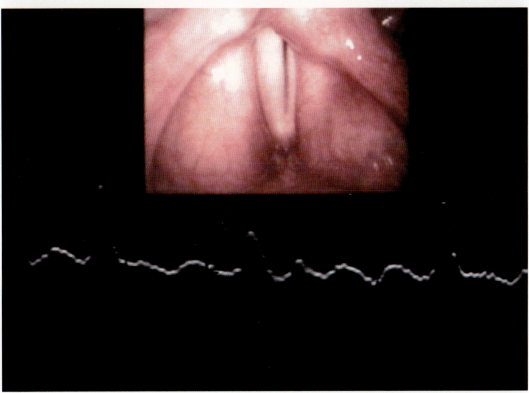

B. Phonation in case shown in **A**. **C.** Phonation with EGG: irregular patterns with a long open vibration phase.

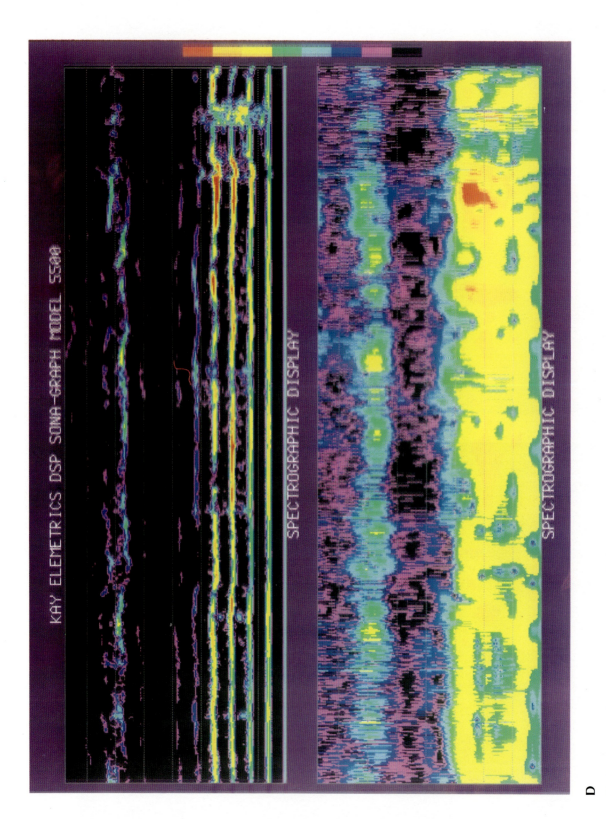

D. Spectrography of case shown in **A–C** showing:
- Reduced register: high pitch.
- Five harmonics.
- Level of noise slightly increases.
- Formants are correct with these harmonics.

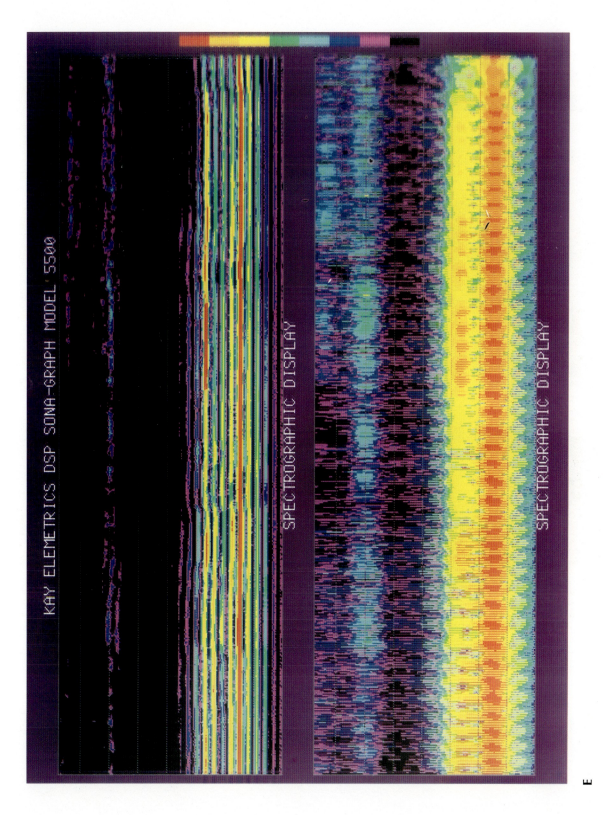

E. Spectrography of case shown in **A–D** is the same as seen in **D** but with low pitch.

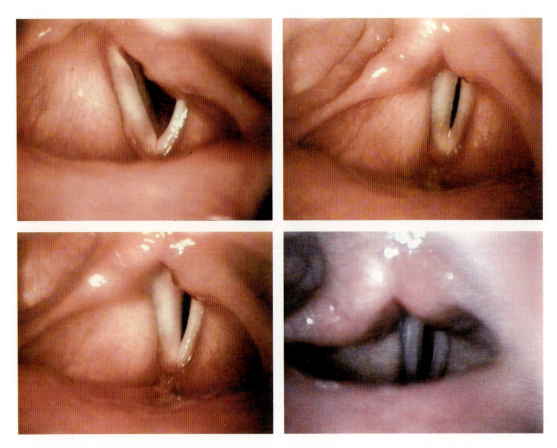

PLATE 4.124: Tele-videoscopy showing paralysis of left vocal fold in adduction:

1	2
3	4

1. Breathing phase.
2. Vocal attack.
3. Vibrations of the vocal folds.
4. End of phonation.

Laryngeal Pathologies: PARALYSIS

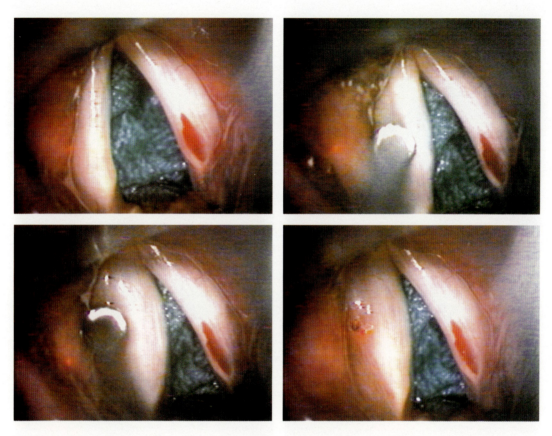

PLATE 4.125: Phonosurgery for increasing the volume of the vocal fold with collagen.

1	2
3	4

1. Larynx exposure: amyotrophy of the left vocal fold.
2. Setting of the needle on the middle third, superior surface.
3. Injection of collagen.
4. Laser is performed to seal the puncture.

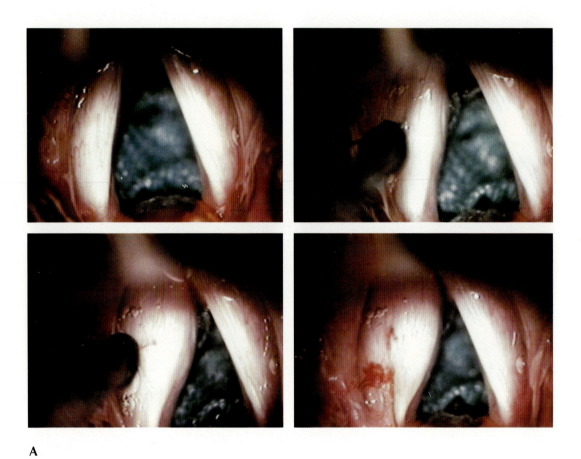

A

PLATE 4.126: **A.** Same technique shown in **Plate 4.125**. Spectrographic data were recorded.

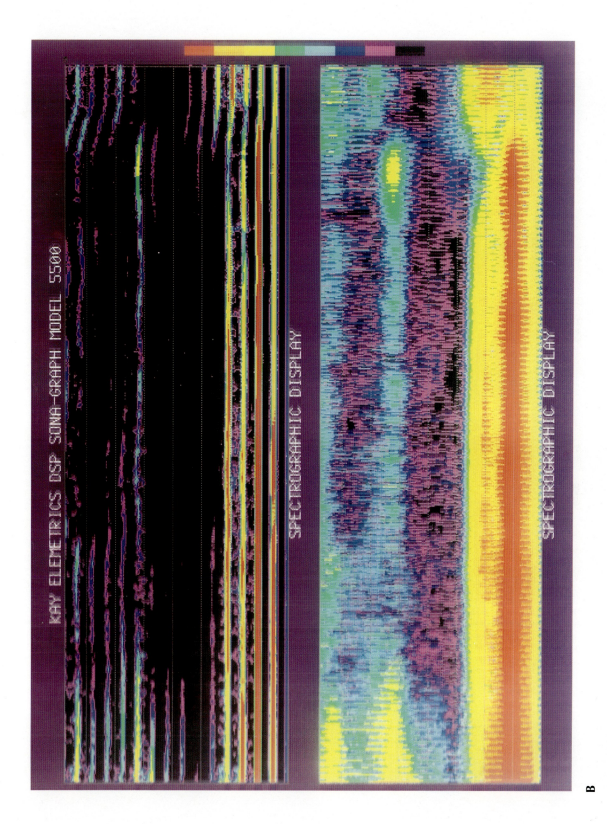

B. Spectrography before surgery for case shown in **A.**

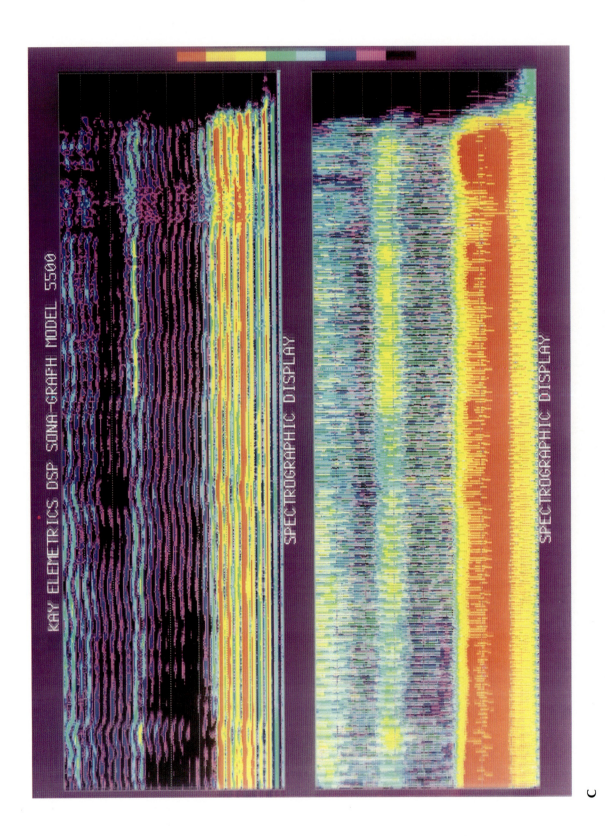

C. Spectrography after surgery for case shown in **A** and **B**.

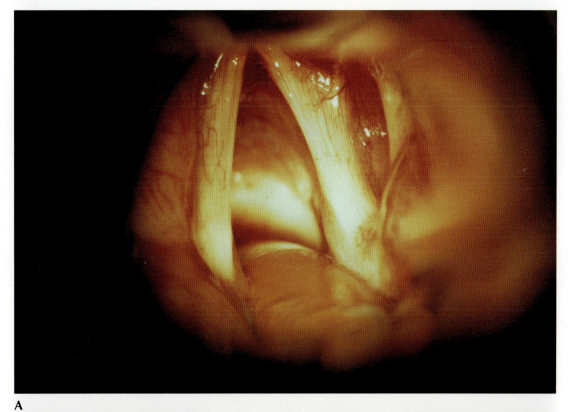

A

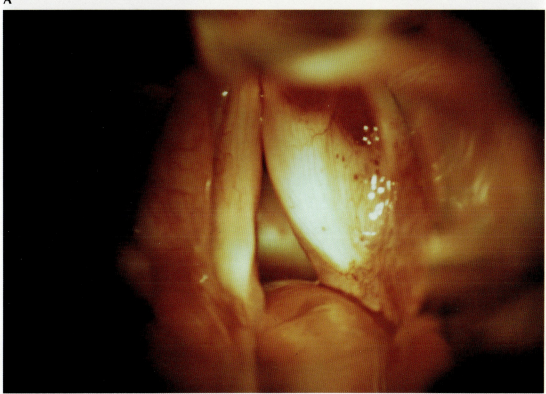

B

PLATE 4.127: **A.** Larynx exposure under laryngoscopy showing paralysis of right vocal fold. **B.** Same case shown in **A** after Teflon injection.

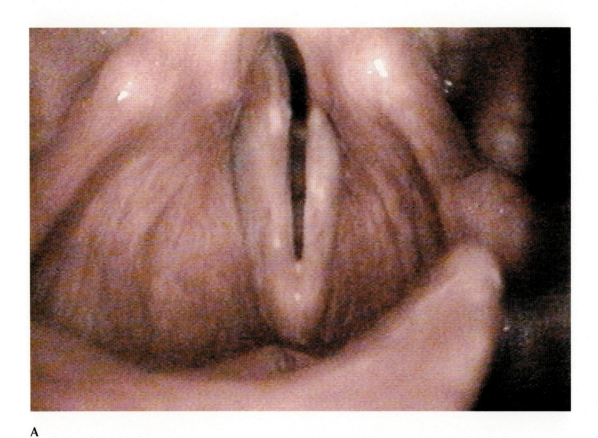

A

PLATE 4.128: **A.** Bilateral paralysis in adduction. During breathing. **B.** Case shown in **A** during phonation. **C.** EGG of case shown in **A** and **B** shows irregular patterns.

Laryngeal Pathologies: PARALYSIS

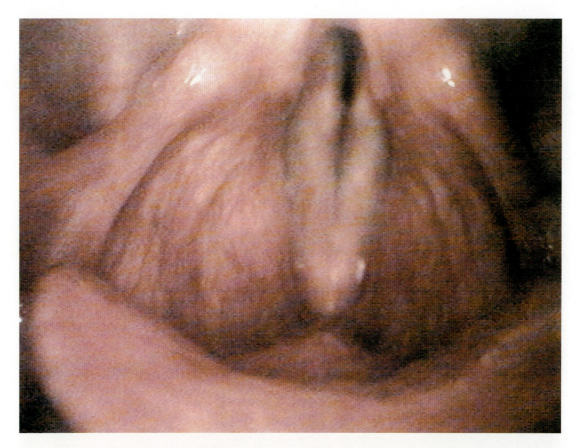

B

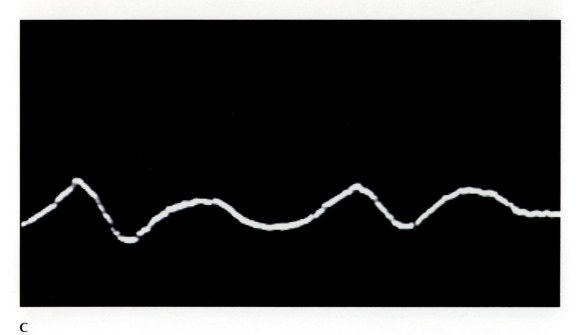

C

351

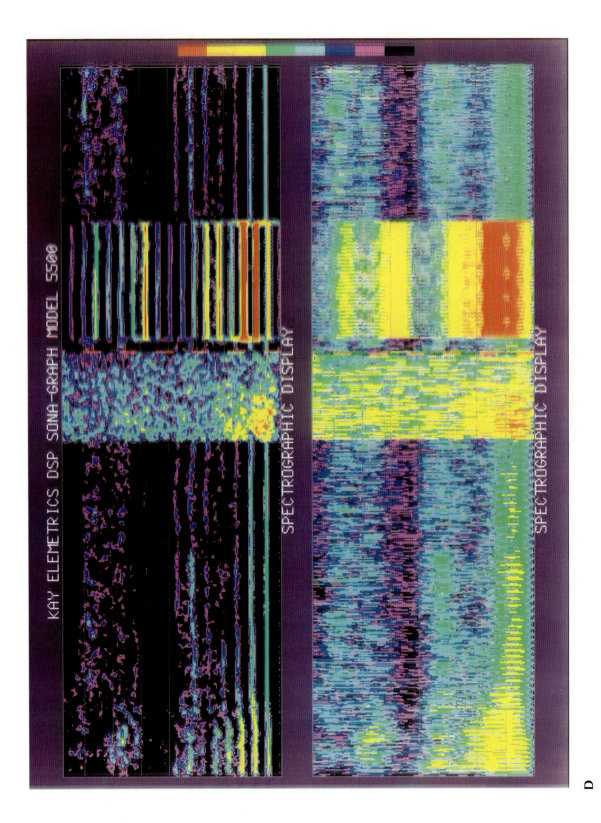

D. Spectrography of case shown in **A–D**. Note: (a) Very narrow register: two harmonics with a high level of noise; (b) stridor during breathing; (c) normal voice; (d) same as (a), formants are synchronized with harmonics. (a), (b), and (c) are the patient's patterns.

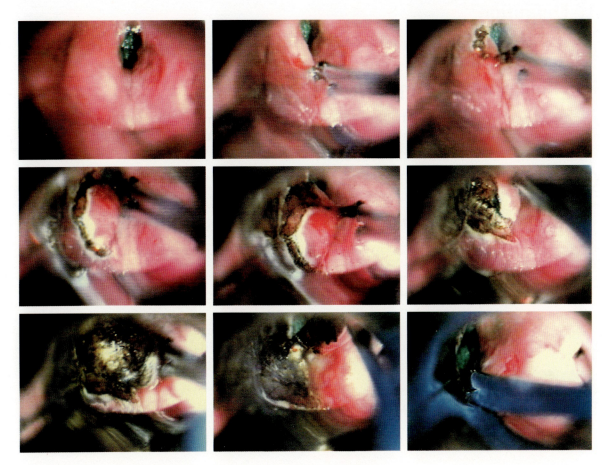

PLATE 4.129: Arytenoidectomy: laser microsurgical procedure.

1. Exposure of the larynx, protection of the subglottic space with the green gauze.
2. A-forceps grasps the arytenoid.
3. Impact: Laser starts: 10 watts, continuous fire.
4. The laser beam goes around the arytenoid mass.
5–8. Removal of the arytenoid mass.
9. End of the surgical procedure.

SUB-ANKYLOSIS OF THE CRICOARYTENOID JOINT

A. Definition

It is an ankylosis of the cricoarytenoid joint.

B. Etiology and Histopathogeny

Besides arthritis, most of the time this condition is due to intubation trauma. In long-standing cases, it is difficult to distinguish from a paralyzed vocal fold.

C. Clinical Approach

1. Primary Symptoms

- When one side is involved, hoarseness and dysphagia are observed.
- When both sides are involved, dyspnea is observed.
- Phonation time is always reduced.
- It must last more than 3 weeks; an acute laryngitis may involve an inflammatory reaction of the cricoarytenoid joints.

2. Tele-Video-Naso-Fiberscope and Telescope

Most of the time, the vocal fold is blocked in an adducted position.

Glottal closure is often incomplete. When both vocal folds are involved, dyspnea—with or without stridor—may occur.

Please note that the vocal muscle is not amyotrophied.

3. Stroboscopy

When vocal fold closure is possible, there is regular vibration because mechanical properties are intact.

4. Electroglottography (EGG)

EGG shows a long open phase and is periodic and regular with a small amplitude.

5. Spectrography

In unilateral ankylosis, reduced register with three to five harmonics and increased noise are observed. In bilateral ankylosis, noise is predominant, voice intensity is weak, and a reduced register with noise is observed.

D. Conclusion

Ankylosis of the cricoarytenoid joint:

1. **In adduction:** The joint should be manipulated under direct laryngoscopy with specially designed forceps (Micro-France).
2. **In abduction:** If manipulation of the cricoarytenoid joint does not work, it will require an injection technique. Collagen or fat may be used after failure of 6 months of voice therapy.
3. **In bilateral adduction pathology:** A laser arytenoidectomy must be performed to avoid a tracheotomy.

Ankylosis of the cricoarytenoid joint requires different treatment depending on the position of the vocal folds in the glottic space.

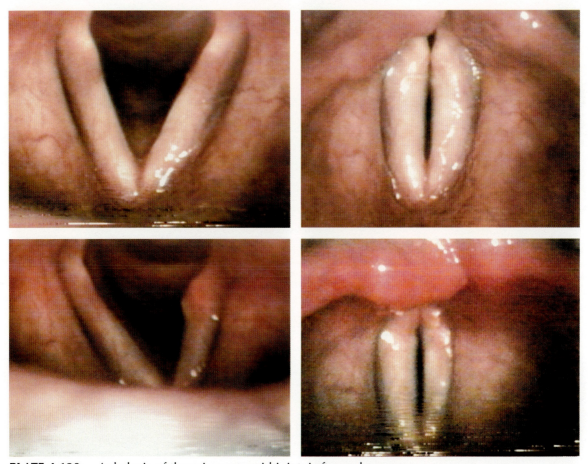

PLATE 4.130: Ankylosis of the cricoarytenoid joint. Left vocal process.

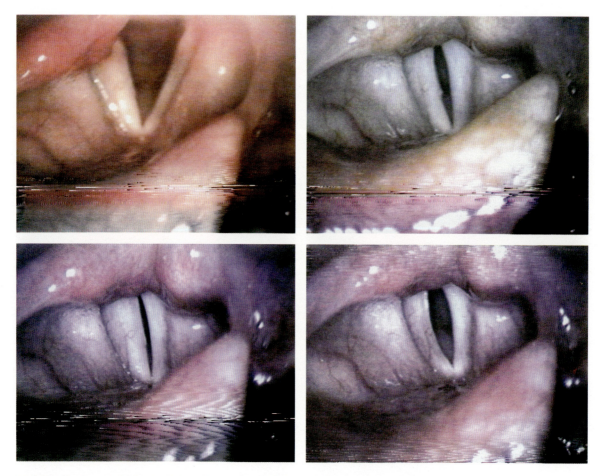

PLATE 4.131: Ankylosis of the cricoarytenoid joint. Right vocal process.

HERNIA OF THE FALSE VOCAL FOLDS OR LARYNGOCELE

A. Definition

A bilateral or unilateral hypertrophy of the false vocal fold, which produces a ventricular dysphonia.

B. Location

False vocal folds are increased on one side; in some cases, on both sides.

C. Etiology and Histopathogeny

1. Etiology and Pathogenesis

Vocal abuse is the main factor for hypertrophy of the false vocal folds. Patients have a hard glottal attack and an antero-posterior squeezing. They "push" on their voice with an inappropriate pitch. The results of such behavior more often produce true vocal fold lesions, although rarely we observe a false vocal fold pathology with a husky voice. If ventricular phonation is due to psychogenic dysphonia, voice therapy must be performed for at least 1 year. If this therapy fails and the patient does not like his or her voice, it may lead to laser surgery.

2. Macroscopic Aspect and Histology

- It shows increased development of columnar, ciliated epithelium, mainly of the glandular cells, with dilatated glandular ducts. Many inflammatory cells are seen in the superficial corium with increased capillaries and adipose stroma.

- Usually, it is not keratinized.

D. Clinical Approach

1. Primary Symptoms

The voice is low in pitch and intensity, more or less hoarse sounding, sometimes cracking or diplophonia.

2. Tele-Video-Naso-Fiberscope and Telescope

- Acoustic data and tele-video-endoscopy will reveal the diagnosis of ventricular phonation and the hernia of the false vocal folds or laryngocele.

- The vocal folds are hidden under the false vocal folds. They may touch if both sides are involved. Videofiberscopy allows more precise observation of the true vocal folds and analysis of the vocal attack.

3. Stroboscopy

This is the most revealing examination.

a. If one false vocal fold is involved:

- The true vocal fold on the same side may or may not vibrate, as if the ventricular mass were touching the epithelium of the vocal fold (vibratory mass).
- The false vocal fold may vibrate also, and may be synchronized or asynchronized with the vocal fold.
- It may totally stop the vibration of the affected larynx.

b. If both false vocal folds are involved.

- The true vocal folds may or may not vibrate.
- Most of the time, the false vocal folds vibrate and prevent the true vocal folds from vibrating.

These signs are fundamental for follow-up after voice therapy.

4. Electroglottography (EGG)

EGG is very irregular and may show supraglottic contact.

5. Spectrography

Loss of harmonics is important, as is loss of formants. Noise levels are very high. During voice therapy, follow-up with spectrography is important to check voice improvement. Harmonics and intensity recover from low to high partial harmonics.

E. Conclusion

This is often a reversible pathology. Voice therapy will help to improve these symptoms. After 1 year of voice therapy, if the patient does not like his or her voice, laser phonosurgery will be performed to remove one or both false vocal folds with very satisfactory results.

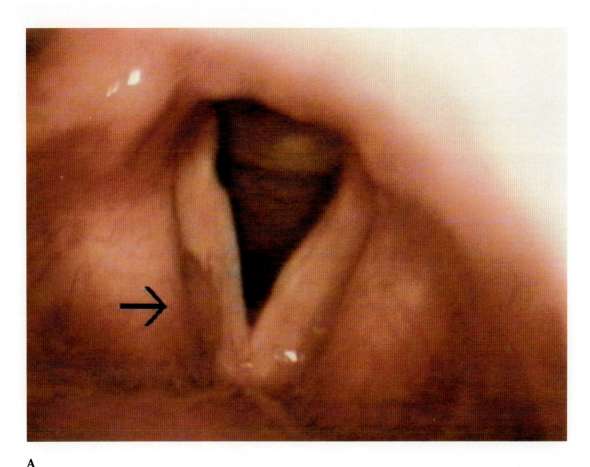

A

PLATE 4.132: **A.** Hernia of the right false vocal fold. Tele-videoscopy. Visible during breathing.

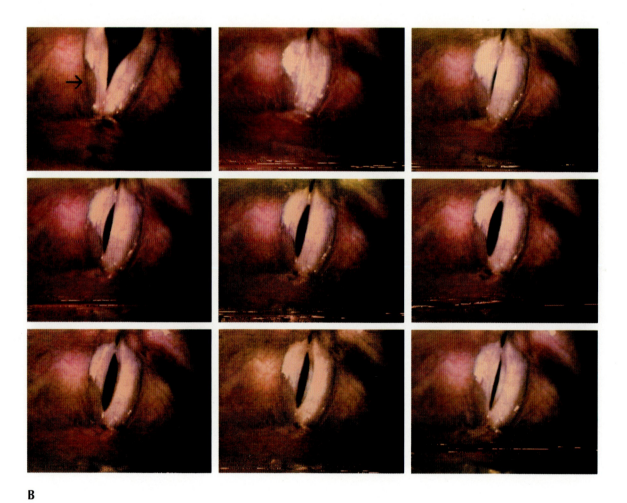

B

B. During stroboscopy (9 steps). It is an hyperfunctional dysphonia. Hernia is purely functional. The mechanical structures are disturbed, as if these false vocal folds touch the true vocal folds and stop the vibratory cycle. The hernia may vibrate also. Voice therapy is performed for 1 year.

Laryngeal Pathologies: LARYNGOCELE

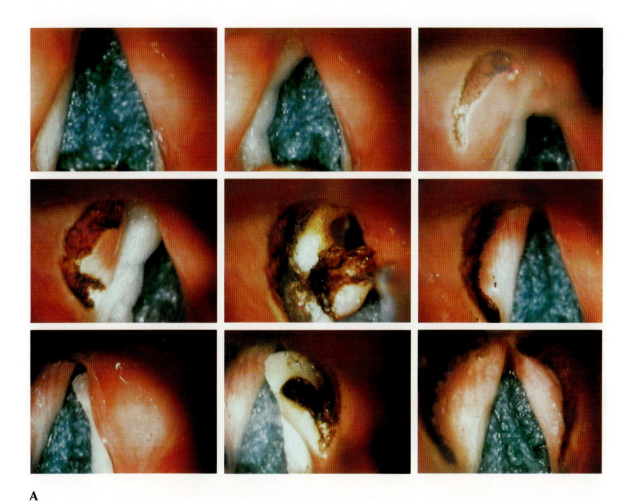

A

PLATE 4.133: **A.** Hernia or hypertrophy of the false vocal folds, which remained after 6 months of voice therapy. Laser microsurgery is performed because the voice is very rough and dysphonia important.

1	2	3
4	5	6
7	8	9

1. Larynx exposure: False vocal folds can be seen well. The true vocal folds are hidden.
2. A small piece of white cotton is put between the true and the false vocal folds inside the ventricle.
3. Laser surgery is performed: 10 watts, continuous mode.
4–5. The A-forceps helps to remove the sample.
6. The true vocal fold is seen well.
7. A small piece of white cotton is put in the right ventricle.
8. Removal of the right false vocal fold.
9. End of surgery: no laser impact on the vocal fold.

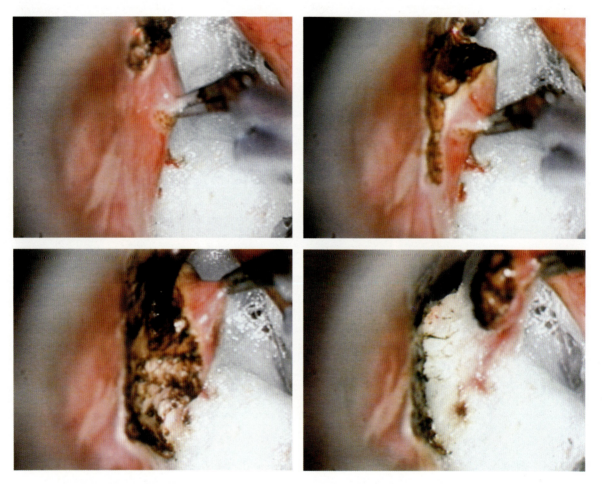

B

B. Removal of the false vocal fold with a magnified vision.

1	2
3	4

1. First impact in the anterior part of the false vocal fold; the A-forceps grasps it toward the glottic space. The cotton protects the vocal fold.
2–3. Removal of the false vocal fold: it is bloodless.
4. End of the procedure.

EPIGLOTTIC AND VALLECULAR CYSTS

A. Definition

It is a cyst lined by squamous or columnar epithelium on the epiglottis.

B. Location

This cyst develops from the lingual surface of the epiglottis and rarely extends to the aryepiglottic fold.

C. Etiology and Histopathogeny

1. Etiology and Pathogenesis

This has not been well explained. It appears after 35 years of age and is as commonly found in men as women.

2. Macroscopic Aspect and Histology

- Cysts are made of a network of capillaries surrounding the plump yellow cyst.
- It is composed of squamous or columnar epithelium on the surface with a yellow, gelatinous glue inside.

D. Clinical Approach

1. Primary Symptoms

A discomfort in the throat with the feeling that the voice is smothered, and there is prominent dysphagia.

2. Tele-Video-Naso-Fiberscope and Telescope

- Video-telescope and video-fiberscope reveal the epiglottic cyst. It is usually single. The cyst can be discovered incidentally or because of pseudo-dysphonia and dysphagia.
- It appears with a lot of capillaries on the surface of a plump, yellow round mass between the epiglottis and the tongue.

3. Stroboscopy, Electroglottography, and Spectrography

All are normal.

E. Conclusion

If the cyst is small, it may not need any treatment.

If the epiglottic cyst is large, laser surgery must be performed. The laryngoscope is placed above the epiglottis smoothly. The laser opens the cyst, the A-forceps grasps it, and the laser will decorticate the surface of the cyst to remove the entire sac.

Results are satisfactory with no recurrence.

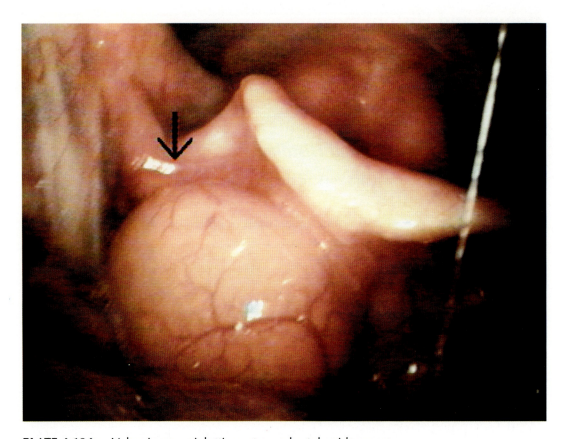

PLATE 4.134: Voluminous epiglottic cyst seen by tele-videoscopy.

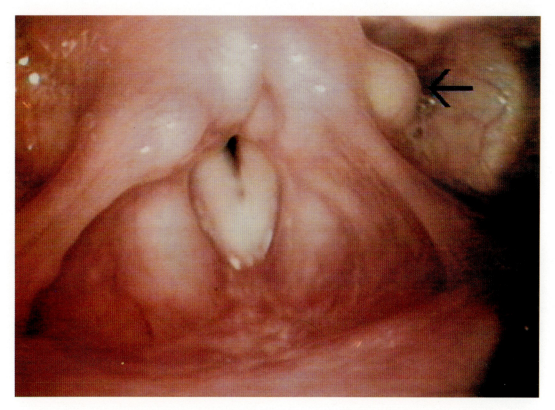

PLATE 4.135: Extralaryngeal cyst located on the posterior and lateral surface of the arytenoids.

LARYNGEAL STENOSIS

A. Definition

Laryngeal stenosis is a narrowing of the lumen with dysphonia and obstruction of the airway.

B. Location

Larynx.

C. Etiology

It occurs in a wide variety of conditions. Beside congenital abnormalities, it appears after trauma or prolonged intubation, and mainly in women.

D. Clinical Approach

Before attempting any laser surgery, it is necessary to determine precisely the level, the nature, and the extension of the stenosis by CT scan of the larynx and the trachea. Severity of the patient's symptoms may lead to a tracheotomy.

A fiber-videoscopy of the larynx and the trachea must be performed to evaluate the precise location of the stenosis.

E. Conclusion

If the stenosis is severe, a tracheostomy may be necessary. If severe dyspnea is not present, and voice is correct, no laser surgery should be undertaken.

Laser surgery may be palliative when a tracheostomy is necessary for the first step. It is curative when only the laser laryngo-endoscopic surgery can be performed (more than 95% of the time).

Laryngeal stenosis is often associated with subglottic stenosis. (see Plates 4.136–4.137)

Two kinds of stenosis may be distinguished:

1. **Diphragmatic stenosis** consists of a ring of scar tissue. If thin, laser surgery may be efficacious; if thick, an external surgical procedure will be necessary (Plate 4.138).
2. **Anterior stenosis** may be improved by laser micro-endolaryngeal technique.

To perform surgery in laryngeal stenosis, the scar tissue must be dry, mature, and not inflammed; and most importantly, the patient must not have any coughing, disease, or reflux. Often, several laser procedures are necessary.

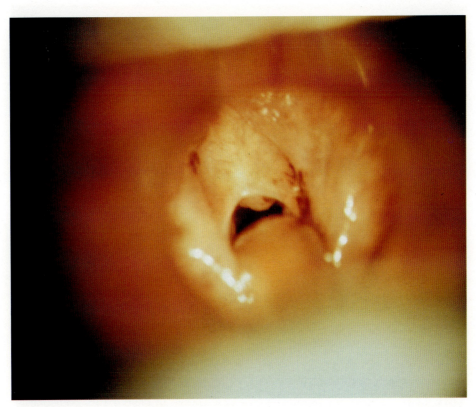

PLATE 4.136: Exposure of a laryngeal synechiae with granuloma on the subglottic space.

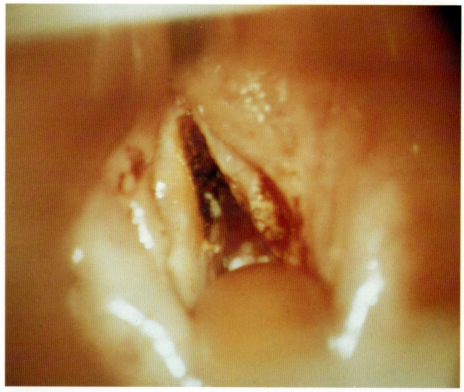
PLATE 4.137: After laser vaporization in case shown in Plate 4.136, cortisone is injected on both sides.

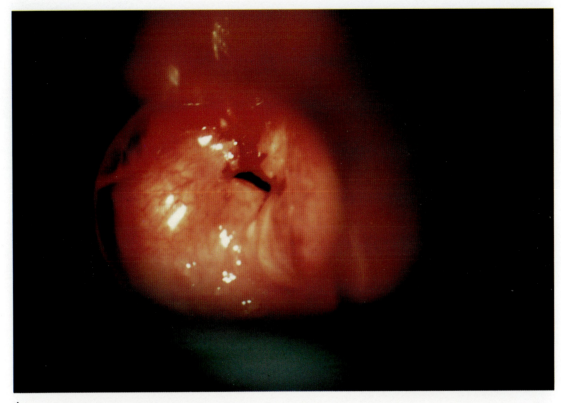

A

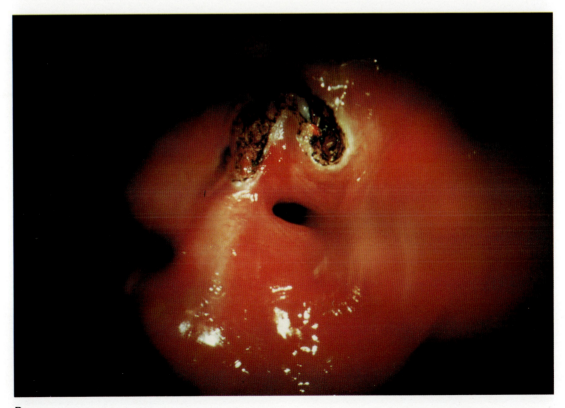

B

PLATE 4.138: **A.** Diaphragmatic stenosis with a ring of scar tissue. **B.** Laser impact on the anterior commissure (10 watts, continuous mode).

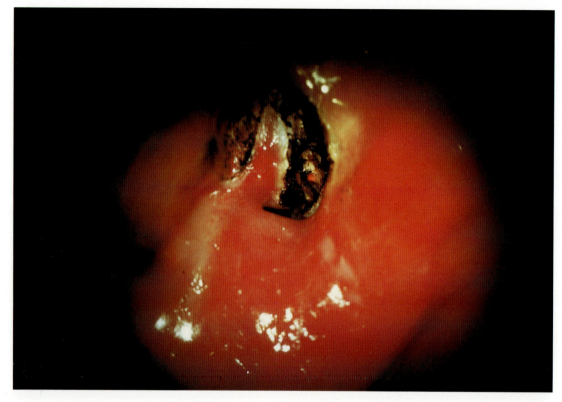

C

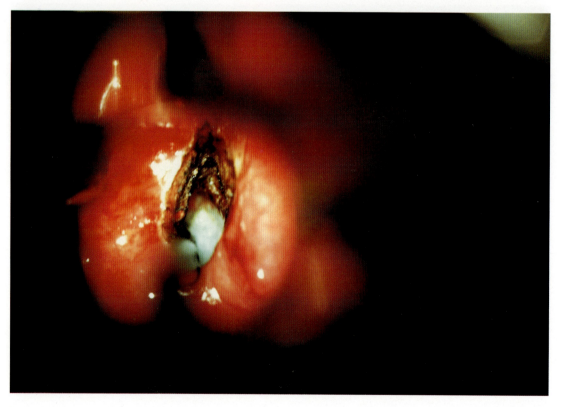

D

C. Laser impact to the posterior commissure. **D.** The glottic space is free of obstruction.

CONGENITAL LARYNGEAL WEB

A. Definition

A web is a process that connects the two vocal folds. It may be congenital or acquired following a trauma by laryngeal surgery, intubation, infection, or other causes.

B. Location

It is located on the anterior commissure. It can be small or involve both the anterior thirds of the vocal process. Webs can be thin or thick, attaching only on the glottic edges, in some cases also in the subglottic area, but rarely on the supraglottic area.

C. Etiology and Histopathogeny

1. Etiology and Pathogenesis

It is congenital.

2. Macroscopic Aspect and Histology

Webs are composed of squamous epithelium and connective tissue and are very thin, and transparent. In some cases, an anomaly of the cricoid cartilage is also observed.

D. Clinical Approach

1. Primary Symptoms

Voice has a high pitch level, weak intensity, and poor timbre.

2. Tele-Video-Naso-Fiberscope and Telescope

Vocal folds are "stopped" by a transparent membrane.

3. Stroboscopy

- Mucosal waves are normal until contact with the web.
- The membrane of the web does not vibrate.

4. Electroglottography (EGG)

- The closure phase is increased.
- Waves are regular, but amplitude is increased.

5. Spectrography

It is normal. The F_0 (fundamental frequency) is higher than usual.

E. Conclusion

There is no reason to operate on a microweb if there are no complaints from the patient. The "plastic pleasure of the surgeon" to see perfect vocal folds is erroneous.

If the congenital web significantly disturbs the voice, laser surgery must be performed, and during the same procedure, an injection of cortisone is given on the anterior third of the vocal fold.

For large webs, the laser used with the microspot is a perfect tool. A power of 1.5 watts is used in continuous fire mode.

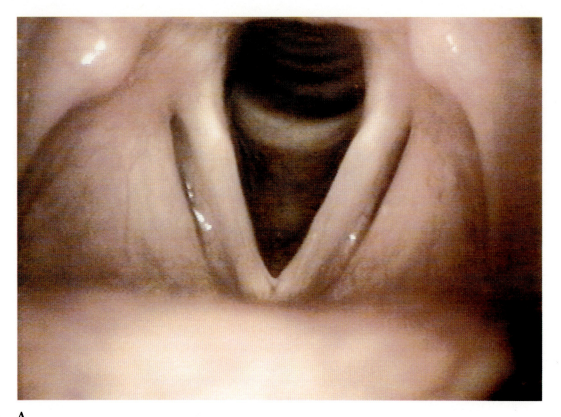

A

PLATE 4.139: **A.** A congenital microweb that did not require surgery.

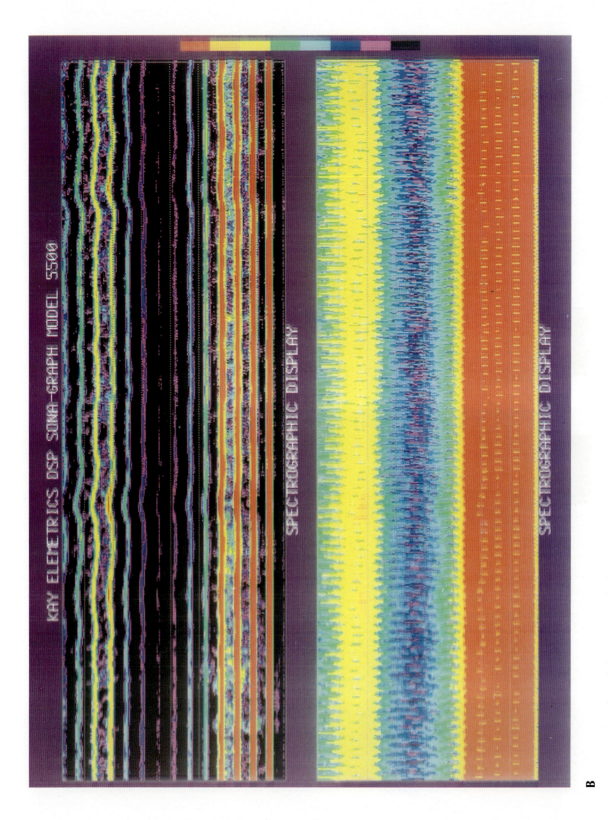

B. Spectrography of the microweb shown in **A**. The voice pattern is normal, all harmonics are present, formants are normal, and noise level is low.

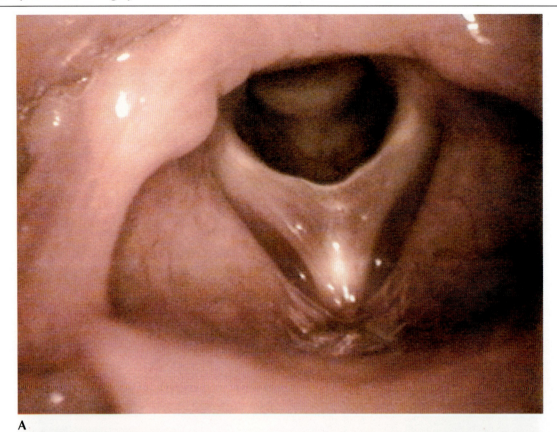

PLATE 4.140: **A.** Tele-videoscopy of congenital web located on the anterior commissure in an 11-year-old child. It is typically thin and transparent. **B.** Tele-videoscopy during phonation with EGG patterns. Closing phase is short with a double step.

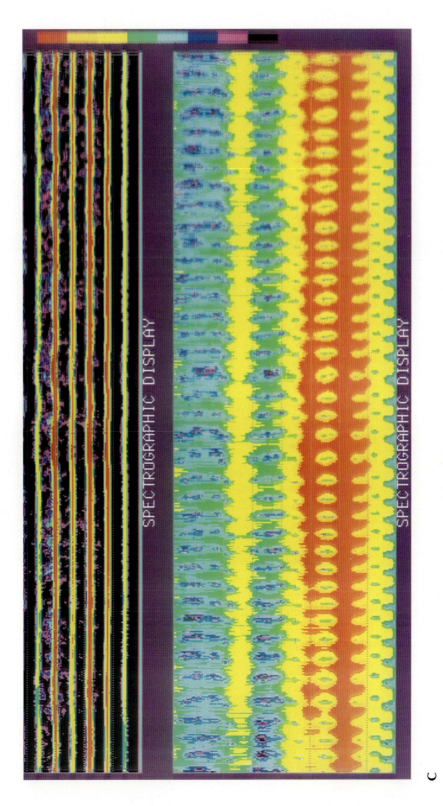

C. Spectography of case shown in **A** and **B** is almost normal. Harmonics and formants are normal. The level of noise is slightly increased. No surgery was performed.

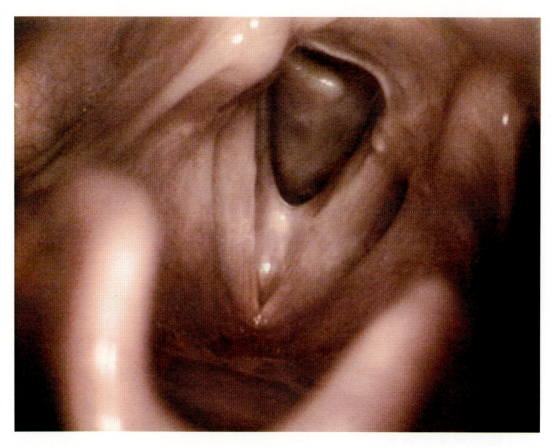

A

PLATE 4.141: **A.** Congenital web with bad voice. Spectrography pattern is necessary. The web extends under the free edges of the vocal fold. **B.** Spectrography of case **A** showing reduced range and few harmonics (6). Formants are synchronized with harmonics.

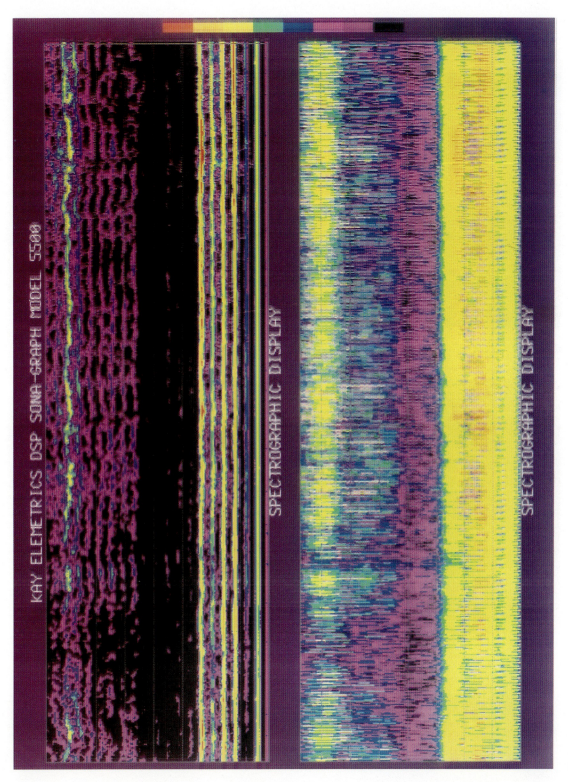

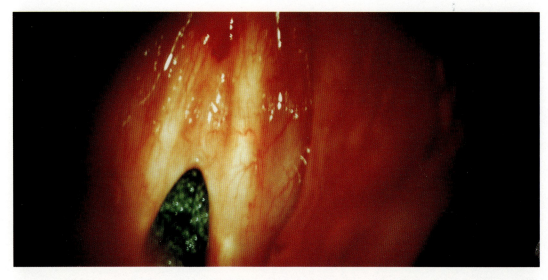

C

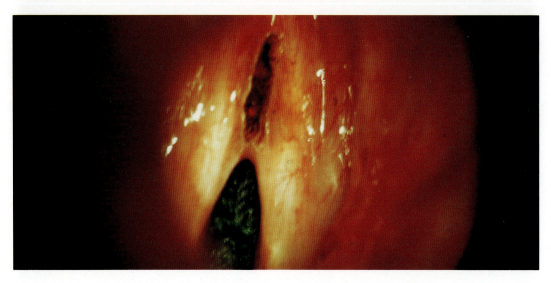

D

C. Exposure of the larynx in case shown in **A** and **B**. **D.** Attack by laser impact on the medial line (see **A–C**). **E.** Cortisone is injected on the anterior third of the vocal fold. End of the surgical procedure: The web is thick near the anterior commissure. This explains why voice is so bad (see **A–D**).

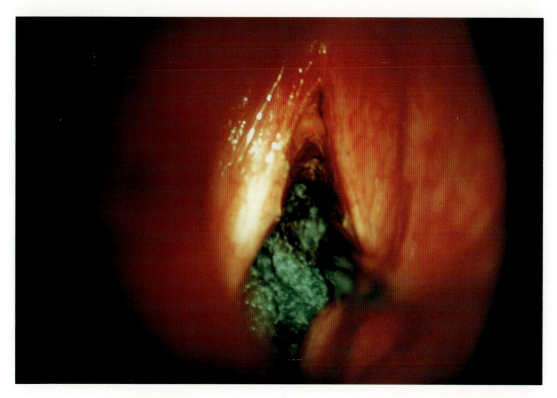

E

ANTERIOR POST-TRAUMATIC WEB

A. Definition

This section is related to "congenital web." We will describe the parameters that differentiate the congenital web from the anterior post-traumatic web.

B. Etiology and Histopathogeny

Anterior webs may arise after exo- or endolaryngeal surgery, intubation, or fractures.

C. Clinical Approach

1. Stroboscopy

In most cases, vocal folds do not vibrate properly. The mucosal trauma affects the web and the vocal vibratory mass. The vocal wave is irregular, aperiodic, and asymmetrical. However, asymptomatic webs are occasionally seen.

2. Electroglottography (EGG)

EGG is irregular with an increased closure phase and a flat pattern, possibly due to compensatory vocal hyperfunction.

3. Spectrography

Harmonics and formants are poorly visualized, the register is reduced, and the intensity is low. Fundamental frequency is variable.

Spectrography provides interesting data for post-surgical follow-up.

D. Conclusion

Removing the web by laser is easy, using the microspot with 1.5 watts and ultrapulse, but keeping it open is another story. Haslinger's technique with a keel and Dedo's technique with a mucosal flap are useful. In our experience, recurrences are less frequent when the microspot laser technique is used.

Laryngeal Pathologies: ANTERIOR POST-TRAUMATIC WEB

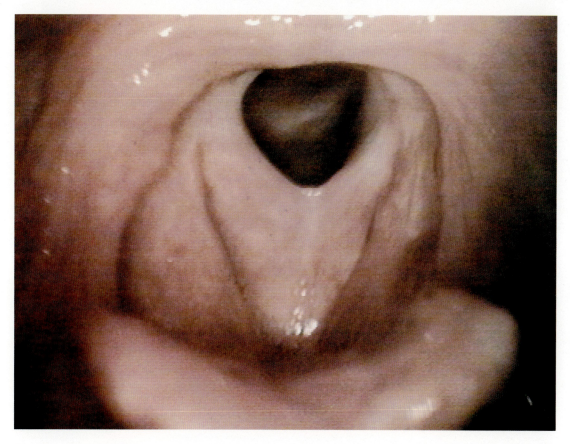

A

PLATE 4.142: **A.** Anterior web after trauma caused by vocal fold stripping for papillomatosis (Tele-videoscope).

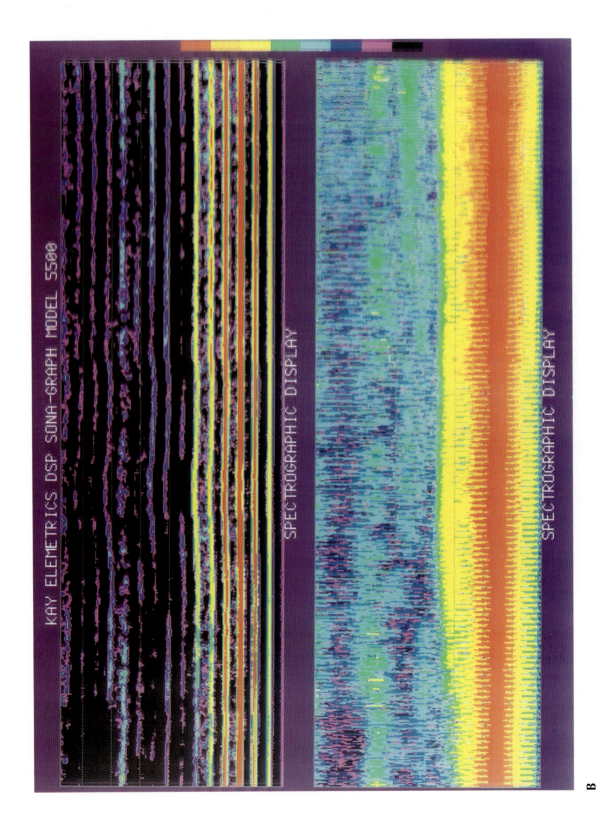

B. Spectrography of the anterior web showing reduced range.

Laryngeal Pathologies: ANTERIOR POST-TRAUMATIC WEB

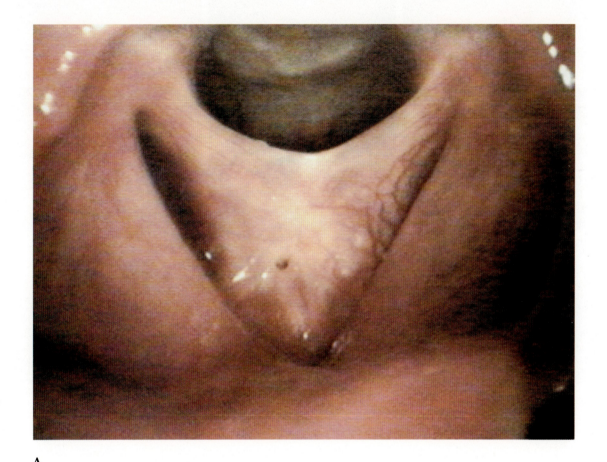

A

PLATE 4.143: **A.** Anterior web after double cordectomy. Tele-videoscope. Leukoplakia can be seen on the right side, under the free border.

Atlas of Laser Voice Surgery

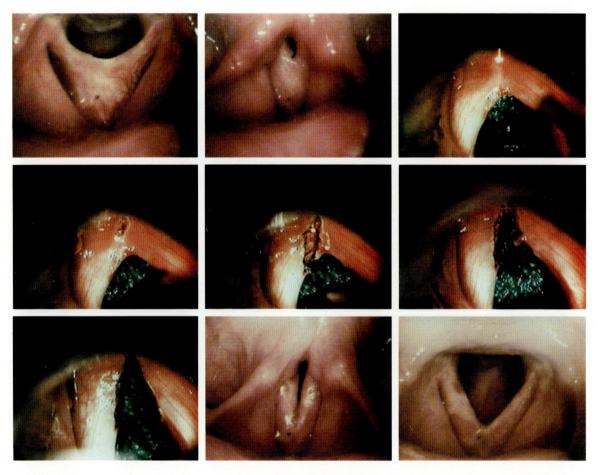

B

B. Aim: To restore the normal glottic anatomy.

1	2	3
4	5	6
7	8	9

1. Tele-videoscopy during breathing: before surgery.
2. Tele-videoscopy during phonation.
3. Laryngoscopy: laser phonosurgery.
4. First impacts with microspot starting from the anterior commissure and on the line of the free border of the left vocal fold.
5. Removal of the synechiae.
6. Glottis is open.
7. Regularization of the free edge: satisfactory per operative result.
8. Tele-videoscopy 3 months later during phonation.
9. During breathing.

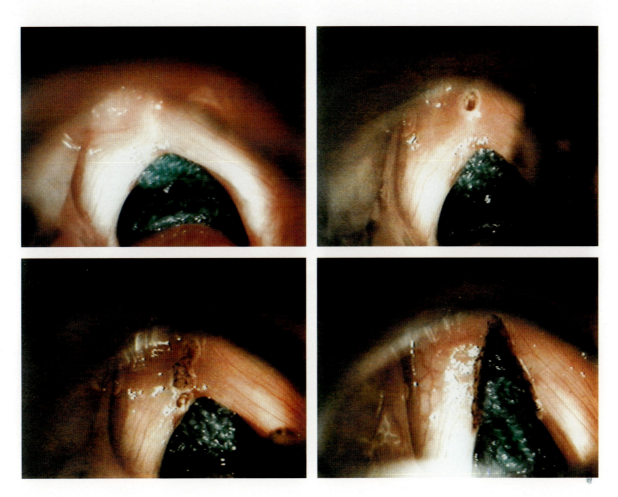

C. Laser web surgery.

1	2
3	4

1. Exposure of the anterior web.
2. First spot of laser fire: 2 watts power, 0.1 second, discontinuous fire using the microspot. We start by shooting on the anterior commissure.
3. From front to back parallel to the free edge of the right vocal fold. (This vocal fold did not vibrate during stroboscopy.)
4. Restoration of the vocal fold anatomy.

Atlas of Laser Voice Surgery

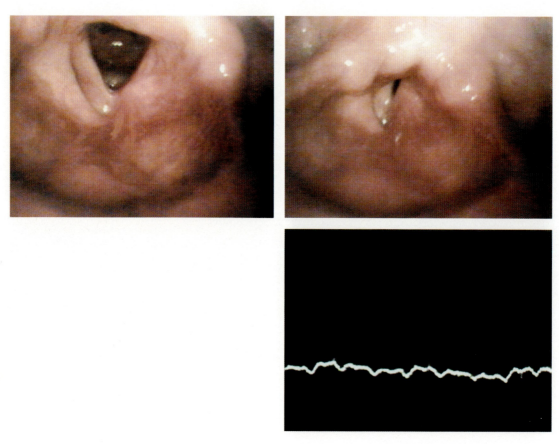

PLATE 4.144

1	2
	3

1. Small anterior healing web after laryngeal surgery with a scar on the left vocal fold. A subglottic granuloma can be seen in breathing phase.
2. In phonation.
3. EGG shows irregular patterns, and the closure phase is increased.

SULCUS VOCALIS

A. Definition

The term "sulcus" has been used since the beginning of this century to define a lesion that appears on indirect laryngoscopy as a whitish fissure running parallel to the free edge of the vocal fold. If this fissure is deep, it seems to divide the vocal fold in two.

Two different anatomical lesions correspond to this generic definition:

1. **Sulcus vocalis** is an invagination of the covering epithelium that extends through the superfical layer of the lamina propria to adhere to the vocal ligament.
2. **Sulcus vergeture** is an atrophic depression situated along the free border of the vocal fold. The term is derived from the French word *vergeture* which describes atrophic modifications of the skin such as striae gravidarum.

B. Location

Sulcus vocalis lies parallel to the free edge of the vocal fold. This fissure is more or less deep and frequently occurs at the level of the middle third of the vocal fold. This malformation is most often seen in females with a long history of dysphonia.

C. Etiology and Histopathogeny

1. Etiology

Sulcus vocalis seems to represent an open epidermal cyst.

Sulcus vergeture seems congenital in some patients but acquired in others. It may also be seen in children.

2. Pathogenesis

The pathogeny of sulcus vocalis is still a matter of debate, some maintaining it is a congenital and hereditary malformation, others that it is an acquired malformation. In our experience, both types exist. After vocal abuse or hematoma of the vocal fold, we have observed the formation of "sulcus" and "vergeture." It looks like the lamina propria becomes thinner and atrophies after a vocal trauma.

This malformation is sometimes associated with severe hyperplasia, chronic laryngitis, and hyperkinetic disorders involving nodule or polyp formation, as well as microvarix or capillary ectasia.

3. Macroscopic Aspect

Sulcus vocalis is a groove lying parallel to the free border of the vocal fold. With the help of a curved microforceps, the mucosa of the superior surface of the fold is laterally retracted, thus releasing the upper lip of the groove and exposing the more or less deep, epithelialized pocket.

The sulcus may be bilateral.

4. Histology

Located in the superficial layer of the lamina propria. Body and transition layers are absent.

   a. **Sulcus vocalis:** The sulcus creates a blind sac with walls formed by stratified squamous epithelium of variable thickness and hyperkeratosis when it approaches the depth of the pocket

   b. **Sulcus vergeture:** The mucosa lining the vergeture is thin and atrophic and tends to adhere to the underlying vocal ligament very closely.

D. Clinical Approach

1. Primary Symptoms

- ☐ The primary voice symptom is breathiness, due to incomplete closure of the vocal folds.
- ☐ The voice typically is loud and may be muffled or husky, particularly in men. The pitch of the voice may be lower than normal.
- ☐ Persistent vocal fatigue and laryngeal pain may prompt consultation in patients who fail to respond to voice therapy.

2. Tele-Video-Naso-Fiberscope and Telescope

When the lesion is sizable, the typical oval appearance of the glottis is suggestive. A sulcus will be seen as a depression or line along the upper medial edge of the vocal fold. The depression may extend the entire length of the vocal fold. The finding of a closure defect along the length of the free margin of both vocal folds associated with stiffness and inflammation may also be suggestive.

3. *Stroboscopy*

It is the main diagnostic tool.

When the sulcus is very subtle, it can only be appreciated by the videostroboscopic examination. Diminished amplitudes of vocal fold movement with little continuity of the mucosal wave across the sulcus are observed. A mucosal wave can usually be seen across the uninvolved superior surface of the fold.

4. *Electroglottography (EGG)*

Electroglottographic recording should show increased perturbation with the possibility of short closure time.

5. *Spectrography*

Phonation and intensity ranges are reduced. It is a narrow range.

Voice in sulcus vocalis performs few harmonics, from F_0 to F_4.

Levels of spectral noise in the voice are elevated.

Frequency, amplitude, harmonics, and noise are disturbed.

E. Conclusion

Surgical management of sulcus vocalis should be conservative. Injection of collagen gives a satisfactory voice. In our experience, laser surgery using the normal spot size is contraindicated. Using the ultrapulse with microspot, a power of 1.5 watts, 0.1 second, in discontinuous mode gives satisfactory results.

These lesions are frequently bilateral.

If surgery is performed, both sides can be done in the same operation.

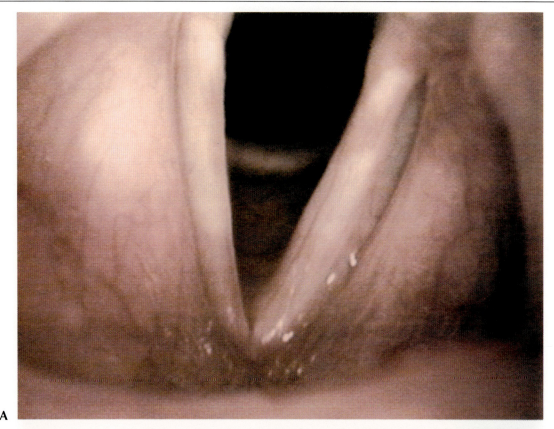

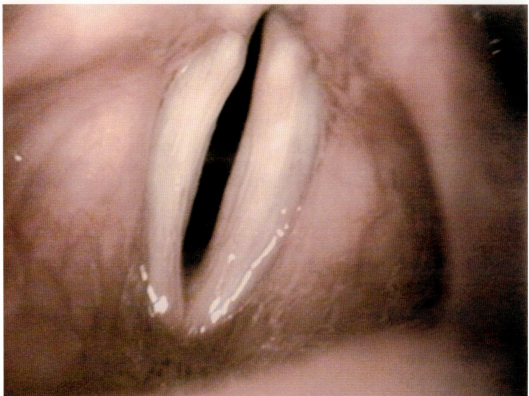

PLATE 4.145: **AIM:** To restore the shape of the free edge of the vocal fold. **A.** Sulcus vocalis of the left vocal fold. Almost all the free edge is involved. During breathing, only the left sulcus vocalis is seen. **B.** Case shown in **A** during phonation. Left and right sulcus vocalis appear.

Laryngeal Pathologies: SULCUS VOCALIS

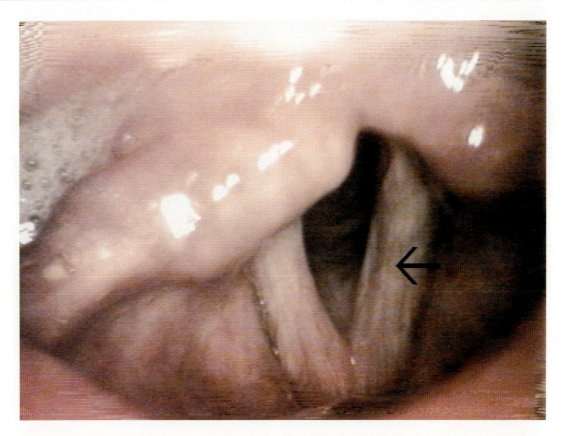

A

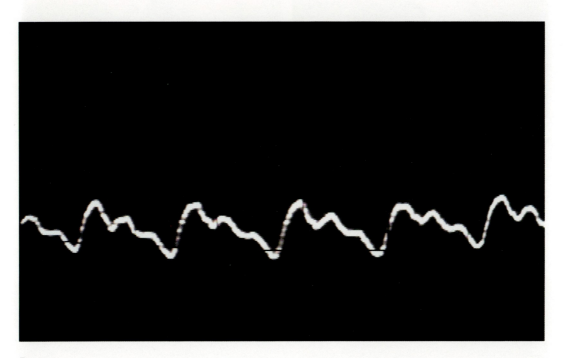

B
PLATE 4.146: **A.** Sulcus vocalis of the left vocal fold. **B.** EGG of case shown in **A.** Closing phase shows three different steps: The real closure time is very short.

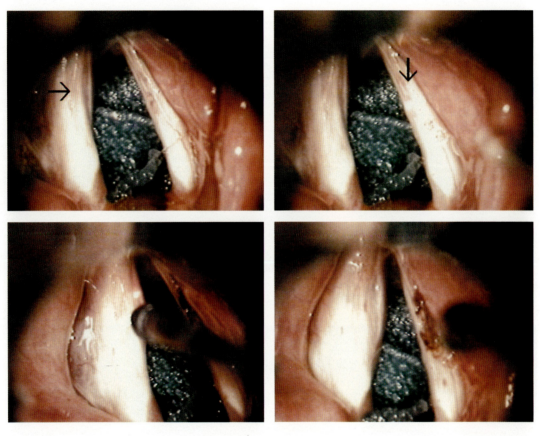

C

Microsurgical procedure: Sulcus vocalis of the left vocal fold—loosening of the epithelium of the right vocal fold: atrophy of the epithelium.

1	2
3	4

1. Larynx exposure: sulcus vocalis of the left vocal fold.
2. Atrophied epithelium of the left vocal fold.
3. Injection of collagen directly on the subepithelial layer.
4. Laser removing the atrophied epithelium.

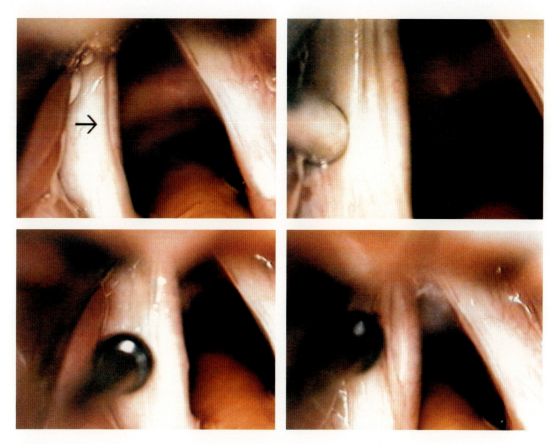

PLATE 4.147: Sulcus vocalis of the left vocal fold.

1	2
3	4

1. Larynx exposure: sulcus vocalis of the anterior and middle thirds of the vocal folds.
2. Magnified vision, pushing the superior surface of the vocal fold with the forceps, smoothly to the trachea. Sulcus vocalis can be seen with a bridge.
3. Injection of the collagen.
4. End of the procedure

CHANGING THE VOCAL PITCH

A. Introduction

Changing the vocal pitch of patients with excessively high or low vocal pitches may require surgery.

Speech therapy, however, is the first step of treatment and should be continued for 1 year. Surgery is performed only for patients who do not improve following speech therapy.

The vocal fold pitch is regulated by four principle parameters (see Chapter 2):

1. The static mass
2. The vibratory mass
3. The length of the vocal folds, on the one hand
4. The subglottic pressure, on the other hand.

Surgery may modify the vocal parameters: the static mass (thyroarytenoid muscle), the vibratory mass (the cover of the vocal fold), the length (thyroarytenoid muscle and, indirectly, the cricothyroid muscles), but will not alter subglottic pressure.

The pitch control mechanism in humans is very intricate. Increasing the tension may elevate the vocal pitch and vice versa.

Any procedure or treatment that affects the vocal fold mass, for example, removing a lesion, injecting collagen, prescribing an androgen treatment, or modifying the laryngeal framework may change the pitch by affecting the respiratory tract or dynamics of the vocal system.

B. Indications

Microsurgery to lower vocal pitch, in our procedure, involves collagen injection on one side to increase the static vocal mass. Results are interesting but temporary. It seems that the best technique remains the Isshiki procedures first described in 1974 and more recently by Tucker (1985).

Laser microsurgery to raise vocal pitch is satisfactory. We first reported five cases at the French E.N.T. Congress in 1993. Five women underwent laser microsurgery. All had abnormally low voices as a side effect of hormonal drugs such as androgens or anabolic steroids. These surgical techniques also may be performed in transsexuals.

Here again, the Isshiki technique remains a very satisfactory procedure.

C. Principles

The parameter on which this procedure acts is the thyroarytenoid muscle without touching epithelium of the free edge of the vocal fold.

D. Techniques

An incision is made parallel to the free edge of the vocal fold by CO_2 laser (microspot, a power of 1.5 watts, discontinuous fire, 0.1 sec.) then some fibers of the thyroarytenoid muscle are removed from front to back. One side is operated. An injection of cortisone is performed on both sides. If the voice is not satisfactory, a second procedure is carried out 3 months later.

E. Conclusion

The technique we have developed, to our knowledge, is an original approach to the surgical modification of pitch. Isshiki techniques remain very satisfactory procedures if the patient accepts an open laryngeal surgery. Our technique is simple with fast healing and, up to now, no side effects have been observed. Spectrography before and after laser surgery will indicate whether the second vocal fold must undergo laser surgery 3 months later. The results offer promise for surgical improvement of pitch via laser surgery.

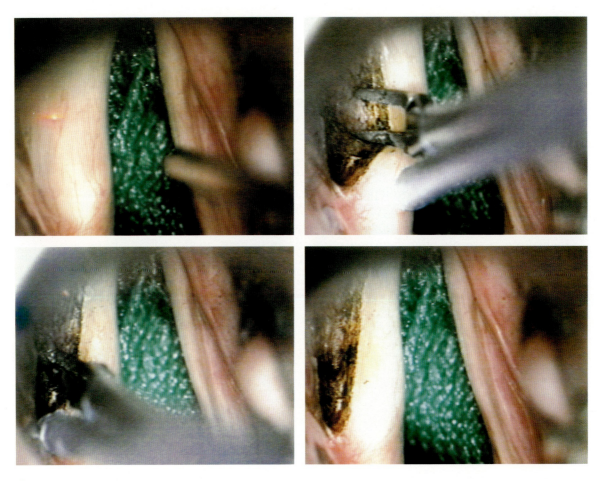

A

PLATE 4.148: A. Laser surgery to alter pitch. The left thyroarytenoid muscle is partially removed.

1	2
3	4

1. Exposure of the larynx: The laser is focused on the left vocal fold. (The right vocal fold was operated on 3 months earlier.)
2. Opening of the vocal muscle.
3. The A-forceps removes a part of the muscle fibers parallel to the other fibers.
4. End of procedure.

B. Tele-videoscopy before surgery. C. Tele-videoscopy 6 weeks after surgery.

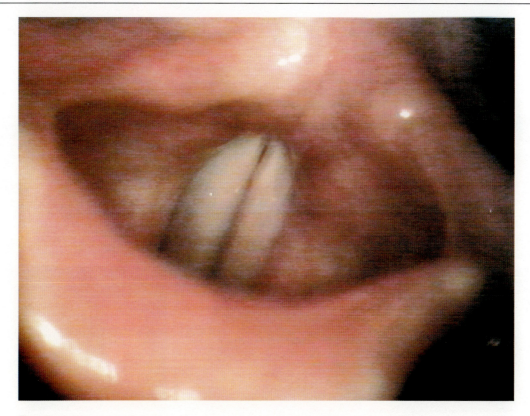

B

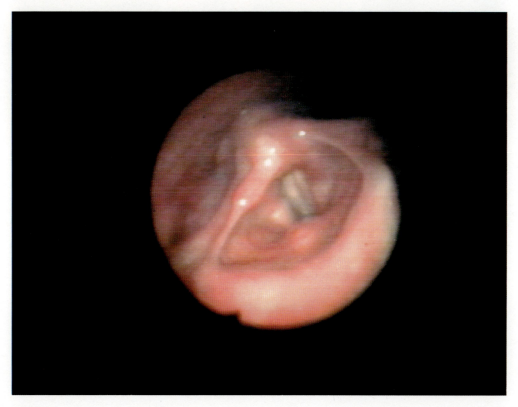

C

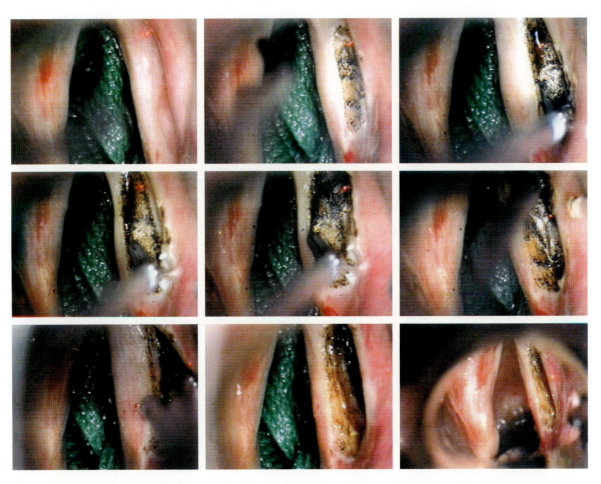

A

PLATE 4.149: **A.** Laser pitch surgery on the right thyroarytenoid muscle.

1	2	3
4	5	6
7	8	9

1. Exposure of the larynx.
2. Incision of the upper surface of the right vocal fold parallel to the free border (8 watts, continuous fire).
3. The A-forceps grasps the vocal fold muscle.
4–5. The fibers of the muscle are pulled.
6. The muscle fibers are removed.
7. The free edge of the vocal fold is not touched.
8. End of the procedure with green gauze still in place.
9. End of the procedure with green gauze removed.

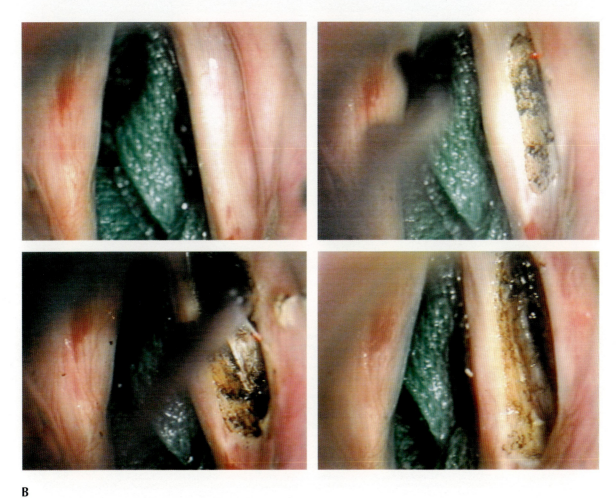

B

Surgery for pitch on the right vocal fold illustrating the four principle steps of the procedure.

1	2
3	4

1. Exposure of the larynx.
2. Incision of the upper surface of the right vocal fold.
3. Excision of the fibers of the muscle.
4. End of the procedure.

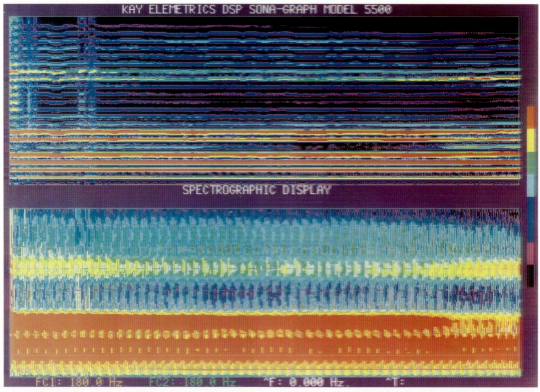

C

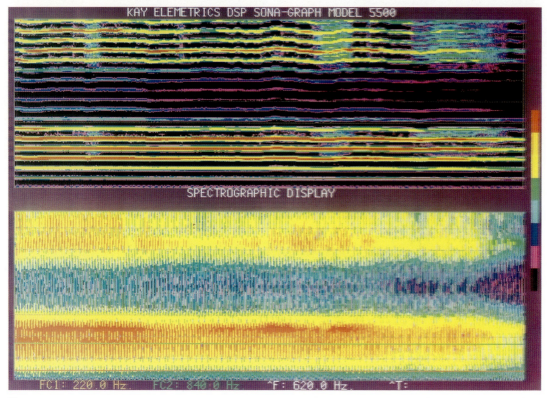

D

C. Spectrography before surgery shows an F_0 of 180 Hz (typically, a male pitch) in a 39-year-old woman.
D. Spectrography 8 weeks after surgery. F_0 is 220 Hz, showing that the female pitch has recovered.

MISCELLANEOUS LESIONS

A. Notches and Scars (Plates 4.150 A–C, 4.151, and 4.152)

Conventional surgical techniques using forceps may be traumatic and remove too much tissue, including epithelium and the vocal ligament, creating notches and scars.

Besides webs, other iatrogenic lesions, such as lesions and scars, may be seen. These lesions produce hoarseness and voice fatigue; and on spectrography, few harmonics and high noise are present.

A notch needs to be treated by fat or collagen injection and vaporization of the bed of the epithelium if it is keratotic.

A scar needs to be treated by laser microsurgery decortication. The epithelium is removed up to the vocal ligament, without touching it. We use the laser beam with only a cutting effect. That is why the microspot is very useful in this pathology.

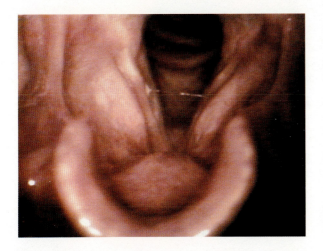

A

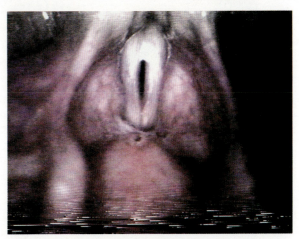

B

PLATE 4.150: **A.** Amyotrophy during breathing. **B.** Amyotrophy during phonation showing bowing of the glottic space.

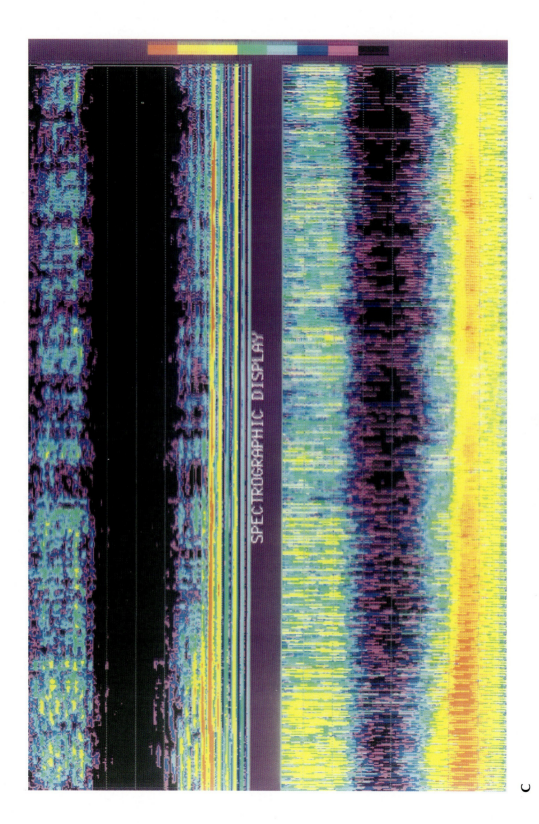

C. Spectrography shows a narrow range. The higher harmonics are lost.

Laryngeal Pathologies: MISCELLANEOUS LESIONS

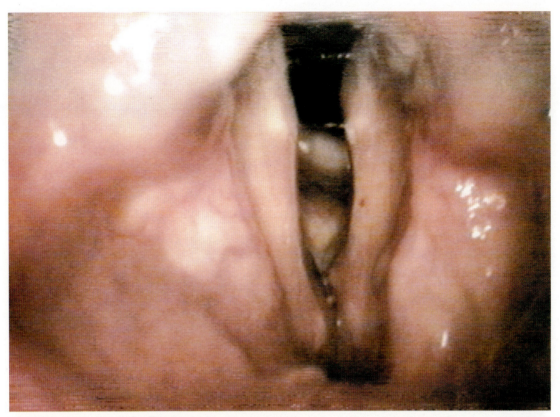

PLATE 4.151: Tele-videoscopy during breathing shows a notch on both sides.

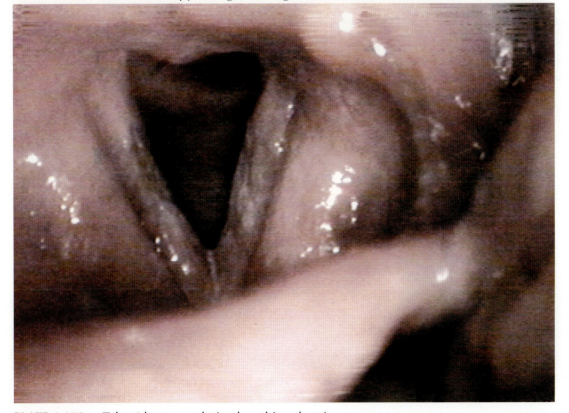

PLATE 4.152: Tele-videoscopy during breathing showing a scar.

B. Atrophy

Atrophy is related to a paralyzed vocal fold in abduction. It can be seen in aged larynx.

In this pathology, we use injection of collagen or fat material (see Paralysis of the Vocal Folds section).

C. Spasmodic Dysphonia

- Laser surgery is interesting by vaporizing the anterior part of the arytenoid where the small branches of the recurrent laryngeal nerve arrive.

- Injection of Botox® (botulinum toxin) is interesting and is performed under local anesthesia through the neck skin.

D. Amyloid Tumors (Plates 4.153 A and B)

Amyloid tumors are very rare. They are benign lesions. They look like a cyst, polyp, or laryngitis. Most amyloid deposits are supraglottic. The epithelium is avascular and yellowish.

Laser microsurgery is a perfect tool to remove such lesions.

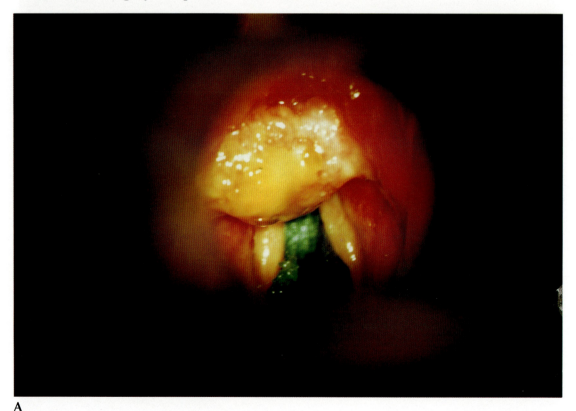

A

PLATE 4.153: **A.** Amyloid tumor of the epiglottis at the anterior commissure before surgery.

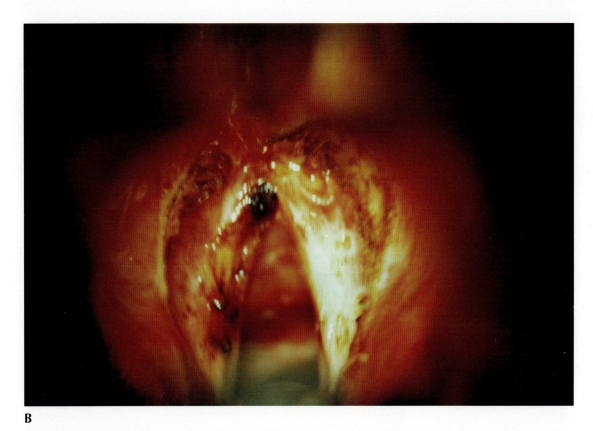

B

B. After surgery using laser with 10 watts power, continuous mode, and normal spot size.

E. Edema After Radiotherapy

Edema can occur after radiotherapy for a period of 2 months to 3 years. It is located on the posterior vocal process.

This edema is treated by laser microvaporization of 7 watts and continuous fire mode.

The results are very satisfactory.

F. Teflon Ablation from the Vocal Folds (Plates 4.154 A–D)

Ablation or removal of Teflon is necessary when granulomas and tumors appear.

To remove Teflon, we use the laser with a power of 20 watts after having performed a flap on the superior surface of the vocal fold. (using the microspot and a power of 1.5 watts). We remove the charred tissue with icy cottonoid—not with suction. Often, several laser procedures are necessary.

Atlas of Laser Voice Surgery

Teflon granulomas are usually located in the ventricle or in the subglottic space. When the vocal fold vibrations and the voice are normal, nothing has to be done, except a regular follow-up by stroboscopy on a videotape. When severe dysphonia appears, laser ablation of the Teflon must be performed.

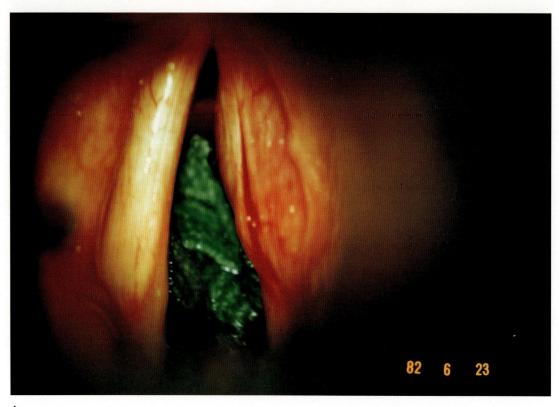

A

AIM: To remove Teflon material and restore the viscoelasticity of the vocal fold.
PLATE 4.154: **A.** Exposure of the larynx and laser incision on the superior surface of the right vocal fold.

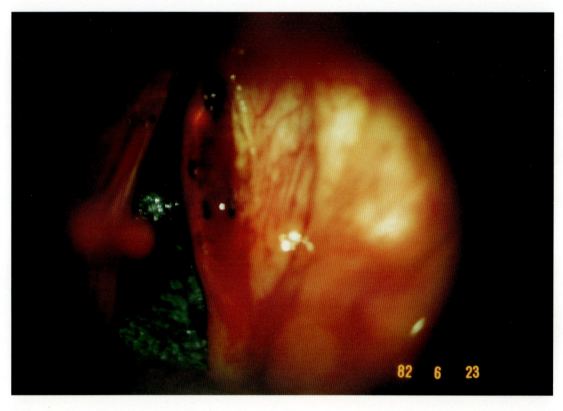

B

B. Penetration of the beam near the vocal ligament using classical laser spot size, power of 20 watts, continuous mode.

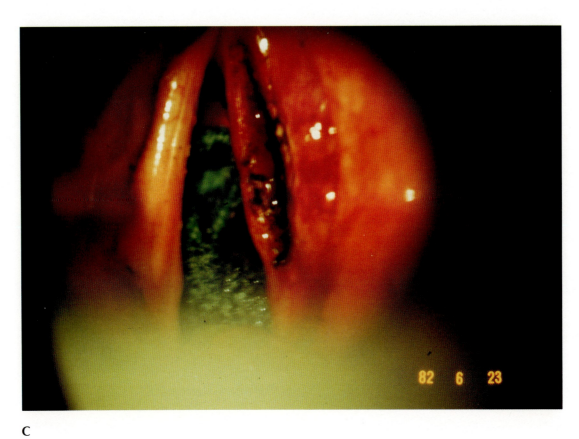

C

C. Removal of the scar tissue and Teflon particles. **D.** Total removal is done. Vocal muscle can be seen.

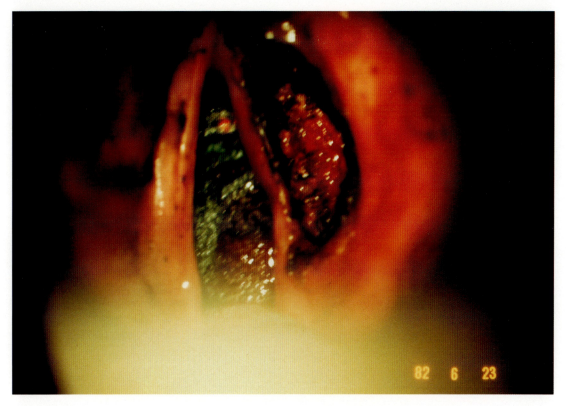
D

Atlas of Laser Voice Surgery

MULTIPLE LESIONS

One lesion can mask another. Despite the plethora of sophisticated techniques available for diagnosis, accurate diagnosis of multiple pathologies still requires the clinical intuition and experience of the physician.

This is illustrated in the following plates.

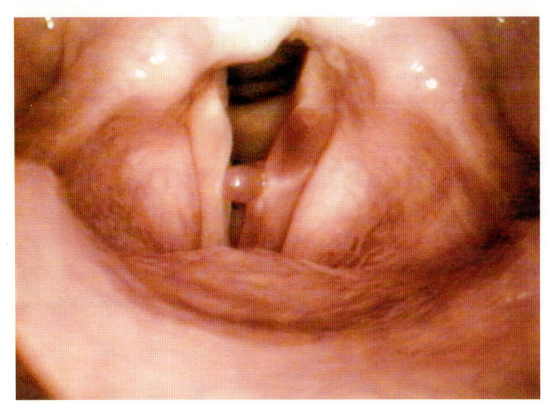

PLATE 4.155: Polyp and hemorrhage of the left vocal fold shown by tele-videoscopy.

Laryngeal Pathologies: MULTIPLE LESIONS

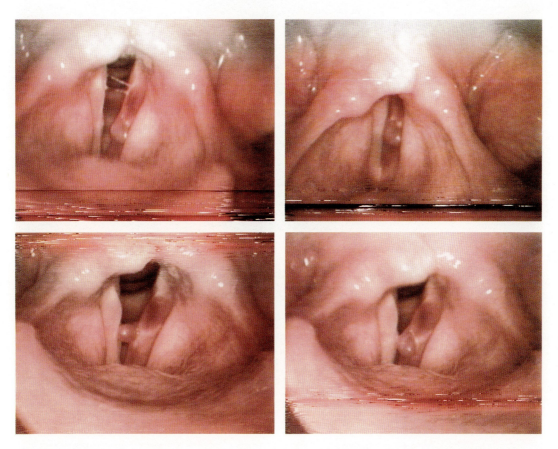

PLATE 4.156: Polyp and hemorrhage of the left vocal fold. Tele-videoscopy during breathing and phonation.

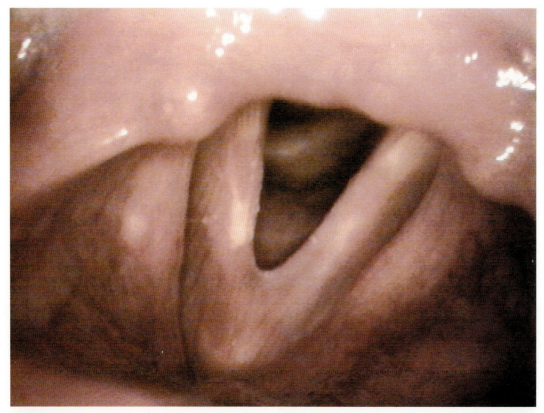

PLATE 4.157: Microweb and keratosis of the right vocal fold.

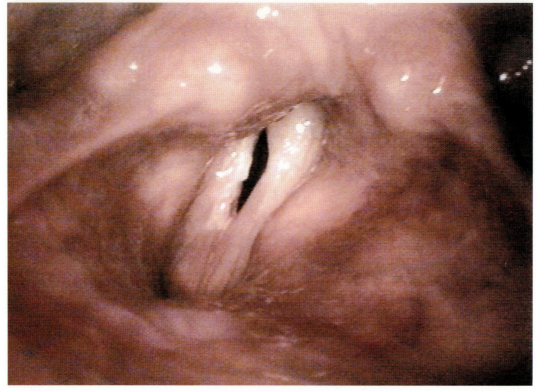

PLATE 4.158: Recurrent laryngeal nerve paralysis, left vocal fold. Keratotic granuloma.

Laryngeal Pathologies: MULTIPLE LESIONS

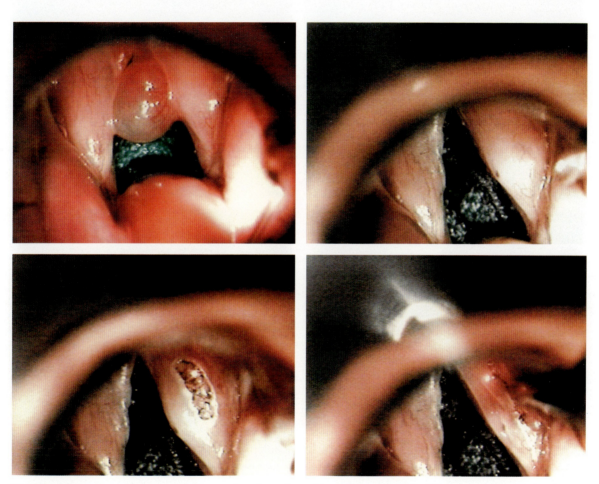

PLATE 4.159: Laser microsurgical procedure for polyp of the right vocal fold with associated Reinke's edema.

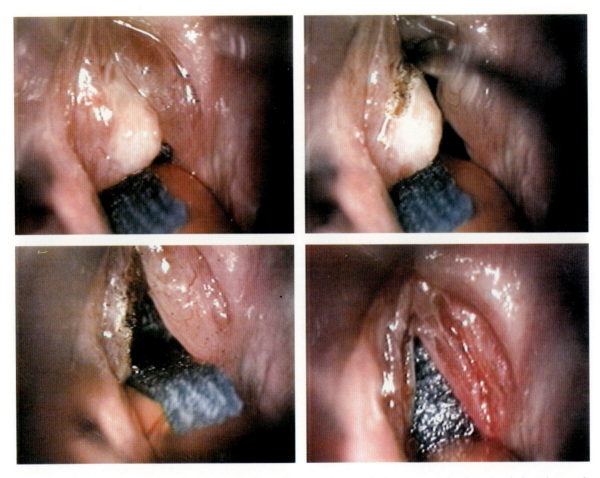

PLATE 4.160: Laser microsurgical procedure for a polyp with benign pachydermia (left side) and Reinke's edema (right side).

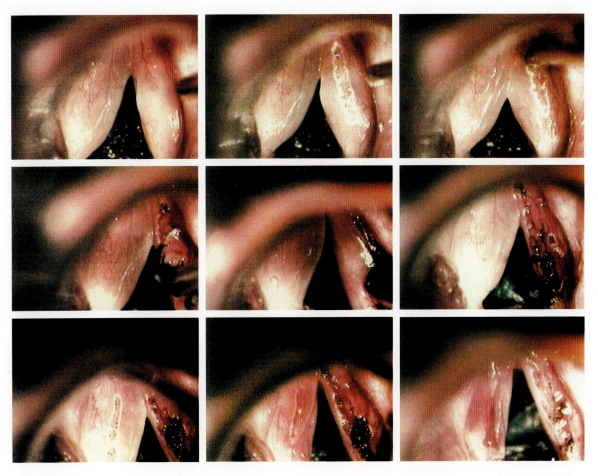

PLATE 4.161: Laser microsurgical procedure for Reinke's space, stage 2. Note in **4** that leukoplakia has to be removed.

1	2	3
4	5	6
7	8	9

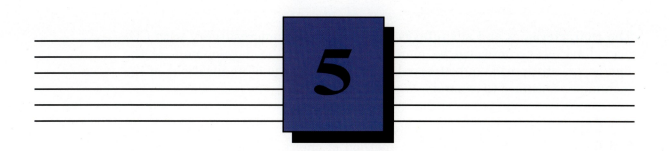

5

Conclusions

Personal Experience

The data reported here on 5,035 cases of CO_2 laser phonosurgery were collected from April 1, 1979 to October 1993.

The characteristics and advantages of endolaryngeal microsurgery with CO_2 laser have been confirmed by many authors. With the development of the microspot, ultrapulse, and superpulse lasers, the range of applications of the technique continues to expand.

On the one hand, using CO_2 laser by just skimming the free edge of the vocal fold for nodules or tiny edema is a method of choice. On the other hand, to remove and analyze samples, use of the microspot, which gives a 100-micron incision, can be performed for polyps, cordectomies, and arytenoidectomies.

The bloodless nature of the procedure and the excellent healing observed in these surgeries, coupled with increased practice of laser phonosurgery and confidence in the reliability of laser removal and laser biopsy samples, have led to wide use of these techniques.

This review of 5,035 patients includes 385 malignant lesions and 4,650 benign lesions. Our experience in laser phonosurgery consisted of treatment of both benign and early malignant lesions. In benign lesions and carcinoma in situ, the goal was to restore the voice by removing the lesion while touching the vibrating vocal mass as little as possible and to avoid recurrences.

Since 1982, preoperative assessment for each patient has included a Dynamic Vocal Exploration (video telescope, stroboscopy, fiberscopy, voice recording, and electroglottography). Since 1987, Dynamic Vocal Exploration has also included spectrography.

All patients were videotaped and a preoperative photograph was made with a video printer. All patients underwent surgery by suspension laryngoscopy, and a CO_2 laser was used. The micro-instruments used were our personal tools (Abitbol Laser Phonosurgery instruments manufactured by Micro France).

Statistics for all cases are reported in Table 5.1.

We distinguish four types of vocal pathologies:

1. Vocal pathology secondary to vocal abuse (see Table 5.2)
2. Vocal pathology secondary to airway obstruction (see Table 5.3)
3. Miscellaneous vocal pathologies (see Table 5.4)
4. Vocal pathology secondary to malignant laryngitis and miscellaneous pathology (see Tables 5.5 and 5.6)

Conclusions

TABLE 5.1: Distribution of 5,035 cases of laser phonosurgery.

Pathology	Number of Cases
Nodules	666
Polyps	1052
Cysts	254
Reinke's edema	912
Benign laryngitis	406
Malignant lesions	385
Dysphonic plica ventricularis	56
Vascular pathology	305
Sulcus vocalis	8
Granuloma	145
Papillomatosis	357
Web	175
Arytenoidectomy	37
Laryngeal stenosis	9
Vocal fold scar	4
Vocal fold paralysis (abduction)	259
Vocal fold pitch	5

TABLE 5.2: Vocal pathologies secondary to vocal abuse and surgical outcomes.

Lesions	Number of Cases	Failures	
Nodules[a]	666	5	
Polyps	1052	9	
Cysts	254	6	
Polypoid fold edema or Reinke's edema	912	44	
Benign laryngitis	406	2	(scars)
Dysphonia plica ventricularis	56	1	
Vascular pathology (microvarix, vascular corditis, telangiectasia hematoma, angiomatosis)	305	2	
Sulcus vocalis	8	5	
Granuloma	145	16	(recurrences)
Posterior	115	15	
Anterior	30	1	

[a]Soft nodules do not undergo micro-surgery and must be treated by voice therapy.

TABLE 5.3: Airway obstruction.

Lesions	Number of Cases	Failures
Papillomatosis	357	Fewer recurrences
Web	179	
Anterior	164	135
Posterior	11	3
Arytenoidectomy	37	6
Laryngeal stenosis	9	5

TABLE 5.4: Miscellaneous vocal fold pathologies.

Lesions	Number of Cases	Failures
Vocal fold scar (stiff vocal mass)	4[a]	1
Abduction paralysis of the vocal fold	259	
Teflon	98	11
Collagen	161	32
Vocal fold pitch	5	0

[a]As seen on stroboscopy during breathing the vocal fold appears normal. During phonation, the scar is revealed.

TABLE 5.5: Distribution of malignant vocal fold pathologies treated.

Lesions	Number of Cases
Cancers	385
In situ	97
T1N0	169
T2N0	119
Site	
Middle third	335
Anterior third	44
Posterior third	6

TABLE 5.6: Results of laser treatment for malignant lesions.

	Cancer Classification								
	CIS			T1N0			T2N0		
Site of Lesion	No. of Cases	No. of Recurrences	Failure Rate	No. of Cases	No. of Recurrences	Failure Rate	No. of Cases	No. of Recurrences	Failure Rate
Middle Third (335)	95	1	1.0%	134	2	1.5%	106	5[a]	4.7%
Anterior Commissure (44)	2	1	50.0%	31	23[b]	74.1%	11	9	81.8%
Posterior Commissure (6)	0	0	0%	4	3[a]	75.0%	2	2	100.0%

[a] 1 morbidity
[b] 2 morbidities

Note: The overall cure rate for lesions located on the middle third was 97.7% (327 of 335 cases). For lesions of the anterior and posterior commissures, this rate dropped to 75% and 17%, respectively.

Indications, Contraindications, Complications, Cautions, Advantages, and Disadvantages

Benign Lesions

Indications for laser phonosurgery are summarized in Table 5.7.

Limits of indications for benign lesions are summarized on Table 5.8.

TABLE 5.7: Indications for laser phonosurgery.

Papillomatosis

Malignant laryngitis: middle third of vocal fold

Polyps, nodules, cysts

Polypoid vocal fold edema or Reinke's edema

Benign laryngitis

Dysphonia plica ventricularis

Vascular pathology (microvarix, corditis, hematoma, angiomatosis)

Arytenoidectomy

Vocal fold pitch

TABLE 5.8: Limits in indications for laser phonosurgery in benign lesions.

Web:
   Anterior (In the past 2 years, good results have been obtained with the use of the microspot.)
   Posterior

Laryngeal stenosis

Vocal fold scar: stiff vocal mass (Microspot has improved the results.)

Vocal fold paralysis (abduction)
   Teflon
   Collagen

Cysts (Microspot has improved the results.)

Granuloma
   Posterior: contact ulcer
   Medium
   Anterior

Sulcus vocalis

Cancer of the Vocal Folds:
Limits in Indications (see Tables 5.5 and 5.6)

In 1920, Lynch performed endoscopic cordectomy for the first time. In 1941, New and Dorton reported that 9 of 11 patients were successfully cured of carcinoma. In 1972, Jako and Strong in Boston started laser microsurgery treatment for vocal fold carcinoma.

In our experience with carcinoma of the vocal folds from 1980 to 1994, 385 previously untreated patients were selected and underwent laser cordectomy for carcinoma of the vocal fold. All patients had a second look laser microsurgery 2 months later. The results reported in Table 5.6 are after 4 to 14 years of follow-up.

Cancer stages included:

- [ ] 97 carcinoma in situ
- [ ] 169 T1N0
- [ ] 119 T2N0

Patient characteristics included:

- [ ] Age: 39–88 years
- [ ] Sex: 346 males and 39 females (9.8% females)

- Habits:
  - 9 nonsmokers (3 females and 6 males). Six of the nine were exposed to carcinogens in the work place
  - 2 nurses working in a laboratory
  - 3 men in a plastic factory and painting factory
  - 4 smokers were working in a plastic factory with Teflon gas.

In the cases of smokers and professional exposure, lesions were bilateral, for example, dysplasia on one side and T1 on the other, T1 and CIS, T1, T2.

Laser cordectomy by microlaryngoscopy procedure was stimulated by the CO_2 laser technique, early recognition of premalignant stage by telestroboscopic exploration, and the improved health education of the general exploration. Stroboscopy is essential for diagnosis: **A small lesion is always suspicious if the aspect of the vibration looks like a surfboard on a wave.** In a large lesion, the entire vocal fold does not vibrate. In all cases, fundamental rules must be followed for laser microlaryngoscopic cordectomy (section carcinomas).

The results for our 385 patients were very interesting. If recurrences were clinical diagnosed, a third microsurgery was performed, and if carcinoma was found, a complementary treatment was achieved. **More than the T.N.M. classification, the location of lesions was fundamental for the prognosis.** (Table 5.6)

335 lesions on middle third location of the vocal fold: 8 recurrences (2.3%)

44 lesions on anterior commissure: 33 recurrences (75%)

6 lesions on posterior commissure: 5 recurrences (81%)

Laser cordectomy is limited by the location and the volume of the tumor on the middle third of the vocal fold and no more advanced stage than T2N0.

Laser microlaryngoscopic surgery of carcinoma of the vocal fold needs early detection by stroboscopic exploration and smear test. These patients also need follow-up by Dynamic Vocal Exploration, stroboscopy, and smear test. All patients also had a second-look laser surgery 2 months later.

Contraindications

In our experience with laser microlaryngoscopy, lesions on the anterior or posterior commissure need a complementary treatment and are contraindications for laser cordectomy; only carcinoma in situ (C.I.S.), T1N0, and T2N0 of the middle third have very satisfactory results. Why?

The distance between the mucosa and the cartilage varies from the front to the back of the vocal fold. That is why a T1 becomes a T3 very rapidly.

> Anterior commissure: 2 mm between mucosa and cartilage
>
> Middle one third: 6 to 10 mm between mucosa, muscle, and cartilage
>
> Posterior commissure: 2 mm between mucosa and cartilage

Limitations of Laser Surgery

Laser phonosurgery is limited by its very design. CO_2 is transmitted through the microscope and acts only in direct firing.

Besides the fact that laser phonosurgery is done under suspension laryngoscopy, general anesthesia, and is limited by this technique, patient morphologies such as a short neck, cervical arthroses, and limited mouth opening (retrognathism) contraindicate its use. These conditions, however, are rare. The volume of lesions such as huge papillomas and pendulum polyps limits intubation but not laser surgery.

In summary, there are three limitations of laser phonosurgery:

1. The laser acts only by direct fire.
2. We can treat only what we can see.
3. The morphology of the patient.

Complications

Complications from laser phonosurgery can be divided into three groups. In our personal experience (see Tables 5.9 and 5.10), they include:

Complications Involving the laser (see Table 5.9)

- Ignition of the tube
- Reflection of the laser on instruments
- Too much or not enough power.

All of these elements can be avoided.

Complications Involving the Phonosurgical Technique
(see Table 5.10):

- Notches, scars, and webs
- Recurrences of benign lesions such as papillomas

TABLE 5.9: Complications observed from the equipment (no morbidity).

The electrocardiogram (observed in extended neck)
Laryngoscopy
   310 cases of bradycardia or tachycardia during surgery
    90 cases with loss of taste lasting 1 to 12 weeks
Laser
   1 case in 1983 (laser caused ignition of the green gauze)
   1 case in 1986 (laser caused ignition of the tube)
   17 cases (laser beam exploded the cuff — we added another green gauze to make the trachea water-tight
Reflection on instruments
   On forceps: 2 cases
   On laryngoscope: 72 cases

TABLE 5.10: Complications observed from the surgical procedures.

Anterior glottic webs: 4
   2 papillomas
   1 polypoid fold, type 3
   1 on resection of the two false vocal folds

Notches (polyps): 2

Scars: 55

(Web between the mucosa and the vocal ligament; see stroboscopy shown in Plate 5.4)
   44 polypoid folds
    3 polyps
    3 nodules
    5 sulcus vocalis

Recurrences
    5 nodules*
    6 polyps
    6 cysts
    2 laryngitis
    2 vascular pathology
   16 granulomas

*Soft nodules undergo no surgery and are treated by voice therapy.

Complications Involving Anesthesia (see Table 5.11)

Cautions

In CO_2 laser surgery, use of caution are fundamental. The correct instruments and perfect laser control are required (see Table 5.12).

Advantages and Disadvantages

There are many, and they are summarized in Tables 5.13 and 5.14.

TABLE 5.11: Complications observed from anesthetic techniques (no morbidity).

Curare allergy:	6 cases (0.1%)
Bradycardia	221 cases (4.0%) changes observed in electrocardiogram (observed in extended neck)

TABLE 5.12: Cautions to observe in laser phonosurgery.

Beam reflection on the instruments or endotracheal tube

Protection of the endotracheal tube
   The tube is wrapped with an aluminum tape (this wrap may scratch the vocal folds).
    Moist green gauze protects the tube and the cuff (or use an Oswal tube)

Protection of the patient's lips with moist gauze

Very good suction

TABLE 5.13: Advantages of laser phonosurgery.

1. Experience with the CO_2 laser
2. No touch surgery
3. No edema
4. No bleeding
5. Less scarring
6. Fast healing
7. No pain

TABLE 5.14. Disadvantages of laser phonosurgery.

1. Lack of experience with the CO_2 laser
2. Smoke and plumes
3. Hemostasis (capillaries <0.6 mm)
4. Direct fire
5. No touch surgery

Conclusions

What to Avoid

- Reflections
- Improper exposure of the larynx
- Accidents

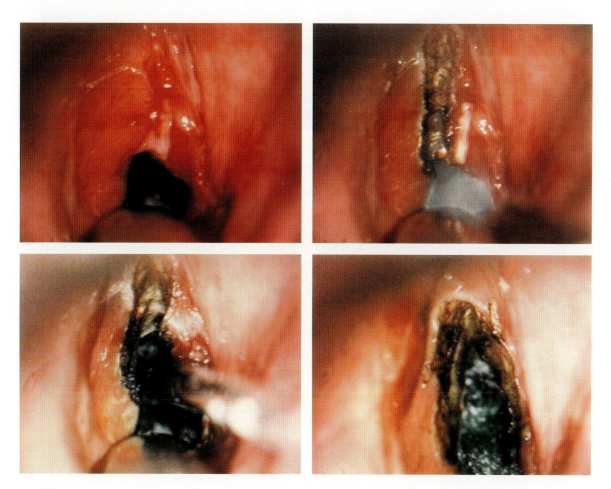

PLATE 5.1:

1	2
3	4

1. Leukoplakia with anterior web.
2. Laser impact from front to back.
3. The laser procedure is going too far on the right vocal fold; the posterior third has been vaporized.
4. End of the procedure shows too much scar tissue on both vocal folds from the anterior commissure to the posterior third.

Atlas of Laser Voice Surgery

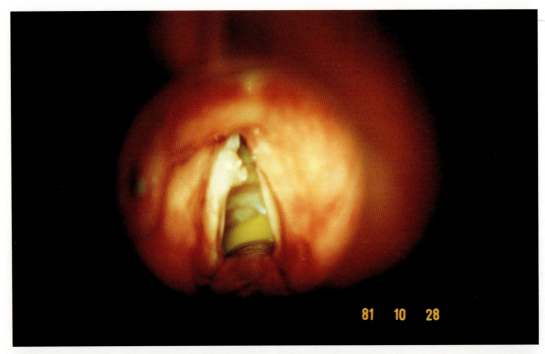

A

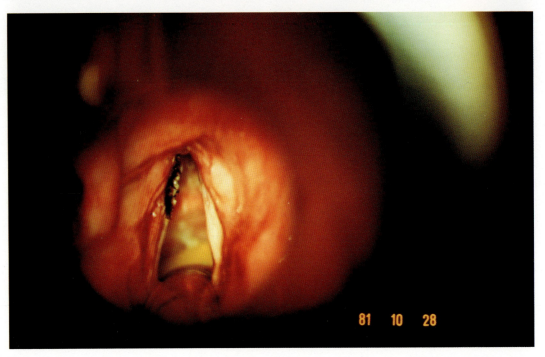

B

PLATE 5.2: **A.** Vocal fold polyp on the left vocal fold. Laser microlaryngoscopy—larynx exposure. **B.** After laser surgery.

MISTAKES:
- The subglottic space is not protected
- The spatula is not far enough to expose the anterior commissure
- A notch and an excessive thermal effect were created on the left vocal fold.

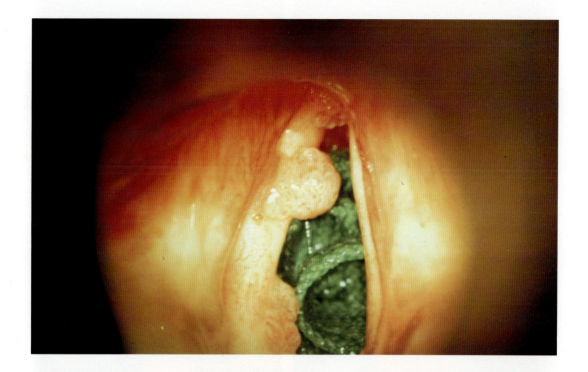

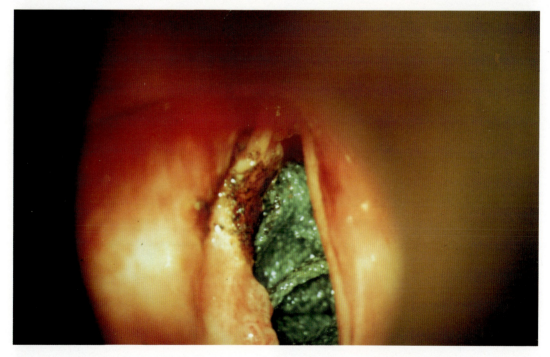

B

PLATE 5.3: **A.** Exposure of the larynx: Papillomas of the left vocal fold reaching the anterior commissure. **B.** During laser microsurgery.
MISTAKES: • The vocal ligament has been touched, instead of a real "decortication."
• The anterior commissure is not well exposed.

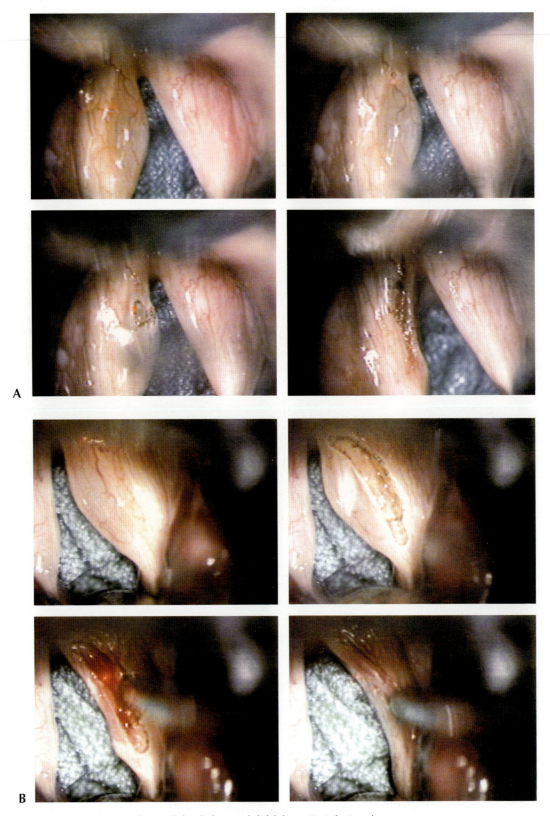

PLATE 5.4: **A.** Lifting of the left vocal fold for a Reinke's edema.
MISTAKES: • Too much mucosa was removed. **B.** The same case shown in **A** on the right vocal fold with no mistakes.

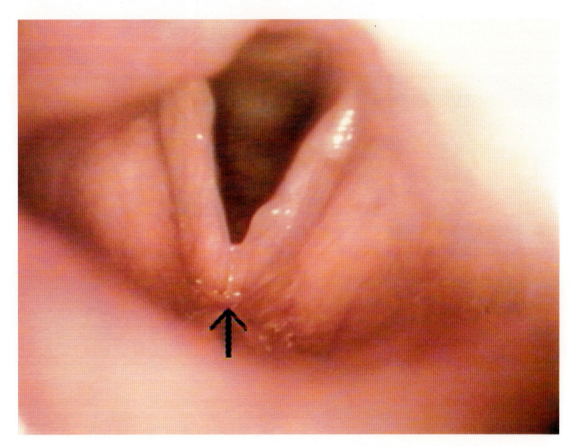

PLATE 5.5: Microweb after Reinke's edema surgery caused by stripping. Tele-videoscope: No surgery.
MISTAKES: • Never do a stripping on the vocal folds.
• Never touch the two vocal folds at the same time if there is a risk of provoking a web.

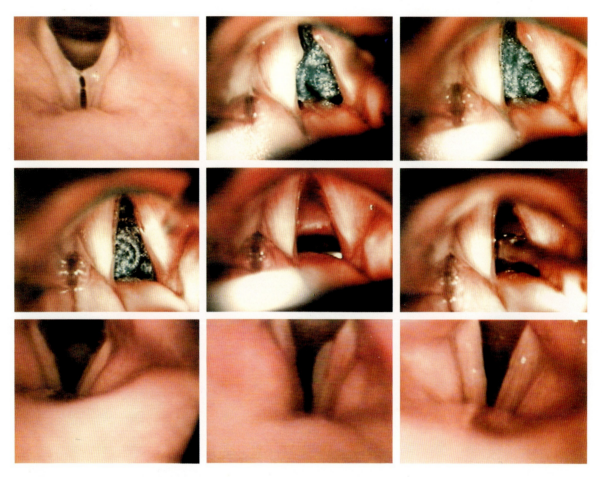

PLATE 5.6: A very interesting case.

1	2	3
4	5	6
7	8	9

1. Tele-videoscopy reveals a cyst on the left vocal fold and a secondary lesion on the right side.
2. Laser surgery is performed under microlaryngoscopy.
3. Removal of the left cyst; 7 watts, continuous mode.
4. Removal of the right side lesion: 7 watts, continuous mode.
5. The green gauze is removed.
6. A normal forceps is on the glottic space to protect the trachea because a tiny scar has to be vaporized on the left side.
   FIRST MISTAKE: Reflection of the laser on the forceps.
7. Tele-videoscopy on the next day.
8. Edema due to the thermic effect of the laser by reflection.
9. After 3 weeks of therapy: healing is complete.

A TEAM OPERATES, NOT A SURGEON

Phonosurgery requires a highly experienced team: anesthetist, surgeon, pathologist, and nurses. Patient collaboration with the team is also important, and voice therapy is one of the key factors in postoperative care.

The surgeon operates not with his eyes but with the laser's eyes. He has to guess all the possible effects of the impact of the laser before making the shot with the laser.

What to Do

If you do not yet know what to do, read the book again!

However, on a more serious note, here is a suggested reading list in the field of the voice. Many aspects of voice and its surgical treatment are described in these books, ranging from voice physiology to phonosurgery. They make an important contribution to laryngology.

Books

Brodnitz, F. (1988) *Keep your voice healthy.* Boston: College-Hill Press.

Bunch, M. (1982) Dynamics of the singing voice. *Disorders of human communication 6.* New York: Verlag-Springer.

Carruth, J. A. S., & Simpson, G. T. (1988). *Lasers in otolaryngology.* London: Chapman & Hall. This book should enable laryngologists to identify proper laser indications with any kind of laser.

Colton, R. H., & Casper, J. K. (1990). *Understanding voice problems: A physiological perspective for diagnosis and treatment.* Baltimore: Williams & Wilkins.

Dedo, H. H. (1990) *Surgery of the larynx and trachea.* Philadelphia, PA: B. C. Decker.

Ford, C. H., & Bless, D. M. (1991). *Phonosurgery: Assessment and surgical management of voice disorders.* New York: Raven Press. This book shows various aspects of phonosurgery with scientific emphasis on voice physiology and neurology of laryngeal system by Dr. Bless, R. Sherrer, D. Garet, and C. R. Larson.

Gould, W. J., & Lawrence, V. L. (1984). *Surgical care of voice disorders: Disorders of human communication 8.* New York: Springer-Verlag.

Gould, W. J., Sataloff, R. T., & Spiegel, J. R. (1993) *Voice surgery.* St. Louis: Mosby. These authors present a very good basic textbook on voice surgery.

Hirano, M. (1981). *Clinical examination of the voice. Disorders of human communication* 5. New York: Springer-Verlag.

Hirano, M., & Bless, D. M. (1993). *Videostroboscopic examination of the larnx.* San Diego, CA: Singular Publishing Group. Information, technique, and pitfalls on videostroboscopy in this clinical text are presented through very interesting and numerous illustrations. The clinicians will find, with no doubt, a useful help in their daily practice.

Hirano, M., & Sato, K. (1993). *Histological color atlas of the human larynx.* San Diego, CA: Singular Publishing Group. This book presents the anatomical structures of human larynx from newborns to adults with excellent color plates.

Hixon, T. (1988). *Respiratory function in speech and song.* San Diego, CA: Singular Publishing Group.

Isshiki, N. (1989). *Phonosurgery: Theory and practice.* New York: Springer-Verlag. An excellent book on voice physiology and the surgical aspects of the laryngeal framework.

Oswal, V. H., Kashima, H. K., & Flood, L. M. (1988). *The CO_2 laser in otolaryngology and head and neck surgery.* London: Butterworths. Laser surgical techniques in Otolaryngology are well described not only on laryngeal surgery but in the other fields of E.N.T.

Rossing, T. D. (1990). *The science of sounds.* New York: Addison-Wesley.

Sataloff, R. T. (1991). *Professional voice: The science and art of clinical care.* New York: Raven Press. Written for physicians, this book is useful to anyone interested in care of the professional voice.

Sataloff, R. T., Bronfenbrenner, A., & Lederman, R. (1991). *Performing arts medicine.* New York: Raven Press.

Titze, I. R., & Scherer, R. C. (1983). *Vocal fold physiology: Biomechanics, acoustics, and phonatory control.* Denver, CO: The Denver Center for the Performing Arts.

Tucker, H. M. (1992). *The larynx* (2nd ed.). New York: Thieme Medical.

Weir, N. (1990). *Otolaryngology: An illustrated history.* London: Butterworths.

Weisberger, E. C. (1991). *Lasers in head and neck surgery.* New York: Igaku-Shoin. This book gives a complete, very clear review of laser applications in the head and neck area.

Journals

Journal of Voice. A quarterly publication available from Raven Press, 1185 Avenue of the Americas, New York, NY 10036.

The NATS Journal. A bimonthly publication of the National Association of Teachers of Singing, Oberlin, OH.

Laser in Medical Science Journal. A quarterly publication available from W. B. Saunders Company Ltd. London.

Journal of Clinical Laser Medicine and Surgery. A bimonthly publication published by Mary Ann Liebert, Inc., New York.

Journal of Medical Speech-Language Pathology. A quarterly publication available from Singular Publishing Group, 4284 41st Street, San Diego, CA 92105

E.N.T. News. A bimonthly publication, V. H. Oswal, Editor, Cleveland, England.

Conclusions

KEY RULES

Excellent experience is needed in laser phonosurgery. In our experience, the 10 commandments for success are:

1. Don't touch the vocal fold unless the patient specifically asks for it (except in cancer)
2. Ensure perfect exposure of the vocal folds and the anterior commissure
3. Avoid touching the free edge of the vocal fold as much as possible
4. Aim for the superior surface of the vocal fold as much as possible.
5. Keep the beam perpendicular to the operated surface.
6. Keep hand speed regular
7. Protect the subglottic space with icy green gauze which must be changed if laser surgery lasts more than 8 minutes
8. Never shoot on charred tissue
9. Use wet cottonwool pledgets to remove charred tissue
10. Ensure an 8-day period of voice rest postsurgery with medical treatment and speech therapy

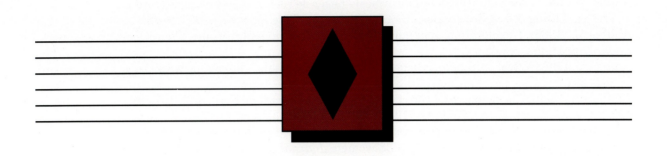

Bibliography

VOICE EXPLORATION

Abitbol, J. (1983). Nouvelle approche chirurgicale Laser de l'oèdme gélatineux des cordes vocales: Lifting des cordes vocales. *Annales Otolaryngologie Français, 100,* 73–76.

Abitbol, J. (1985). L'exploration dynamique vocale par télévidéofibroscopie. *Encyclopedia Universalis, 18,* 485.

Abitbol, J. (1988) Vocal cord hemorrhages in voice professionals. *Journal of Voice, 2*(3), 261–266.

Abitbol, J. (1989). Hormonal vocal cord cycle in women. *Journal of Voice, 3*(2), 157–162.

Abitbol, J., de Brux, G., & Miller, G. (1989). Does a hormonal vocal cord cycle exist in women? Study of vocal premenstrual syndrome in voice performers by videostroboscopy, glottography and cytology on 38 women. *Journal of Voice, 3,* 157–162.

Alberti, P. W. (1978). The diagnostic role of laryngeal stroboscopy. *Otolaryngology Clinics of North America, 11,* 347–354.

American Cancer Association. (1983). *ACA staging and end results manual for staging of cancer* (2nd ed.). Philadelphia: J. B. Lippincott.

Appelman, D. R. (1967). *The science of vocal pedagogy.* London: Indiana University Press.

Arnold, G. E. (1962). Vocal nodules and polyps: Laryngeal tissue reaction to habitual hyperkinetic dysphonia. *Journal of Speech and Hearing Disorders, 27,* 205–217.

Arnold, G. E., Winckel, F., & Wyke, B. D. (1982). *Meribeth Bunch dynamics of the singing voice.* New York/Vienna: Springer-Verlag.

Aronson, A. E. (1985). *Clinical voice disorders* (2nd ed.). New York: Thieme.

Baer, T., Lofqvist, A., & McGarr, N. (1983). Laryngeal vibrations: A comparison between high-speed filming and glottographic techniques. *Journal of the Acoustical Society of America, 73,* 1304–1308.

Baken, D. C. (1962). Laryngeal problems in singers. *Laryngoscope, 72,* 902–908.

Baken, R. J. (1987). *Clinical measurement of speech and voice.* San Diego: College-Hill Press.

Baken, R. J., & Daniloff, R. G. (Eds.). (1990). *Readings in clinical spectrography of speech.* San Diego: Singular Publishing Group.

Baken, R. J., & Isshiki, N. (1977). Arytenoid displacement by simulated intrinsic muscle contraction. *Folia Phoniatrica, 29,* 206–216.

Baken, R. J., & Orlikoff, R. F. (1987). The effect of articulation on fundamental frequency in singers and speakers. *Journal of Voice, 1,* 68–76.

Balestieri, F., & Watson, C. (1982). Intubation granuloma. *Otolaryngologic Clinics of North America, 15,* 567–579.

Ballantyne, J., & Groves, J. (1971). *Diseases of the ear, nose and throat* (3rd ed.). London: Butterworths.

Bastian, R. W. (1985). Laryngeal biofeedback for voice modification. In V. Lawrence (Ed.), *Transcript of the Fourteenth Symposium on Care of the Professional Voice* (pp. 330–333). New York: The Voice Foundation.

Bastian, R. W. (1986). Benign mucosal disorders, saccular disorders and neoplasms. In C. Cummings, J. Fredrickson, L. Harker, C. Krause, & D. Schuller (Eds.), *Otolaryngology—Head and Neck surgery* (Vol. 3, pp. 1965–1987). St. Louis: C. V. Mosby.

Benjamin, B., & Croxson, G. (1985). Vocal cord granulomas. *Annals of Otology, Rhinology and Laryngology, 94,* 538–541.

Biever, D. M., & Bless, D. M. (1989). Vibratory characteristics of the vocal folds in young adult and geriatric women. *Journal of Voice, 3,* 120–131.

Bless, D. M., & Abbs, J. H. (Eds.). (1983). *Vocal fold physiology: Contemporary research and clinical issues*. San Diego, CA: College-Hill Press.

Bless, D. M., & Brandenburg, J. H. (1983). *Stroboscopic evaluation of "functional" voice disorders*. Paper presented at the Triologic Society meeting, Madison, WI.

Bless, D. M., Hirano, M., & Feder, R. J. (1987). Videostroboscopic evaluation of the larynx. *Ear, Nose and Throat Journal, 66*(7), 289–296.

Boone, D. R. (1987). *Human communication and its disorders*. Englewood Cliffs, NJ: Prentice-Hall.

Bouchayer, M., Cornut, G., Witzig, E., Loire, P., Roch, J., & Bastian, R. (1985). Epidermoid cysts, sulci and mucosal bridges of the true vocal cord: A report of 157 cases. *Laryngoscope, 95*, 1087–1094.

Boudin, G., Duron, B., Ossart, M., & Abitbol, J. (1984). Electromyographie larynge technique—premiers résultats. *Journale Français Otorhinolaryngologie, 33*(1), 46–48.

Bourdial, J. (1970). Les troubles de la voix provoques par la therapeutique hormonale androgene. *Annales Otolaryngologie (Paris), 87*, 725–734.

Brewer, D. W., Brodnitz, F., Gould, W. J., Lawrence, V. L., Monaghan, J., Pratt, D., Titze, I. R., & Vaughan, C. (1979). Medical care for professional voice: Panel discussion. In V. Lawrence (Ed.), *Transcripts of the Seventh Symposium: Care of the Professional Voice* (pp. 3–38). New York: The Voice Foundation.

Brewer, D. W., & McCall, G. (1974). Visible laryngeal changes during voice therapy: Fiberoptic study. *Annals of Otology, Rhinology and Laryngology, 83*, 423–427.

Brodnitz, F. (1971). Hormones and the human voice. *Bulletin of the New York Academy of Medicine, 47*, 183–187.

Brodnitz, F. (1975). The age of the castrato voice. *Journal of Speech and Hearing Disorders, 40*, 291–295.

Casper, J. C., & Brewer, D. W. (1985). Selected therapy techniques and laryngeal physiological changes in patients with vocal fold immobility. In V. Lawrence (Ed.), *Transcripts of the Fourteenth Symposium: Care of the Professional Voice* (Part II, pp. 318–323). New York: The Voice Foundation.

Casper, J. C., Colton, R. H., Brewer, D. W., & Woo, P. (1989). *Investigation of selected voice therapy technqiues*. Paper presented at the Eighteenth Annual Symposium: Care of the Professional Voice, Philadelphia, PA.

Chodzko-Zajko, W. J., & Ringer, R. L. (1987). Physiologic aspects of aging. *Journal of Voice, 1*, 18–26.

Coleman, R. J., Mabis, J. H., & Hinson, J. K. (1977). Fundamental frequency-sound pressure level profiles of adult male and female voices. *Journal of Speech and Hearing Research, 20*, 197–204.

Colton, R. H. (1988). Physiological mechanisms of vocal frequency control. The role of tension. *Journal of Voice, 2*, 208–220.

Colton, R. H., Sagerman, R., Chung, C., Young, Y., & Reed, G. (1978). Voice change after radiotherapy. *Radiology, 127*, 821–824.

Cornut, G., Bouchayer, M., & Parent, F. (1986). Value of videostroboscopy in indicating phonosurgery. *Acta Otorhinolaryngologica (Belgium), 40*(2), 436–442.

Damste, P. H. (1967). Voice changes in adult women caused by virilizing agents. *Journal of Speech and Hearing Disorders, 32*, 125–132.

Dedo, H. H. (1976). Recurrent laryngeal nerve section for spastic dysphonia. *Annals of Otology, Rhinology and Laryngology, 85*, 451–459.

Dedo, H. H. (1990). *Surgery of the larynx and trachea*. Philadelphia: B. C. Dekker.

Dedo, H. H., & Izdebski, K. (1981). Surgical treatment for spastic dysphonia. *Contemporary Surgery, 18*, 75–90.

Dedo, H. H., & Izdebski, K. (1983). Problems with surgical (RLN section) treatment of spastic dysphonia. *Laryngoscope, 93*, 263–271.

Dedo, H. H., Izdebski, K., & Townsend, J. J. (1977). Recurrent laryngeal nerve histopathology in spastic dysphonia. *Annals of Otology, Rhinology and Laryngology, 86*, 808–812.

Dedo, H. H., Townsend, J., & Izdebski, K. (1978). Current evidence for the organic etiology of spastic dysphonia. *Otolaryngology, 86*, 806–812.

DeJonckere, P. H., & Lebacq, J. (1985). Electroglottography and vocal nodules: An attempt to quantify the shape of the signal. *Folia Phoniatrica, 37*, 195–200.

Dordain, M. (1972). Etude statistique de l'influence des contraceptifs hormonaux sur la voix. *Folia Phoniatrica, 24*, 86–96.

Eroschenko, V. P. (1993). *Difiore's atlas of histology with functional correlation* (7th ed.). Philadelphia/London: Lea & Febiger.

Fant, G. (1968). *Acoustic theory of speech production*. The Hague: Mouton.

Feder, R. (1986). On standardizing the laryngeal examination. *Archives of Otolarygology—Head and Neck Surgery, 112*, 112–145.

Feder, R. J., & Michell, M. J. (1984). Hyperfunctional, hyperacidic and intubation granulomas. *Archives of Otolaryngology, 110*, 582–584.

Fink, B. R. (1975). *The human larynx: A functional study*. New York: Raven Press.

Flach, M., Schwickardi, H., & Simen, R. (1968). Welchen Einfluss haben Menstruation und Schwangerschafft auf die augsgebildete gesangsstimme? *Folia Phoniatrica, 21*, 199–210.

Frachet, B., Morgon, A., & Legent, F. (1992). *Pratique phoniatrique en O.R.L.* Paris: Masson.

Frokjaer-Jenson, B., & Prytz, S. (1976). Registration of voice quality. *Bruel and Kjüer Technical Review, 3*, 3–17.

Fujimura, O. (1981). Body-cover theory of the vocal fold and its phonetic implications. In K. Stevens & M. Hirano (Eds.), *Vocal fold physiology* (pp. 271–288). Tokyo: University of Tokyo Press.

Fujimura, O. (1988). *Vocal fold physiology. Volume 2: Voice production, mechanisms and functions*. New York: Raven Press.

Gates, G. A., & Montalbo, P. J. (1987). The effect of low dose beta blockade on performance anxiety in singers. *Journal of Voice, 1*, 105–108.

Gates, G. A., Saegert, J., Wilson, H., Johnson, L., Sheppard, A., & Hearne, E. A. (1985). Effects of beta blockage on singing performance. *Annals of Otology, Rhinology and Laryngology, 94*, 570–574.

Gompel, C. (1978). *Atlas of diagnostic cytology:* New York: John Wiley.

Gould, W. J. (1984). The clinical voice laboratory—clinical application of voice research. *Annals of Otology, Rhinology and Laryngology, 93*(4, pt. 1), 346–350.

Gould, W. J., Kojima, H., & Lambiase, A. (1979). A technique for stroboscopic examination of the vocal folds using fiberoptics. *Archives of Otolaryngology, 105*(5), 285.

Gracco, C., & Kahane, J. C. (1989). Age-related changes in the vestibular folds of the human larynx: A histomorphometric study. *Journal of Voice, 3*, 204–212.

Hanson, D. G., Gerratt, B. R., & Ward, P. H. (1983). Glottographic measurement of vocal dysfunction: A preliminary report. *Annals of Otology, Rhinology and Laryngology, 92*, 413–420.

Hirano, M. (1974). Morphological structure of the vocal cord as a vibrator and its variations. *Folia Phoniatrica, 26*, 89–94.

Hirano, M. (1975). Phonosurgery: Basic and clinical investigations. *Otologia (Fukuoka), 21*, 239–442.

Hirano, M. (1981). *Clinical examination of voice: Disorders of human communication*. New York/Vienna: Springer-Verlag.

Hirano, M. (1983). Epithelial hyperplasia of the larynx. In M. Hirano (Ed.), *Illustrated handbook of clinical otolaryngology* (Vol. 4, pp. 100–101). Tokyo: Medical View.

Hirano, M. (1988a). Behavior of the laryngeal muscles of the late William Vennard. *Journal of Voice, 2*, 291–300.

Hirano, M. (1988b). Endolaryngeal microsurgery. In G. M. English (Ed.), *Otolaryngology* (Chapter 43, pp. 1–22). Philadelphia: J. B. Lippincott.

Hirano, M., Koike, Y., & von Leden, H. (1968). Maximum phonation time and air usage during phonation. *Folia Phoniatrica, 20*, 185–201.

Hirano, M., Kurita, S., Kyokawa, K., & Sato, K. (1986). Posterior glottis: Morphological study in excised human larynges. *Annals of Otology, Rhinology and Laryngology, 95*, 576–581.

Hirano, M., Kurita, S., Matsuo, K., & Nagata, K. (1981). Vocal fold polyp and polypoid vocal fold (Reinke's edema). *Journal of Research in Singing, 4*, 33–44.

Hirano, M., Kurita, S., & Nakashima, T. (1983). Growth, development and aging of the human vocal fold. In D. M. Bless & J. W. Abbs (Eds.), *Vocal fold physiology* (pp. 22–43). San Diego, CA: College-Hill Press.

Hirano, M., Kurita, S., & Saguchi, S. (1988). Vocal fold tissue of a 104-year old lady. *Bulletin of the Research Institute of Logopedics and Phoniatrics, 22*, 1–5.

Hirano, M., & Sato, K. (1993). *Histological color atlas of the human larynx*. San Diego, CA: Singular Publishing Group.

Hollien, H. (1960). Vocal pitch variation related to changes in vocal fold length. *Journal of Speech and Hearing Research, 3*, 150–156.

Hollien, H. (1987). Old voices: What do we really know about them? *Journal of Voice, 1*, 2–17.

Hollien, H., & Colton, R. H. (1969). Four laminographic studies of vocal fold thickness. *Folia Phoniatrica, 21*, 179–198.

Isshiki, N. (1964). Regulatory mechanism of voice intensity variation. *Journal of Speech and Hearing Research, 7*, 17–19.

Isshiki, N. (1966). Approach to the objective diagnosis of hoarseness. *Folia Phoniatrica (Basel), 18*, 393–400.

Isshiki, N., Tanabe, M., Ishizaka, K., & Board, C. (1977). Clinical significance of asymmetrical tension of the vocal cords. *Annals of Otology, Rhinology and Laryngology, 86*, 1–9.

Izdebski, K., Dedo, H. H., & Shipp, T. (1981). Postoperative and follow-up studies of spastic dysphonia patients treated by recurrent nerve section. *Otolaryngology—Head and Neck Surgery, 89*, 96–101.

Jako, G. J. (1972). Laser surgery of the vocal cords. An experimental study with carbon dioxide lasers on dogs. *Laryngoscope, 89*, 2204–2216.

Kahane, J. (1981). Anatomic and physiologic changes in the aging peripheral speech mechanism. In D. Beasley & G. Davis (Eds.), *Aging communication processes and disorders* (pp. 22–45). New York: Grune & Stratton.

Kahane, J. (1982). Anatomy and physiology of the organs of the peripheral speech mechanism. In N. J. Lass, L. V. McReynolds, J. L. Northern, & D. E. Yoder (Eds.), *Speech, language and hearing* (Vol. 1, pp. 109–155). Philadelphia: W. B. Saunders.

Kahane, J. C. (1987). Connective tissue changes in the larynx and their effects on voice. *Journal of Voice, 1*, 27–30.

Kahane, J. C. (1988). Histologic structure and properties of the human vocal folds. *Ear, Nose and Throat Journal, 67*, 322–330.

Kahane, J., & Mayo, R. (1989). The need for aggressive pursuit of healthy childhood voices. *Language, Speech and Hearing Services in Schools, 20*, 102–107.

Karnell, M. P. (1989). Synchronized videostroboscopy and electroglottography. *Journal of Voice, 3*((1), 68–75.

Kitzig, P. (1985). Stroboscopy—a pertinent laryngeal examination. *Journal of Otolaryngology, 14*, 151–157.

Kleinsasser, O. (1968). *Microlaryngoscopy and endolaryngeal microsurgery*. Philadelphia, PA: W. B. Saunders.

Kleinsasser, O. (1987). *Surgery in unilateral vocal fold paralysis*. Paper presented at the International Symposium on Phonosurgery, Cairo, Egypt.

Koike, Y., Ohta, F., & Monju, T. (1969). Hormonal and non-hormonal actions of endocrines on the larynx. *Excerpta Medica International Congress Series, 206*, 339–343.

Lacina, O. (1968). The influence of menstruation on the voice of female singer. Premenstrual laryngopathy. *Folia Phoniatrica (Basel), 20*, 13–24.

Leroi-Gourhan, A. (1964). *Le geste et la parole: La mémoire et les rythmes*. Paris: Albin Michel.

Luchsinger, R., & Arnold, G. E. (1965). *Voice, speech language clinical communicology: Its physiology and pathology*, Belmont, CA: Wadsworth.

Martin, F. G. (1983). Drugs and the voice. In V. Lawrence (Ed.), *Transcripts of the Twelfth Symposium: Care of the Professional Voice* (pp. 124–132). New York: The Voice Foundation.

Martin, F. G. (1984). The influence of drugs on the voice (Part II). In V. Lawrence (Ed.), *Transcripts of the Thirteenth Symposium: Care of the Professional Voice* (pp. 191–201). New York: The Voice Foundation.

Martin, F. G. (1988). Tutorial: Drugs and vocal function. *Journal of Voice, 2*, 338–344.

Mathew, O. P., & Sant'Ambrogio, G. (1988). *Respiratory function of the upper airway*. New York: Marcel Dekker.

Meyer-Breiting, E., & Burkhardt, A. (1988). *Tumours of the larynx*. New York/London: Springer-Verlag.

Moore, D. M., Berle, S., Hanson, D. G., & Ward, P. H. (1987). Videostroboscopy of the canine larynx: The effects of asymmetric laryngeal tension. *Laryngoscope, 97*(5), 543–553.

Moore, G. P., Cannon, K. A., & Wilson, L. I. (1979). Vocal fold vibration in the presence of vocal nodules. In V. Lawrence (Ed.), *Transcripts of the Eighth Symposium: Care of the Professional Voice* (pp. 24–31). New York: The Voice Foundation.

Moore, P., & Von Leden, H. (1958). Dynamic variations of the vibratory pattern of the normal larynx. *Folia Phoniatrica, 10*, 205–238.

Morris, M. D., & Morris, B. D. (1990). Dysphonia and bulimia: Vomiting laryngeal injury. *Journal of Voice, 4*(1), 76–80.

Morris, R. J., & Brown, W. S. (1987). Age-related voice measures among adult women. *Journal of Voice, 1*, 38–43.

Morrison, M. D., & Morris, B. D. (1990). Dysphonia and bulimia: Vomiting and laryngeal injury. *Journal of Voice, 4*(1), 76–80.

Murry, T. (1978). Speaking fundamental frequency characteristics associated with voice pathologies. *Journal of Speech and Hearing Disorders, 43*, 374–379.

Murry, T. (1982). Phonation: Remediation. In N. Lass, L. V. McReynolds, J. Northern, & D. E. Yoder (Eds), *Speech, language and hearing* (Vol. 2, pp. 489–498). New York: W. B. Saunders.

Murry, T., & Doherty, E. T. (1980). Selected acoustic characteristics of pathological and normal speakers. *Journal of Speech and Hearing Research, 23*, 361–369.

Murry, T., & Large, J. (1978). Frequency perturbation in singers. In V. Lawrence (Ed.), *Transcripts of the Seventh Symposium: Care of the Professional Voice* (pp. 36–39). New York: Voice Foundation.

Musehold, A. (1898). Stroboskopische und photographische Studien über die Stellung der Stimmlippen im Brust- und Falsetto-Register. *Arkiv Laryngologie und Rhinologie (Berlin), 7*, 1–21.

Nielson, V. M., Hojslet, P. E., & Karlsmose, M. (1986). Surgical treatment of Reinke's edema (long-term results). *Journal of Laryngology and Otology, 100*, 187–190.

Oertel, M. J. (1895a). Das laryngoscopische Untersuchung. *Arkiv Laryngologie und Rhinologie (Berlin), 3*, 1–16.

Oertel, M. J. (1895b). Ueber eine neue laryngostroboscopische Untersuchungsmethode. *Munchen Medjinische Wochenschrift, 42*, 233–236.

Powell, L. S. (1934). Larynstroboscope. *Archives of Otolaryngology, 19*, 708–710.

Proctor, D. F. (1980). *Breathing, speech and song*. New York/Vienna: Springer-Verlag.

Ross Dickson, D., & Maue-Dickson, W. (1982). *Anatomical and physiological bases of speech*. Boston: Little, Brown.

Roubeau, C., Chevrie-Muller, C., & Arabia-Guidel, C. (1983). Electroglottographic study of the changes of voice registers. *Folia Phoniatrica, 39*, 280–289.

Saez, S., & Francoise, S. (1975). Recepteurs d'angrogenes: Mise en evidence dans la fraction cytosolique de muqueuse normale et d'epitheliomas pharyngolarynges humains. *CR Academie de Science (Paris), 280*, 935–938.

Saito, S. (1977). Phonosurgery: Basic study of the mechanism of phonation and endolaryngeal microsurgery. *Otologia (Fukuoka), 23*, 171–384.

Saito, S., Fukuda, H., Kitahara, S., & Kowara, N. (1978). Stroboscopic observation of vocal fold vibration with fiberoptics. *Folia Phoniatrica (Basel), 30*(4), 241–244.

Sataloff, R. T. (1981). Professional singers: The science and art of clinical care. *American Journal of Otolaryngology, 2*, 251–266.

Sataloff, R. T. (1987a). Clinical evaluation of the professional singer. *Ear, Nose, and Throat Journal, 66*, 267–277.

Sataloff, R. T. (1987b). Common diagnoses and treatments in professional singers. *Ear, Nose, and Throat Journal, 66*, 278–288.

Sataloff, R. T. (1987c). The aging voice. *NATS Journal, 44*(1), 20–21.

Sataloff, R. T. (1987d). The professional voice: I. Anatomy and history. *Journal of Voice, 1*(1), 92–104.

Sataloff, R. T. (1987e). The professional voice: II. Physical examination. *Journal of Voice, 1*(2), 191–201.

Sataloff, R. T. (1987f). The professional voice: III. Common diagnoses and treatments. *Journal of Voice, 1*(3), 283–292.

Sataloff, R. T. (1991). *Professional voice: The science and art of clinical care*. New York: Raven Press.

Sataloff, R. T. Branfenbrenner, A. G. & Lederman, R. J. (1991). *Textbook of performing arts medicine*. New York: Raven.

Sataloff, R. T., Spiegel, J. R., & Carroll, L. M. (1988). Strobovideolaryngoscopy in professional voice users: Results and clinical value. *Journal of Voice, 1*(4), 359–364.

Sato, S. (1977). Phonosurgery, basic study on the mechanism of phonation and endolaryngeal microsurgery. *Otologia (Fukuoka), 23*, 171–384.

Scherer, R. C., Gould, W. J., Titze, I. R. et al. (1988). Preliminary evaluation of selected acoustic and glottographic measures for clinical phonatory function analysis. *Journal of Voice, 2*(1), 230–244.

Schiff, M. (1967). The influence of estrogens on connective tissue. In G. Asboe-Hansen (Ed.), *Hormones and connective tissue* (pp. 282–341). Copenhagen: Munksgaard Press.

Schonharl, E., (1960). *Die Stroboskopie in der Praktischen Laryngologie*. Stuttgart: Georg Thieme Verlag.

Schonharl, E. (1966). New stroboscope with automatic regulation of frequency and recent results of its application to study of vocal cord vibrations in dysphonias of various origins. *Revue of Laryngology, 77*(Suppl.), 476–481.

Sellars, I. E., & Keen, E. N. (1978). The anatomy and movements of the cricoarytenoid joint. *Laryngoscope, 88*, 667–674.

Shipp, T. (1987). Vertical laryngeal position: Research findings and application for singers. *Journal of Voice, 1*, 217–219.

Shipp, T., Izdebski, K., Schutte, H. R., & Morrissey, P. (1988). Subglottal air pressure in spastic dysphonia speech. *Folia Phoniatrica, 40*, 105–110.

Spiegel, J. R., Sataloff, R. T. Cohn, J. R., & Hawkshaw, M. (1988). Respiratory dysfunction in singers: Medical assessment, diagnosis and treatment. *Journal of Voice, 2*(1), 40–50.

Strong, M. S., & Kako, G. J. (1972). Laser surgery in the larynx: Early clinical experience with continuous CO_2 laser. *Annals of Otology, Rhinology and Laryngology, 81*, 791–798.

Sundberg, J. (1974). Articulatory interpretation of the "singing formant." *Journal of the Acoustical Society of America, 55*, 838–844.

Sundberg, J. (1987). *The science of the singing voice*. Dekalb: Northern Illinois University Press.

Sundberg, J., & Askenfelt, A. (1983). Larynx height and voice source: A relationship. In D. M. Bless & J. Abbs (Eds.), *Vocal fold physiology: Contemporary research and clinical issues* (pp. 307–316). San Diego, CA: College-Hill Press.

Takahashi, H., & Koike, Y. (1975). Some perceptual dimensions and acoustical correlates of pathologic voices. *Acta Otolaryngologica, 338*, 1–24.

Tanaka, H., & Gould, W. (1985). Vocal efficacy and aerodynamic aspects of voice disorders. *Annals of Otology, Rhinology and Laryngology, 94*, 29–33.

Tarneaud, J. (1933). Study of the larynx and of voice by stroboscopy. *Clinique, 28*, 337–341.

Tarneaud, J. (1941). *Traité pratique de phonologie et de phoniatrie: La voix, la parole, le chant*. Paris: Libraire Maloine.

Tarneaud, J. (1946a). *Importance de la constitution d'un nodule*. Paris: Libraire Maloine.

Tarneaud, J. (1946b). *La chant, sa destruction et sa construction*. Paris: Libraire Maloine.

Titze, I. (1981). Heat generation in the vocal folds and its possible effect on vocal endurance. In V. Lawrence (Ed.), *Transcripts of the Tenth Symposium: Care of the Professional Voice* (pp. 52–59). New York: The Voice Foundation.

Titze, I. R. (1988). A framework for the study of vocal register. *Journal of Voice, 12*, 59–62.

Titze, I. R. (1989). On the relation between subglottal pressure and fundamental frequency in phonation. *Journal of the Acoustical Society of America, 85*, 901–906.

Titze, I. R. (1990). Interpretation of the electroglottographic signal. *Journal of Voice, 4*(1), 1–9.

Titze, I. R. (1993). *Vocal fold physiology: Frontiers in basic science*. San Diego, CA: Singular Publishing Group.

Titze, I. R., Jiange, J., & Drucker, D. G. (1987). Preliminaries to the body-cover theory of pitch control. *Journal of Voice, 1*, 314–319.

Titze, I. R., Luschei, E. S., & Hirano, M. (1989). Role of the thyroarytenoid muscle in regulation of fundamental frequency. *Journal of Voice, 1*, 213–224.

Titze, I. R., & Scherer, R. C. (1983). *Vocal fold physiology: Biomechanics, acoustics and phonatory control*. Denver, CO: The Denver Center for the Performing Arts.

Tucker, H. M. (1978). Human laryngeal reinnervation: Long term experience with nerve-muscle pedicle technique. *Laryngoscope, 88*, 598–604.

Tucker, H. M. (1980). Vocal cord paralysis—etiology and management. *Laryngoscope, 90*, 585–590.

Tucker, H. (1985). Anterior commissure laryngoplasty for adjustment of vocal fold tension. *Annals of Otology, Rhinology and Laryngology, 94*, 547–549.

Tucker, H. M. (1992). *The larynx* (2nd ed.). New York: Thieme Medical.

Tucker, H. M., & Rusnov, M. (1981). Laryngeal reinnervation for unilateral vocal fold paralysis: Long term results. *Annals of Otology, Rhinology and Laryngology, 90*, 457–459.

Von Leden, H. (1961). The electric synchron-stroboscope: Its value for the practicing laryngologist. *Annals of Otology, Rhinology and Laryngology, 70*, 881–893.

Vuorenkoski, V., Lenko, H. L., Tjernlund, P., et al. (1978). Fundamental voice frequency during normal and abnormal growth and after androgen treatment. *Archives of Disabled Children, 53*, 201–209.

Ward, P. H., Sander, J. W., Goldman, R., & Moore, G. P. (1969). Diplophonia. *Annals of Otology, Rhinology and Laryngology, 78*, 771–777.

Weir, N. (1990). *Otolaryngology: An illustrated history*. London: Butterworths.

Welch, D. F., Sergeant, D. C., & MacCurtain, F. (1989). Zeroradiographic-electrolaryngographic analysis of male vocal register. *Journal of Voice, 3*, 224–256.

Wicart, A. (1931). *Le chanteur*. Paris: Author.

Woo, P., Colton, R., & Shangold, L. (1987). Phonatory airflow analysis in patients with laryngeal disease. *Annals of Otology, Rhinology and Laryngology, 96*, 549–555.

Yana, D. (1969). Stroboscopy of the larynx: Apropos of a new stroboscope; the strobo-rama type L6. *Annales Otolaryngologie Chirurgie Cervicofaciale, 86*(9), 589–592.

FILMOGRAPHY

Abitbol, J. (1983). *Larynx exploration*. Prix au Festival du Film de Bichat. New York: Voice Foundation.

Abitbol, J. (1984). *Larynx print*. Premier prix du Festival International du Film et du Livre Medical 1985. New York: Voice Foundation.

Abitbol, J. (1986). *Vocal wave*. Prix au Festival de Deauville. New York: Voice Foundation.

Abitbol, J. (1987). *Performers and voice fatigue*. New York: Voice Foundation.

Hirano, M. Glottic reconstruction following vertical partial laryngectomy and vibration at the new glottis.

Hirano, M. Microsurgery of the larynx.

Hirano, M. Vocal cord vibration.

Isshiki, N. Thyroplasty.

Other videotapes on voice are available from the Voice Foundation (Chairman: R. T. Sataloff).

LASER PHONOSURGERY AND ANESTHESIA

Abitbol, J. (1984). Limitations of the laser in microsurgery of the larynx. In V. L. Lawrence (Ed.), *Transactions of the Twelfth Symposium: Care of the Professional Voice* (pp. 297–301). New York: The Voice Foundation.

Abitbol, J., Mathae, G., & Battista, C. (1988). Preliminary report on detection of papilloma viruses types 6, 11, 16 and 18 in laryngeal benign and malignant lesions. *Journal of Voice, 2*(4), 334–337.

Abramson, A. L., Dilorenzo, T. P., & Steinberg, B. M. (1990). Is papilloma virus detectable in the plume of laser treated laryngeal papilloma? *Archives of Otolaryngology—Head and Neck Surgery, 116*(5), 604–607.

Abramson, A. L., Steinberg, B. M., & Winkler, B. (1987). Laryngeal papillomatosis: Clinical, histopathologic and molecular studies. *Laryngoscope, 97*(6), 678–685.

Anand, V. K., Herbert, J., Robbett, W. F., & Zelman, W. H. (1987). Safe anesthesia for endoscopic laryngeal laser surgery. *Lasers in Surgical Medicine, 7*(3), 275–277.

Baggish, M. S., & Elbakry, M. (1989). The effects of laser smoke on the lungs of rats. *American Journal of Obstetrics and Gynecology, 156*(5), 1260–1265.

Bandieramonte, G., Chiesa, F., Lupi, M., & Marchesini, R. (1987). Laser microsurgery in oncology: Indications, techniques, and results of 5 years experience. *Lasers in Surgical Medicine, 7*(6), 478–486.

Bellina, J. H., Stejemholm, R. L., & Kurpel, J. E. (1981). Biochemical analysis of carbon dioxide plume emission from irradiated tumors. In J. H. Bellina (Ed.), *Gynecologic laser surgery*. New York: Plenum Press.

Benjamin, B., & Parsons, D. S. (1988). Recurrent respiratory papillomatosis: A 10 year study. *Journal of Laryngology and Otology, 102*(11), 1022–1028.

Benjamin, B., Robb, P., Clifford, A., & Eckstein, R. (1991). Giant Teflon granuloma of the larynx. *Head and Neck, 13*(5), 453–456.

Bennett, S., Bishop, S. G., & Lumphkin, S. M. (1989). Phonatory characteristics following surgical treatment of severe polypoid degeneration. *Laryngoscope, 99*(5), 525–532.

Best, D. J., & Toohill, R. J. (1991). Micro-trapdoor flap repair of laryngeal and tracheal stenosis. *Annals of Otology, Rhinology and Laryngology, 100*(5), 420–423.

Carruth, J. A. (1987, September 22). Laser. *ENT Practitioner*, pp. 1206–1207.

Carruth, J. A. (1990) The role of laser in otolaryngology. *Annales Chirurgie Gynaecologie, 79*(4), 216–224.

Carruth, J. A., Morgan, N. J., Nielsen, M. S., Phillipps, J. J., & Wainwright, A. C. (1986). The treatment of laryngeal stenosis using the CO_2 laser. *Clinical Otolaryngology, 11*(3), 145–148.

Carruth, J. A. S., & Simpson, G. T. (1988). *Lasers in otolaryngology*. London: Chapman and Hall.

Casiano, R. R., Cooper, J. D., Lundy, D. S., & Chandler, J. R. (1991). Laser cordectomy for T1 glottic carcinoma: A 10 year experience and videostroboscopic findings. *Otolaryngology—Head and Neck Surgery. 104*(6), 488–492.

Catlin, F. I., & Smith, R. J. (1987). Acquired subglottic stenosis in children. *Annals of Otology, Rhinology and Laryngology, 96*(5), 488–492.

Chandler, J. R. (1989). Clinical observation regarding laser surgery for early glottic cancer. [Letter]. *Archives of Otolaryngology—Head and Neck Surgery, 115*(9), 1134.

Chaput, M., Ninane, J., Gosseye, S., Moulin, D., Hamoir, M., Claus, D., Francis, C., Richard, F., Vermylen, C., & Cornu, G. (1989). Juvenile laryngeal papillomatosis and epidermoid carcinoma. *Journal of Pediatrics, 114*(2), 269–272.

Chisea, F., Tradati, N., Costa, L., Podrecca, S., Borachi, P., Garramoe, R., Sala, L., Bartoli, C., & Molinari, R. (1991). CO_2 laser surgery in laryngeal cancer: Three years results. *Tumori, 77*(2), 151–154.

Cohen, S. R., & Thompson, J. W. (1986). Lymphangiomas of the larynx in infants and children: A survey of pediatric lymphangioma. *Annals of Otology, Rhinology and Laryngology, 127*(Suppl.), 1–20.

Cotton, R. T., & Tewfik, T. L. (1985). Laryngeal stenosis following carbon dioxide laser in subglottic hematoma. Report of three cases. *Annals of Otology, Rhinology, and Laryngology, 94*(5, pt. 1), 494–497.

Courtine, J. C., (1991). *Moyens de protection les effets nocifs du rayon laser en O.R.L.* Presentation at the Sixth International Reunion.

Cragle, S. P., & Brandenburg, J. H. (1993). Laser cordectomy or radiotherapy: Cure rates, communication and cost. *Otolaryngology—Head and Neck Surgery, 108*(6), 648–654.

Crockett, D. M., McCabe, B. F., & Shive, C. J. (1987). Complications of laser surgery for recurrent respiratory papillomatosis. *Annals of Otology, Rhinology, and Laryngology, 96*(6), 639–644.

Crockett, D. M., & Reynolds, B. H. (1990). Laryngeal laser surgery. *Otolaryngology Clinics of North America, 23*(1), 49-66.

Crumley, R. L. (1993). Endoscopic laser medial arytenoidectomy for airway management in bilateral laryngeal paralysis. *Annals of Otology, Rhinology, and Laryngology, 102*(2), 81–84.

Davis, R. K., Kelly, S. M., & Hayes, J. (1991). Endoscopic CO_2 laser excisional biopsy of early supraglottic cancer. *Laryngoscope, 101*(6, pt. 1), 680–683.

De Bery-Borowiecki, B. (1990). CO_2 laser surgery in therapy of laryngeal carcinoma. *Otolaryngology Poland, 44*(3), 154–155.

Dedo, H. H. (1991). Laser therapy for early cancer of the vocal cords. *Western Journal of Medicine, 154*(6), 719.

Dejonckere, P. H., Franceschi, D., & Scholtès, J. L. (1985). Extensive granuloma pyogenicum as a complication of endolaryngeal argon laser surgery. *Lasers in Surgical Medicine, 5*(1), 41–46.

Dennis, D. P., & Kashima, H. (1989). Carbon dioxide laser posterior cordectomy for treatment of bilateral vocal cord paralysis. *Annals of Otology, Rhinology, and Laryngology, 98*(12, pt. 1), 930–934.

Dhara, S. S., & Butler, P. J. (1992). High frequency jet ventilation for microlaryngeal laser surgery. An improved technique. *Anaesthesia, 47*(5), 421–424.

Di Bartolomeo, J. R., & Ellis, M (1982). The argon laser in otology. *Laryngoscope, 90*, 1789–1796.

Duncavage, J. A., Ossof, R. H., & Toohill, R. J. (1985). Carbon dioxide laser management of laryngeal stenosis. *Annals of Otology, Rhinology, and Laryngology, 94*(6, pt. 1), 565–569.

Duncavage, J. A., Piazza, L. S., Ossof, R. H., & Toohill, R. J. (1987). The micro trapdoor technique for the management of laryngeal stenosis. *Laryngoscope, 97*(7, pt. 1), 825–828.

Elner, A., & Fex, S. (1988). Carbon dioxide laser as primary treatment of glottic TIS and TIA tumours. *Acta Otolaryngologica (Stockholm), 449*(Suppl.), 135–139.

Elo, J., & Mate, Z. (1988). Combined therapy with isoprinosine and CO_2 laser. *Archives of Oto-rhino-laryngology, 244*(6), 342-345.

Epstein, B. E., Lee, D. J., Kashima, H., & Johns, M. E. (1990). Stage T1 glottic carcinoma: Results of radiation therapy or laser excision. *Radiology, 176*(2), 567–570.

Feinstein, I., Szachowicz, E., Hilger, P., & Stimson, B. (1986). Laser therapy of dysphonia plica ventricularis. *Annals of Otology, Rhinology, and Laryngology, 96*(1, pt. 1), 56–57.

Ford, C. N., & Bless, D. M. (1986). A preliminary study of injectable collagen in human vocal fold augmentation. *Otolaryngology—Head and Neck Surgery, 94*, 104–112.

Ford, C. N., & Bless, D. M. (1988). Collagen injected in the scarred vocal fold. *Journal of Voice, 1*(1), 116–118.

Freche, C., & Jakobowitz, M. (1988). The carbon dioxide laser in laryngeal surgery. *Ear, Nose and Throat Journal, 67*(6), 436, 438–440, 445.

Fried, M. P. (1984). *The larynx*. Philadelphia: W. B. Saunders.

Goldman, L. (1981). *The biomedical laser: Technology and clinical applications.* New York/Heidelberg: Springer-Verlag.

Gould, W. J., & Lawrence, V. L. (1984). *Surgical care of voice disorders.* New York: Springer-Verlag.

Gould, W. J., Sataloff, R. T., & Spiegel, A. R. (in press). *Voice surgery.* St. Louis: C. V. Mosby.

Green, D. A. (1987). Vocal quality after endoscopic laser surgery. *Archives of Otolaryngology — Head and Neck Surgery, 113*(11), 1238.

Gregor, R. T. (1988). The use of carbon dioxide laser in dealing with fibrous structures of the larynx and trachea. *Journal of Otolaryngology, 17*(1), 16–18.

Guerry, T. L., Silverman, S., Jr., & Dedo, H. H. (1986). Carbon dioxide laser resection of superficial oral carcinoma: Indication, technique and results. *Annals of Otology, Rhinology, and Laryngology, 96*(6, pt. 1), 547–555.

Hallmo, P., & Naess, O. (1991). Laryngeal papillomatosis with human papillomavirus DNA contracted by a laser surgeon. *European Archives of Otorhinolaryngology, 248*(7), 425-427.

Halstead, L. A., & Bowles, J. T. (1989). Management of post-intubation and post-traumatic airway stenosis. *JCS Medical Association, 85*(9), 447–449.

Hampal, S., & Hawthorne, M. (1990). Hypopharyngeal inverted papilloma. *Journal of Laryngology and Otology, 104*(5), 432–434.

Haraf, D. J., & Weichselbaum, R. R. (1988). Treatment selection in T1 and T2 vocal cord carcinoma. *Oncology (Williston Park), 2*(10), 41–50.

Harari, P. M., Blatchford, S. J., Coulthard, S. W., & Casady, J. R. (1991). Intubation granuloma of the larynx: Successful eradication with low-dose radiotherapy. *Head and Neck, 13*(3), 230–233.

Hearty, G. B. (1987). Current management of lesions of the pediatric larynx. *Annals of Otology, Rhinology, and Laryngology, 96*(1, pt. 1), 122–123.

Herdman, R. C. D., Charlton, A., Hinton, A. E., & Freemont, A. J. (1993). An in vitro comparison of the Erbium: YAG laser and the carbon dioxide laser in laryngeal surgery. *Journal of Laryngology and Otology, 107*(10), 908–911.

Hirano, M., & Hirade, Y. (1988). CO_2 laser for treating glottic carcinoma. *Acta Otolaryngologica (Stockholm), 458* (Suppl. 458), 154–157.

Hirano, M., Hirade, Y., & Kawasaki, H. (1985). Vocal function following carbon dioxide laser surgery for glottic carcinoma. *Annals of Otology, Rhinology, and Laryngology, 94*(3), 232–235.

Hirano, M., & Sato, K. (1993). Laser surgery for epithelial hyperplasia of the vocal fold. *Annals of Otology, Rhinology, and Laryngology, 102*(2), 85–91.

Hoare, T. J., Jayne, D., Rhys Evans, P., Croft, C. B., & Howard, D. J. (1989). Wegener's granulamotosis, subglottic stenosis and antineutrophil cytoplasma antibodies. *Journal of Laryngology and Otology, 103*(12), 1187–1191.

Hurbis, C. G., & Holinger, L. D. (1990). Laryngeal amyloidosis in a child. *Annals of Otology, Rhinology, and Laryngology, 99*(2, pt. 1), 105–107.

Ikeda, M., Takahashi, H., Karaho, Y, Kithara, S., & Ilnouye, T. T. (1991). Amelanotic melanoma metastic to the epiglottis. *Journal of Laryngology and Otology, 105*(9), 776–779.

Ilnouye, T. T. (1985). Application of CO_2 laser to the carcinoma of the larynx. *Auris Nasus Larynx, 12*(Suppl. 2), S178–S181.

Ilnouye, T. T., & Tanabe, T. (1988). CO_2 laser management of laryngeal carcinoma. *Acta Otolaryngologica (Stockholm), 458*(Suppl.), 158–162.

Isshiki, N. (1989). *Phonosurgery: Theory and practice.* New York: Springer-Verlag.

Isshiki, N., Taira, T., & Tanabe, M. (1983). Surgical alteration of the vocal pitch. *Journal of Otolaryngology, 12*, 335–340.

Ito, H., Suzuki, K., Hoshino, T., & Nozue, M. (1991). Total laryngeal stenosis in cicatricial pemphigoid. *Auris Nasus Larynx, 18*(2),163–167.

Kaplan, I. (1975). *Laser surgery I-II.* Tel Aviv: Ot Paz.

Kaplan, I. (1979). *Laser surgery III (Part 1).* Tel Aviv: Ot Paz.

Kashima, H., Kessis, T., Mounts, P., & Shah, K. (1991). Polymerase chain reaction identification of human papillomavirus DNA in CO_2 laser plume from recurrent respiratory papillomatosis. *Otolaryngology—Head and Neck Surgery, 104*(2), 191–195.

Koch, W. M., Hybels, R. L., & Shashay, S. M. (1987). Carbon dioxide laser in removal of polytef paste. *Archives of Otolaryngology—Head and Neck Surgery, 113*(6), 661–664.

Koufman, J. A. (1986). The endoscopic management of early squamous carcinoma of the vocal fold with the carbon dioxide surgical laser: Clinical experience and a proposed subclassification. *Otolaryngology—Head and Neck Surgery, 95*(5), 531–537.

Krespi, Y. P., & Meltzer, C. J. (1989). Laser surgery for vocal cord carcinoma involving the anterior commissure. [Comments]. *Annals of Otology, Rhinology, and Laryngology, 98*(2), 105–109.

Kull, M., Samarutel, J., & Nurm, V. (1993). Double frequency jet ventilation for endolaryngeal laser surgery. *Lasers in Medical Science, 8*(2), 141–146.

Kuriloff, D. B., Finn, D. G., & Kimmelman, C. P. (1988). Pharyngoesophageal hair growth. The role of laser epilation. *Otolaryngology—Head and Neck Surgery, 98*(4), 342–345.

Leonard, R. J., Gallia, L. J., & Charpied, G. (1992). Recovery of vocal fold mucosa from laser incision. *Journal of Voice, 6*(3), 286–291.

Lim, R. Y. (1985). Laser arytenoidectomy. *Archives of Otolaryngology, 111*(4), 262–263

Lim, R. Y. (1991). Endoscopic CO_2 laser arytenoidectomy for post-intubation glottic stenosis. *Otolaryngology—Head and Neck Surgery, 105*(5), 662–666.

Lim, R. Y., & Kenny, C. L. (1986). Precaution and safety in carbon dioxide laser surgery. *Otolaryngology—Head and Neck Surgery, 95*(2), 239–241.

Lofgren, L. A. (1988). Treatment of severe subglottic stenosis in children with the CO_2 laser: A preliminary report on a few successful cases. *Acta Otolaryngologica (Stockholm), 449,* 101–103.

Lumpkin, S. M., Bishop, S. G., & Bennett, S. (1987). Comparison of surgical techniques in the treatment of laryngeal polypoid degeneration. Published erratum. *Annals of Otology, Rhinology, and Laryngology, 96*(4), 386 and 96(3, pt. 1), 254–257.

Mallios, C., Scheck, P. A. E., Medici, G., Robers, C., & Knegt, P. (1993). Laser surgery of the larynx using a metal insufflation catheter for ventilation of the lungs (28). *Anaesthesia, 48*(4), 359–361.

McGuirt, W. F. (1987). Laryngeal carcinoma in situ: A therapeutic dilemma. *Southern Medical Journal, 80*(4), 447–449.

McGuirt, W. F., & Browne, J. D. (1991). Management decisions in laryngeal carcinoma in situ. *Laryngoscope, 101*(2), 125–129.

McGuirt, W. F., & Koufman, J. A. (1987). Endoscopic laser surgery: An alternative in laryngeal cancer surgery. *Archives of Otolaryngology — Head and Neck Surgery, 113*(5), 501–505.

McIlwain, J. C., & Shepperd, H. W. (1986). Laser treatment of primary amyloidosis of the larynx. *Journal of Laryngology and Otology, 100*(9), 1079–1080.

Milford, C. A., & O'Flynn, P. E. (1991). Management of verrucous carcinoma of the larynx. *Clinical Otolaryngology, 16*(2), 160–162.

Milutinovic, Z. (1990). Advantages of indirect video-stroboscopic surgery of the larynx. *Folia Phoniatrica (Basel), 42*(2), 77–82.

Monsonego, J. (1990). Papillomaviruses in human pathology: Recent progress in epidermoid precancers. *Serono Symposia* (Vol. 78). New York: Raven Press.

Morgan, A. H., Norris, J. W., & Hicks, J. N. (1985). Palliative laser surgery for melanoma metastic to the larynx: Report of two cases. *Laryngoscope, 95*(7, pt. 1), 794–797.

Motta, G., Villari, G., Pucci, V., & De Clemente, M. (1987). CO_2 laser in laryngeal microsurgery. *Surgery, 72*(3), 175–178

Motta, G., Villari, G., Jr., Ripa, G., & Salerno, G. (1986). The CO_2 laser in the laryngeal microsurgery. *Acta Otolaryngologica, 433*(Suppl.), 1–31.

Myssiorek, D., & Persky, M. (1989). Laser endoscopic treatment of laryngoceles and laryngeal cysts. *Otolaryngology—Head and Neck Surgery, 100*(6), 538–541.

Nigam, A., Campbell, J. B., & Das Gupta, A. R. (1990). Radiation induced tumours of the pharynx—can they be avoided? *Journal of Laryngology and Otology, 104*(2), 129–130.

Ossof, R. H., & Duncavage, J. A. (1988). Adult subglottiscope for laser surgery. *Annals of Otology, Rhinology, and Laryngology, 97*(5, pt. 1), 552–553.

Ossof, R. H., Duncavage, J. A., & Dere, H. (1991a). Microsubglottoscopy: An expansion of operative microlaryngoscopy. *Otolaryngology—Head and Neck Surgery, 104*(6), 842–848.

Ossof, R. H., Duncavage, J. A., & Dere, H. (1991b). Soft tissue complications of laser surgery for recurrent respiratory papillomatosis. *Laryngoscope, 101*(11), 1162–1166.

Ossof, R. H., Duncavage, J. A., Shapshay, S. M., Krespi, Y. P., & Sisson, G. A., Sr. (1990). Endoscopic laser arytenoidectomy revisited. *Annals of Otology, Rhinology, and Laryngology, 99*(10, pt. 1), 764–771.

Ossof, R. H., & Matar, S. A. (1989). The advantages of laser treatment of tumors of the larynx. *Oncology (Williston Park), 2*(9), 58–61, 64–66.

Ossof, R. H., Tucker, J. A., & Werkhaven, J. A. (1991). Neonatal and pediatric microsubglottiscope set. *Annals of Otology, Rhinology, and Laryngology, 100*(4, pt. 1), 325–326.

Ossof, R. H., Werkhaven, J. A., Raif, J., & Abraham, M. (1991). Advanced microspot for the CO_2 laser. *Otolaryngology—Head and Neck Surgery, 105*(3), 411–415.

Oswal, V. H., Kashima, H. K., & Flood, L. M. (1988). *The CO_2 laser in otolaryngology and head and neck surgery*. London: Butterworths.

Parker, D. A., & Das Gupta, A. R. (1987). An endoscopic silastic keel for anterior glottic web. *Journal of Laryngology and Otology, 101*(10), 1055–1061.

Perkins, R. C. (1980). Laser stapedotomy for otosclerosis. *Laryngoscope, 90*, 228–241.

Prasad, U. (1986). CO_2 surgical laser in the management of bilateral vocal cord paralysis. *Journal of Laryngology and Otology, 99*(9), 891–894.

Rabinov, R. C., Castro, D. J., Calcaterra, T. C., Fu, Y. S., Anderson, C. T. M., Bates, E., Soudani, J., & Saxton, R. (1993). Subglottic plasmacytoma: The use of jet ventilation and contact nd: YAG laser for tissue diagnosis. *Journal of Clinical Laser Medicine and Surgery, 11*(3), 131–134.

Remacie, M., Declaye, X., & Mayne, A. (1989). A subglottic haemangioma in the infant: Contribution by CO_2 laser. *Journal of Laryngology and Otology, 103*(10), 930–934.

Remacle, M., Lawson, G., Sasserath, M., & Claremunt, R. (1993). Treatment of sulcus glottidis by association of CO_2 laser and collagen. *Journale Français Otologie, Rhinologie et Laryngologie, 42*(1), 29–32.

Remson, K., Lawson, W., Patrel, N., & Biler, H. F. (1985). HF laser lateralization for bilateral cord abductor paralysis. *Otolaryngology—Head and Neck Surgery, 93*(5), 645–649.

Roa, R. A., Atkins, J. P., Jr., Cunnane, M. F., & Keane, W. M. (1990). Papillary adenocarcinoma of the larynx: A case report. *Otolaryngology—Head and Neck Surgery, 99*(6), 601–603.

Robison, P. M., & Weir, A. M. (1987). Excision of benign laryngeal lesions: Comparison of carbon dioxide laser with conventional surgery. *Journal of Laryngology and Otology, 101*(2), 1254–1257.

Rontal, M., & Rontal, E. (1990). Endoscopic laryngeal surgery for bilateral midline vocal cord obstruction. *Annals of Otology, Rhinology, and Laryngology, 99*(8), 605–610.

Rossing, T. D. (1990). *The science of sound.* New York: Addison-Wesley.

Rothfield, R. E., Myers, E. N., & Johnson, J. T. (1991). Carcinoma in situ and microinvasive squamous cell carcinoma of the vocal cords. *Annals of Otology, Rhinology, and Laryngology, 100*(10), 793–796.

Ruff, T., & Bellens, E. E. (1985). Sarcoidosis of the larynx treated with CO_2 laser. *Journal of Otolaryngology, 14*(4), 245–247.

Saito, R., Date, R., Una, K., Ueda, S., Quijano, M., & Ogura, Y. (1985). Treatment of juvenile laryngeal papilloma with a combination of laser surgery and interferon. *Auris Nasus Larynx, 12*(2),117–124.

Sataloff, R. T., Feldman, M., Darby, K. S. et al. (1987). Arytenoid dislocation. *Journal of Voice, 1*(4), 368–377.

Sataloff, R. T., Mayer, D. P., & Spiegel, J. R. (1988). Radiologic assessment of laryngeal Teflon injection. *Journal of Voice, 2*(1), 93–95.

Sataloff, R. T., Spiegel, J. R., Hawkshaw, M., & Jones, A. (1992). Laser surgery of the larynx: The case for caution. *Ear, Nose and Throat Journal, 7*(11), 593–595.

Savage, M. M., Crockett, D. M., & McCabe, B. F. (1988). Lipoid proteinosis of the larynx: A cause of voice change in the infant and young child. *International Journal of Pediatric Otorhinolaryngology, 15*(1), 33–38.

Seid, A. B., Park, S. M., Kearns, M. J., & Guggenheim, S. (1985). Laser division of the aryepiglottic folds for severe laryngomalacia. *International Journal of Pediatric Otorhinolaryngology, 10*(2), 153–158.

Selkin, S. G. (1988). Photodocumentation of laser microsurgery: Preoperative, intraoperative, and postoperative techniques for still and video photographs. *Otolaryngology—Head and Neck Surgery, 95*(3, pt. 10), 259–272.

Shapshay, S. M., Hybels, R. L., & Bohigian, R. K. (1990). Laser excision of early vocal cord carcinoma: Indications, limitations, and precautions. *Annals of Otology, Rhinology, and Laryngology, 99*(1), 46–50.

Shapshay, S. M., Rebeiz, E. E., Bohigian, R. K., & Hybels, R. L. (1990). Benign lesions of the larynx: Should the laser be used? *Laryngoscope, 100*(9), 953–957.

Shapshay, S. M., Ruah, C. B., Bohigian, R. K., & Beamis, J. F., Jr. (1988). Obstructing tumors of the subglottic larynx and cervical trachea: Airway management and treatment. *Annals of Otology, Rhinology, and Laryngology, 97*(5, pt. 1), 487–492.

Shapshay, S. M., Wallace, R. A., Kveton, J. F., Hybels, R. L., & Bohigian, R. K. (1988). New microspot micromanipulator for carbon dioxide laser surgery in otolaryngology. Early clinical results. *Archives of Otolaryngology—Head and Neck Surgery, 114*(9), 1012–1015.

Shapshay, S. M., Wallace, R. A., Kveton, J. F., Hybels, R. L., & Setzer, S. E. (1988). New microspot micromanipulator for CO_2 laser application in otolaryngology—head and neck surgery. *Otolaryngology—Head and Neck Surgery, 98*(2),179–181.

Silver, C. E., & Moisa, I. I. (1990). The role of surgery in the treatment of laryngeal cancer. Published erratum in *CA Cancer Journal Clinic, 40*(4), 242 and *40*(3), 134–149.

Simpson, G. T., & Shapshay, S. M. (1983). *The use of lasers in otolaryngologic surgery.* Philadelphia: W. B. Saunders

Smalley, P. J. (1990). Laser. *Otolaryngology Nursing Clinics of North America, 25*(3), 645–656.

Spiegel, J. R., Sataloff, R. T., & Gould, W. J. (1988). The treatment of vocal fold paralysis with injectable collagen: Clinical concerns. *Journal of Voice, 1*(1), 119–121.

Steiner, W. (1988). Experience in endoscopic laser surgery of malignant tumours of the upper aero-digestive tract. *Advances in Otorhinolaryngology, 39*, 135–144.

Steiner, W. (1993). Results of curative laser microsurgery of laryngeal carcinomas. *Annals of Otolaryngology—Head and Neck Medicine and Surgery, 14*(2), 116–121.

Stern, J. C., & Lucente, F. E. (1989). Carbon dioxide laser excision of earlobe keloids. A prospective study and critical analysis of existing data. *Archives of Otolaryngology—Head and Neck Surgery, 115*(9), 1107–1111.

Talbot, A . R. (1990). Laryngeal amyloidosis. *Journal of Laryngology and Otology, 104* (2), 147-149.

Tapia, R. G., Pardo, J., Marigil, M., & Pacio, A. (1984). Effects of the laser upon Reinke's space and the neural system of the vocalis muscle. In V. L. Lawrence (Ed.), *Transactions of the Twelfth Symposium: Care of the Professional Voice* (pp. 289–291). New York: The Voice Foundation.

Thode, S. A. (1986). Laryngo-tracheal laser surgery and general anesthesia. *Lasers in Surgery and Medicine, 6*(3), 369–372

Triglisa, J. M., Portaspana, T., Cannoni, M., & Pech, A. (1991). A subglottic cyst in a newborn. *Journal of Laryngology and Otology, 105*(3), 222–223.

Tsui, S. L., Woo, D. E., & Lo, J. R. (1991). Anaesthetic management of a 2-month-old infant for laser resection of vocal cord granuloma. *British Journal of Anaesthesia, 66*(1), 134–137.

Tsuji, D. H., Fukuda, H., Kawasaki, Y., Kawaida, M., & Kanzaki, J. A. (1989). A clinical study on T1 glottic cancer treated by laser technique. *Keio Journal of Medicine, 38*(4), 413–418.

Tucker, H. M., Harvey, J. E., & Ogura, J. H. (1970). Vocal cord remobilization in the canine larynx. *Archives of Otolaryngology, 92,* 530–533.

von Leden, H., & Moore, P. (1961). The mechanics of the cricoarytenoid joint. *Archives of Otolaryngology, 73,* 63–72.

von Leden, H., Yanagihara, N., & Kukuk-Werner, E . (1967). Teflon in unilateral vocal cord paralysis. *Archives of Otolaryngology, 85*(6),110–118.

von Leden, H. (1978, June). Panel discussion on voice therapy. Presentation at the Seventh Symposium on Care of the Professional Voice, The Julliard School, New York.

Voucth, G. (1981). *Anesthésie et laser—Experience de la chirurgie sous rayon laser en O.R.L.* Presentation at Loeme Reunion Internationale Nord.

Webb, W. R., & Besson, A. (1991). *Thoracic surgery: Surgical management of chest injuries.* St. Louis: Mosby Year Book.

Wegrzynowicz, E. S., Jensen, N. F., Pearson, K. S., Wachtel, R. E., & Scamman, F. L. (1992). Airway fire during jet ventilation for laser excision of vocal cord papillomata. *Anesthesiology, 76*(3), 468–469.

Weisberger, E. C. (l991). *Laser in head and neck surgery.* New York/Tokyo: Igaku Shoin.

Wenig, B. L., & Abramson, & A. L. (1988). Congenital subglottic hemangiomas: A treatment update. *Laryngoscope, 98*(2), 190–192.

Wetmore, S. J., Key, J. M., & Suen, J. Y. (l985) Complications of laser surgery for laryngeal papillomatosis. *Laryngoscope, 95*(7, pt. 1), 798-801.

Wetmore, S. J., Key, J. M., & Suen, J. Y. (l986). Laser therapy for T1 glottic carcinoma of the larynx. *Archives of Otolaryngology—Head and Neck Surgery, 112*(8), 863–855.

Williams, S. R., Van Hasselt, C. A., Aun, C. S. T., Tong, M. C. F., & Carruth, J. A. S. (1993). Tubeless anesthetic technique for optimal carbon dioxide laser surgery of the larynx. *American Journal of Otolaryngology—Head and Neck Medicine and Surgery, 14*(4), 271–274.

Williamson, R. (1989). Anaesthesia for carbon dioxide laser laryngeal surgery in infants. [Letter]. *Anaesthesia, 44*(9), 793

Wolfensberger, M., & Dont, J. C. (1990). Endoscopic laser surgery for early glottic carcinoma: A clinical and experimental study. *Laryngoscope, 100*(10, pt. 1). 1100–1105.

Woo, K. S., Van Hasselt, C. A., & Waldrom, J. (1990). Laser resection of localized subglottic amyloidosis. *Journal of Otolaryngology, 19*(5), 337–338.

Zeiteis, S. M., Vaughan, C. W., Domanowski, G. F., Fuleihan, N. S., & Simpson, G. T. (1990). Second laser epiglottectomy: Endoscopic technique and indications. *Otolaryngology—Head and Neck Surgery, 103*(3), 337–343.

Zohar, Y., & Strauss, M. (1989). Laser surgery for vocal cord carcinoma involving the anterior commissure. [Letter and Comment]. *Annals of Otology, Rhinology, and Laryngology, 98*(10), 836–837.

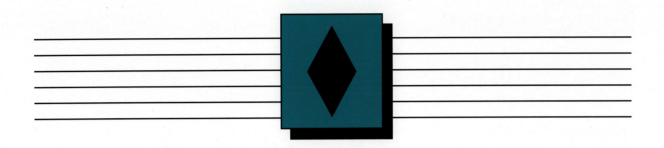

Index

A

Aerodynamic and respiratory studies, 101–103
Amyloid tumors, 404
Anesthetic techniques, 118–122
   agents, 121
     complications from, 426
     preoperative and operative procedures, 121–122
     ventilation, 119–121
Articulation, 71
Aryepiglottic folds, 52
Atrophy, 408
Audiometric tests, 103

B

Bataille, Charles, 78
Bohr, Nils, 4

C

Capillary ectasia, 221–241
Carcinoma, 300–335
Cartilages, 66–68
   cricoid, 52
Chemical hazards, 18–19
Cysts, 173–195, 363–365

D

Dye lasers, 23
Dynamic Vocal Exploration, 99–100

E

Edema
   radiotherapy, after, 409
   Reinke's, 250–280
Edison, Thomas, 78
Einstein, Albert, 3–6
Electrical hazards, 19
Electroglottography (EGG), 86–94
Electromyography (EMG), 100–101
Epiglottis, 49–51
   cysts of, 363–365
Epithelium, 52–54
Eye hazards, 18

F

False vocal folds, 51, 68
Fiberscopy, 81–84
Frequency, fundamental, 76

G

Garcia, Manuel, 78
Glottis, 68
Granulomas, 196–206

H

Hernia of false vocal folds, 357–362
Hertz, 3

K

KTP lasers, 23

L

Lamina propria, 54–55
   aged, 56
Laryngitis, chronic, 281–299
Laryngocele, 357–362
Laryngoscopy, indirect, 80–81
Larynx, 41–106
   anatomy and physiology of, 71–78
   embryology of, 42–70
   normal voice, 78–106
   web of, 371–379
Lasers
   advantages over traditional surgery, 32–33
   argon type, 33
   characteristics of, 23
   CO_2 type, 23–33
   history of, 2–3

Lasers *(continued)*
   laryngeal surgery and, 41–106
   Nd-Yag type, 33–39
   phonosurgical history, 21–23
   safety considerations, 18–21, 123–124
   technology of, 4–7
   tissue interaction with, 7–18
   types of, 7, 23–39
Lesions
   miscellaneous, 401–409
   multiple, 410–415
Ligaments, 64–66
Lungs, 71

M

Maximum phonation time, 102
Maxwell, J.C., 2–3
Mean airflow rate, 102
Membranes, 64–66
Microlaryngoscopy, 108–124
   anesthetic techniques, 118–122
   complications, 118
   procedures, 114–116
Mitochondria, 55–56
Mucosa, laryngeal, 49–58
Muscles, 58–63

N

Nodules, 126–153
Notches and scars, 401–403

P

Papillomas, 207–220
Paralysis of vocal folds, 336–362
Phonation
   normal, 76
   quotient, 102
Phonosurgery
   complications, 123–124, 424–426
   defined, x
   history of, x-xvii
   indications and cautions, 108–109, 421–426
   instruments 109–113
   limitations, 424
   procedures, 116–118
   statistical analyses, 418–426
Pitch, 76
   changing, 394–400
Planck, Max, 3
Plato, 2
Polyps, 154–172
Post-traumatic web, 380–386
Pythagoras, 2

R

Radiography, 103
Radiotherapy, edema following, 405
Reinke's edema, 250–280

S

Safety, CO_2 laser surgery and, 123–124
Skin hazards, 18
Smear tests, 103
Sound, speech and, 75–76
Spectrography, 94–99
Statistical analyses, 418–426
Stroboscopy, 84–86
Sulcus vocalis, 387–393
Supraglottal cavity, 68

T

Tarneaud, Jean, 78
Teflon
   ablation of, 405–406
   injection of, 338
Televideoscopy, 81
Tumors, amyloid, 404

V

Vallecular cysts, 363–365
Vascular pathology, 221–241
Ventricles, 51
   laryngeal, 70
Vocal folds, 52
   atrophy of, 404

Vocal Folds *(continued)*
    hemorrhage of, 242–249
    malignant tumors of, 300–335
    paralysis of, 336–362
    Teflon ablation from, 405–406
    vibration of, 74–75
Vocal pitch, changing, 394–400
Vocal tract resonance, 71, 72–73

Vocalis muscle, 55
Voice, intensity of, 76

W

Web
    anterior post-traumatic, 380–385
    congenital laryngeal, 371–379